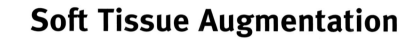

Soft Tissue Augmentation

Procedures in Cosmetic Dermatology

Series Editor: Jeffrey S. Dover MD FRCPC
Associate Editor: Murad Alam MD

Botulinum Toxin, second edition

Alastair Carruthers MA BM BCh FRCPC FRCP(Lon) and
Jean Carruthers MD FRCSC FRC (OPHTH) FASOPRS
ISBN 978-1-4160-4213-6

Soft Tissue Augmentation, second edition

Jean Carruthers MD FRCSC FRC (OPHTH) FASOPRS and
Alastair Carruthers MA BM BCh FRCPC FRCP(Lon)
ISBN 978-1-4160-4214-3

Cosmeceuticals

Zoe Diana Draelos MD
ISBN 978-1-4160-0244-4

Lasers and Lights: Volume I

Vascular • Pigmentation • Scars • Medical Applications
David J. Goldberg MD JD
ISBN 978-1-4160-2386-9

Lasers and Lights: Volume II, second edition

Rejuvenation • Resurfacing • Treatment of Ethnic Skin •
Treatment of Cellulite
David J. Goldberg MD JD
ISBN 978-1-4160-4212-9

Photodynamic Therapy, second edition

Mitchel P. Goldman MD
ISBN 978-1-4160-4211-2

Liposuction

C. William Hanke MD MPH FACP and
Gerhard Sattler MD
ISBN 978-1-4160-2208-4

Scar Revision

Kenneth A. Arndt MD
ISBN 978-1-4160-3131-4

Chemical Peels

Mark Rubin MD
ISBN 978-1-4160-3071-3

Hair Transplantation

Robert S. Haber MD and Dowling B. Stough MD
ISBN 978-1-4160-3104-8

Treatment of Leg Veins

Murad Alam MD and Tri H. Nguyen MD
ISBN 978-1-4160-3159-8

Blepharoplasty

Ronald L. Moy MD and Edgar F. Fincher
ISBN 978-1-4160-2996-0

Advanced Face Lifting

Ronald L. Moy MD and Edgar F. Fincher
ISBN 978-1-4160-2997-7

Procedures in Cosmetic Dermatology

Series Editor: Jeffrey S. Dover MD FRCPC
Associate Editor: Murad Alam MD

Soft Tissue Augmentation

Second edition

Edited by

Jean Carruthers MD FRCSC FRC (OPHTH) FASOPRS
Clinical Professor, Department of Ophthalmology and Visual Sciences,
University of British Columbia, Vancouver, BC, Canada

Alastair Carruthers MA BM BCh FRCPC FRCP (Lon)
Clinical Professor, Department of Dermatology and Skin Science,
University of British Columbia, Vancouver, BC, Canada

Series Editor
Jeffrey S Dover MD FRCPC
Associate Professor of Clinical Dermatology, Yale University School of Medicine,
Adjunct Professor of Medicine (Dermatology), Dartmouth Medical School,
Director, SkinCare Physicians, Chestnut Hill, MA, USA

Associate Editor
Murad Alam MD
Chief, Section of Cutaneous and Aesthetic Surgery,
Department of Dermatology, Northwestern University, Chicago, IL, USA

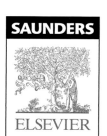

SAUNDERS

ELSEVIER

SAUNDERS
ELSEVIER

An imprint of Elsevier Inc.

First edition 2005
Second edition 2008
ISBN: 978-1-4160-4214-3

British Library Cataloguing in Publication Data
A catalogue record for this book is available from the British Library

Library of Congress Cataloging in Publication Data
A catalog record for this book is available from the Library of Congress

Note
Neither the Publisher nor the Editors and Authors assume any responsibility for any loss or injury and/or damage to persons or property arising out of or related to any use of the material contained in this book. It is the responsibility of the treating practitioner, relying on independent expertise and knowledge of the patient, to determine the best treatment and method of application for the patient.

The Publisher

Commissioning Editors: Claire Bonnett/Karen Bowler
Development Editor: Anne Bassett
Project Manager: Anne Dickie
Design Direction: Charlotte Murray
Illustration Manager: Merlyn Harvey
Illustrator: Jennifer Rose

ELSEVIER your source for books, journals and multimedia in the health sciences
www.elsevierhealth.com

Working together to grow
libraries in developing countries

www.elsevier.com | www.bookaid.org | www.sabre.org

 ELSEVIER   BOOK AID International   Sabre Foundation

The publisher's policy is to use **paper manufactured from sustainable forests**

Printed in China

Last digit is the print number: 9   8   7   6   5   4   3   2

Contents

Series Preface   vii
Series Preface First Edition   viii
Preface   ix
List of Contributors   xi

1   Background Information on the use of Esthetic Fillers   1
        Hayes B. Gladstone, Brian Somoano

2   Fillers Esthetics   11
        Stephen R. Tan, Richard G. Glogau

3   Injectable Collagens   19
        Seth L. Matarasso

4   Hylans and Soft Tissue Augmentation   31
        Rhoda S. Narins, Jason Michaels, Joel L. Cohen

5   Management of the Lips and Mouth Corners   51
        Jean Carruthers, Vic A. Narurkar

6   Augmentation with Autologous Fat   63
        Lisa M. Donofrio

7   Fillers Working by Fibroplasia
        Introduction   83
        A Artefill   Alastair Carruthers, Jean Carruthers   84
        B Radiesse   Jean Carruthers, Alastair Carruthers   87
        C Silicone   Chad L. Prather, Derek H. Jones   90
        D Poly-L-lactic Acid Stephen H. Mandy   101

8   Nasolabial Folds   105
        Gary D. Monheit, Betty Davis

9   Pain Control in Cosmetic Facial Surgery   127
        Kevin Smith, Joseph Niamtu, Jean Carruthers

10   Injectable Fillers in Skin of Color   143
        Pearl E. Grimes, Julius W. Few

11   Complications of Soft Tissue Augmentation   151
        Sue Ellen Cox, Naomi Lawrence

Contents

12   ◉   **Synthetic Fillers**

     A   **Carboxymethyl Cellulose,**   Philippa Lowe, Samuel Falcone,
        Polyethylene Oxide Dermal Filler   Richard Berg, Nicholas J. Lowe   **161**

     B   **BioAlcamid**   David J. Goldberg   **167**

     C   **Bioinblue**   Jean Carruthers, Alastair Carruthers   **173**

Index   **175**

Series Preface
Procedures in Cosmetic Dermatology

Four years ago we began a project to produce "Procedures in Cosmetic Dermatology", a series of high quality, and practical, up-to-date, illustrated manuals on procedures in cosmetic dermatology. Our plan was to provide dermatologists and dermatologic surgeons with detailed books accompanied by instructional DVD's containing all the information they needed to master most, if not all of the leading edge cosmetic dermatology techniques. Thanks to the efforts of our superb book editors, chapter authors, and the tireless and extraordinary publishing staff at Elsevier, the series has been more successful than any of us could have hoped. Over the past 3 years, thirteen volumes have been introduced, which have been purchased by thousands of physicians all over the world. Originally published in English, many of the texts have been translated into different languages including Italian, French, Spanish, Chinese, Polish, Korean, Portuguese, and Russian.

Our commitment to you is to convey information that is practical, easy to use, and up to date. Since new devices and minimally invasive techniques are continually being refined in this rapidly changing area, the time has now come to inaugurate second editions of these books. During the next few years updated texts will be released. The most time-sensitive books will be revised first, and others will follow.

This series is an ever evolving project. So in addition to second editions of current books, we will be introducing entirely new books to cover novel procedures that may not have existed when the series began. Enjoy and keep learning.

Jeffrey S. Dover MD FRCPC and **Murad Alam** MD

Series Preface
Procedures in Cosmetic Dermatology

While dermatologists have been procedurally inclined since the beginning of the specialty, particularly rapid change has occurred in the past quarter century. The advent of frozen section technique and the golden age of Mohs skin cancer surgery has led to the formal incorporation of surgery within the dermatology curriculum. More recently technological breakthroughs in minimally invasive procedural dermatology have offered an aging population new options for improving the appearance of damaged skin.

Procedures for rejuvenating the skin and adjacent regions are actively sought by our patients. Significantly, dermatologists have pioneered devices, technologies and medications, which have continued to evolve at a startling pace. Numerous major advances, including virtually all cutaneous lasers and light-source-based procedures, botulinum exotoxin, soft-tissue augmentation, dilute anesthesia liposuction, leg vein treatments, chemical peels, and hair transplants, have been invented, or developed and enhanced by dermatologists. Dermatologists understand procedures, and we have special insight into the structure, function, and working of skin. Cosmetic dermatologists have made rejuvenation accessible to risk-averse patients by emphasizing safety and reducing operative trauma. No specialty is better positioned than dermatology to lead the field of cutaneous surgery while meeting patient needs.

As dermatology grows as a specialty, an ever-increasing proportion of dermatologists will become proficient in the delivery of different procedures. Not all dermatologists will perform all procedures, and some will perform very few, but even the less procedurally directed amongst us must be well-versed in the details to be able to guide and educate our patients. Whether you are a skilled dermatologic surgeon interested in further expanding your surgical repertoire, a complete surgical novice wishing to learn a few simple procedures, or somewhere in between, this book and this series is for you.

The volume you are holding is one of a series entitled 'Procedures in Cosmetic Dermatology.' The purpose of each book is to serve as a practical primer on a major topic area in procedural dermatology.

If you want to make sure you find the right book for your needs, you may wish to know what this book is and what it is not. It is not a comprehensive text grounded in theoretical underpinnings. It is not exhaustively referenced. It is not designed to be a completely unbiased review of the world's literature on the subject. At the same time, it is not an overview of cosmetic procedures that describes these in generalities without providing enough specific information to actually permit someone to perform the procedures. And importantly, it is not so heavy that it can serve as a door-stop or a shelf filler.

What this book and this series offer is a step-by-step, practical guide to performing cutaneous surgical procedures. Each volume in the series has been edited by a known authority in that subfield. Each editor has recruited other equally practical-minded, technically skilled, hands-on clinicians to write the constituent chapters. Most chapters have two authors to ensure that different approaches and a broad range of opinions are incorporated. On the other hand, the two authors and the editors also collectively provide a consistency of tone. A uniform template has been used within each chapter so that the reader will be easily able to navigate all the books in the series. Within every chapter, the authors succinctly tell it like they do it. The emphasis is on therapeutic technique; treatment methods are discussed with an eye to appropriate indications, adverse events, and unusual cases. Finally, this book is short and can be read in its entirety on a long plane ride. We believe that brevity paradoxically results in greater information transfer because cover-to-cover mastery is practicable.

We hope you enjoy this book and the rest of the books in the series and that you benefit from the many hours of clinical wisdom that have been distilled to produce it. Please keep it nearby, where you can reach for it when you need it.

Jeffrey S. Dover MD FRCPC and Murad Alam MD

Preface

It is indeed an enormous pleasure to present this 2008 Filler Volume.

The Food and Drug Administration (FDA) in the United States has currently approved 16 injectables for esthetic indications (ArteFill) Botox, Captique, CosmoDerm/Plast, Cymetra, Elevess, Fascian, Hylaform, Hylaform Plus, Juvéderm Ultra, Juvederm Ultra Plus, Restylane, Radiesse and ZyDerm/Plast; other products currently seeking approval for esthetic soft tissue augmentation include Evolence, Perlane and Sculptra.

Others are approved in Europe, Canada and South America and will be coming to the US market in the foreseeable future – for example Aquamid.

The American Society for Aesthetic Plastic Surgery states that the number of dermal filler procedures grew from approximately 350,000 in 1997, when only a 3-month filler was available, to almost 1,500,000 in 2005 after the introduction of 6-month fillers.

With so many new products of differing longevity of response available it becomes increasingly important to know all about the features and composition and mechanism of action of each filler as, like people, they each have their own specific properties and tissue responses. We also recognize the immense importance of perfect technique – including injecting gently and slowly and deliberately, at the correct level, in the correct volume and the correct frequency with the correct filler alone or in combination – for example with Botox™.

The greatest pleasure as an educator is to teach students who are receptive and industrious and who have the desire to be better and know more than the teacher! In like vein, the greatest pleasure as an editor is to receive manuscripts from expert colleagues who are passionate and detail oriented and who understand how to present such complicated material with clarity and elegance but with practicality.

Alastair and I hope that you enjoy reading these excellent chapters as much as we have enjoyed working to put this 'Filler Share-Ware' together for you.

Jean Carruthers and Alastair Carruthers

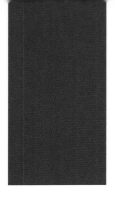

To the women in my life

My grandmothers, Bertha and Lillian

My mother, Nina

My daughters, Sophie and Isabel

And especially to my wife, Tania

For their never-ending encouragement, patience, support, love, and friendship

To my father, Mark – a great teacher and role model

To my mentor, Kenneth A. Arndt for his generosity, kindness, sense of humor, joie de vivre, and above all else curiosity and enthusiasm

At Elsevier, Sue Hodgson who conceptualized the series and brought it to reality and Claire Bonnett for polite, persistent, and dogged determination.

Jeffrey S. Dover

Elsevier's dedicated editorial staff has made possible the continuing success of this ambitious project. The new team led by Claire Bonnett, Anne Bassett and the production staff have refined the concept for the second edition while maintaining the series' reputation for quality and cutting-edge relevance. In this, they have been ably supported by the graphics shop, which has created the signature high quality illustrations and layouts that are the backbone of each book. We are also deeply grateful to the volume editors, who have generously found time in their schedules, cheerfully accepted our guidelines, and recruited the most knowledgeable chapter authors. And we especially thank the chapter contributors, without whose work there would be no books at all. Finally, I would also like to convey my debt to my teachers, Kenneth Arndt, Jeffrey Dover, Michael Kaminer, Leonard Goldberg, and David Bickers, and my parents, Rahat and Rehana Alam.

Murad Alam

Contents

Series Preface vii
Series Preface First Edition viii
Preface ix
List of Contributors xi

1 Background Information on the use of Esthetic Fillers 1
Hayes B. Gladstone, Brian Somoano

2 Fillers Esthetics 11
Stephen R. Tan, Richard G. Glogau

3 Injectable Collagens 19
Seth L. Matarasso

4 Hylans and Soft Tissue Augmentation 31
Rhoda S. Narins, Jason Michaels, Joel L. Cohen

5 Management of the Lips and Mouth Corners 51
Jean Carruthers, Vic A. Narurkar

6 Augmentation with Autologous Fat 63
Lisa M. Donofrio

7 Fillers Working by Fibroplasia
Introduction 83
A Artefill Alastair Carruthers, Jean Carruthers 84
B Radiesse Jean Carruthers, Alastair Carruthers 87
C Silicone Chad L. Prather, Derek H. Jones 90
D Poly-L-lactic Acid Stephen H. Mandy 101

8 Nasolabial Folds 105
Gary D. Monheit, Betty Davis

9 Pain Control in Cosmetic Facial Surgery 127
Kevin Smith, Joseph Niamtu, Jean Carruthers

10 Injectable Fillers in Skin of Color 143
Pearl E. Grimes, Julius W. Few

11 Complications of Soft Tissue Augmentation 151
Sue Ellen Cox, Naomi Lawrence

Contents

12   Synthetic Fillers
   A **Carboxymethyl Cellulose,**   Philippa Lowe, Samuel Falcone,
      Polyethylene Oxide Dermal Filler Richard Berg, Nicholas J. Lowe   161
   B **BioAlcamid**   David J. Goldberg   167
   C **Bioinblue**   Jean Carruthers, Alastair Carruthers 173

Index   175

List of Contributors

Richard Berg PhD
FzioMed Inc., San Luis Obispo, CA USA

Alastair Carruthers MA BM BCh FRCPC FRCP (Lon)
Clinical Professor, Division of Dermatology, University of British Columbia, Vancouver, BC, Canada

Jean Carruthers MD FRCSC FRC (OPHTH) FASOPRS
Clinical Professor, Department of Ophthalmology, University of British Columbia, Vancouver, BC, Canada

Joel L. Cohen MD FAAD
Assistant Clinical Professor, University of Colorado, Department of Dermatology, Director Aboutskin Dermatology and DermSurgery, Denver, CO, USA

Sue Ellen Cox MD
Dermatologic Surgeon, Medical Director of Aesthetic Solutions, Associate Clinical Professor Dermatology Department at University of North Carolina, Chapel Hill, NC, USA

Betty Davis MD
Fellow in Dermatologic Surgery, Total Skin and Beauty Dermatology Center and Department of Dermatology, University of Alabama at Birmingham, Birmingham, AL, USA

Lisa M. Donofrio MD
Associate Clinical Professor, Department of Dermatology, Yale University School of Medicine, New Haven, CT, USA

Samuel Falcone PhD
FzioMed Inc, San Luis Obispo, CA, USA

Julius W. Few MD FACS
Associate Professor of Surgery, Division of Plastic Surgery, Director of the Esthetic and Breast Surgery Fellowship, Worthwestern University Feinberg School of Mechcine IL, USA

Hayes B. Gladstone MD
Director, Division of Dermatologic Surgery Department of Dermatology, Stanford University School of Medicine, Stanford, CA, USA

Richard G. Glogau MD
Clinical Professor of Dermatology, University of California Medical Centre, San Francisco, CA, USA

David J. Goldberg MD
Director, Skin Laser & Surgery Specialists of New York and New Jersey; Clinical Professor of Dermatology, Mount Sinai School of Medicine, New York, NY; Clinical Professor of Dermatology, New Jersey Medical School, Newark, NJ, USA

Pearl E. Grimes MD
Director, Vitiligo & Pigmentation Institute of Southern California, Los Angeles, CA; Clinical Professor, Division of Dermatology, David Geffen School of Medicine at University of California, Los Angeles, CA, USA

Derek H. Jones MD
Division of Dermatology, David Geffen School of Medicine, University of California at Los Angeles, Los Angeles, CA, USA

Naomi Lawrence MD
Head, Procedural Dermatology Cooper-Health, Marlton, NJ, USA

Nicholas J. Lowe MD FRCP
Clinical Professor, University of California School of Medicine, Los Angeles, CA, USA; Consultant Dermatologist, Cranley Clinic, London, UK; Clinical Research Specialist, Santa Monica, CA, USA and London, UK

Philippa Lowe MD
Cranley Clinic, London, UK

Stephen H. Mandy MD FAAD
Volunteer Professor of Dermatology, University of Miami, Miami, FL, USA

Seth L. Matarasso MD
Clinical Professor of Dermatology, University of California School of Medicine, San Francisco, CA, USA

Jason Michaels MD
Associate Clinical Professor, University of Nevada School of Medicine, Aspire Cosmetic MedCenter of Las Vegas Skin and Cancer Clinics, Las Vegas, NV, USA

Gary D. Monheit MD FAAD FACS
Associate Clinical Professor, Department of Dermatology and Ophthalmology, University of Alabama at Birmingham, Birmingham, AL, USA

Rhoda S. Narins MD PC
Director, Dermatology Surgery and Laser Centre, Manhattan and White Plains, NY; Clinical Professor of Dermatology, New York University Medical School, New York, NY, USA

Vic A. Narurkar MD FAAD
Director and Founder Bay Area Laser Institute, San Francisco, CA; Assistant Clinical Professor of Dermatology, University of California David School of Medicine, Sacramento, CA, USA

Joseph Niamtu III DMD
Private Practice, Oral/Maxillofacial & Cosmetic Facial Surgery Richmond, VA, USA

Chad L. Prather MD
Department of Dermatology, Louisiana State University Health Sciences Center, New Orleans, LA, USA

Kevin Smith BA BSc MD FRCPC
Consultant Dermatologist, Niagara Falls, ON, Canada

Brian Somoano MD
Resident in Dermatology, Stanford University Medical Centre, Stanford, CA, USA

Stephen R. Tan MD FRCPC
Director of Dermatologic Surgery, Health Partners Medical Group and Clinics, Minneapolis, MN, USA

1 Background Information on Use of Esthetic Fillers

Hayes B. Gladstone, Brian Somoano

HISTORY

Human beings have used personal cosmetic enhancements for thousands of years. Initially, these applications consisted of topical inks derived from plants and animal sources. The advent of surgical procedures became possible in the second half of the 19th century due to the development of local and general anesthesia; esthetic procedures were able to become much more invasive. Initially, fat was grafted to fill volume after trauma. In the 20th century, autologous fat became the most common filler. However, cutting out fat and transplanting it still represented a major procedure, and in most cases it did not have lasting effects.

With the slowly increasing demand for cosmetic procedures beginning in the 1970s, research into collagen production produced a bovine formulation that could be placed in a syringe and injected. Dermatologists and plastic surgeons helped develop this product, though perhaps because of its more minimally invasive nature, dermatologists such as Sam Stegman and Arnold Klein took the lead in its clinical use.

The temporary nature of bovine collagen and the requirement for double skin testing led to the development and testing of other fillers in Europe and Asia in the 1990s. Public demand was fueled by aging baby boomers demanding procedures with no down-time; media hype surrounding 'lunchtime' cosmetic procedures placed fillers on center stage along with botulinum toxin (Botox). Fillers could be used as sculpting agents to dramatically change a person's appearance in a mere 15 minutes. Today, there are a number of fillers to choose from, each with its own strengths, drawbacks and indications. The development of these substances continues, often at a dizzying pace, so it is important for the esthetic specialist physician to understand the indications and uses of these fillers so that he or she can best serve the patient's needs.

PATIENT ESTHETIC EVALUATION

Though there are different cultural/ethnic norms of beauty, there are certain qualities which seem globally to transcend these differences in determining what is perceptually pleasing. Esthetically pleasing features include symmetry, smooth convex contours, and even, homogeneous skin tone and texture. These features may become disrupted by natural disease such as acne or by environmental agents such as sun exposure or trauma, or merely by the inevitable and natural process of aging. Scars caused by acne or trauma leave depressions of varying depth. Depressions of an entire cosmetic unit may be caused by morphea or that of lipodystrophy secondary to infection with the human immunodeficiency virus (HIV) (Fig. 1.1). Fine rhytides, particularly in the perioral region can be caused by excessive actinic damage. Loss of maxillary and mandibular bone, subcutaneous fat and dermal collagen result in wider lower facial depressions and perioral grooves such as the melolabial and melomental folds. Any line of facial expression becomes accentuated with age, muscular hyperactivity and volume loss. The previous generations of esthetic physicians have depended on the algorithm of surgical skin redraping and tightening. In the modern esthetic world, restoration of facial volume and contour has become the first line of treatment before surgical correction is entertained.

Restoration of facial symmetry and volume, as well as a smooth contour and homogeneous skin tone are the newer goals of the cosmetic surgeon. Leonardo da Vinci divided the face into thirds from the hairline to the chin. Horizontally, the face is approximately the width of five eyes. All of these esthetic divisions must be taken into consideration in making an esthetic treatment plan.

The upper, mid and lower face must be in harmony. This is particularly true of the transitions between the different facial zones. In order to achieve these objectives, a comprehensive approach must be taken, and multiple modalities utilized. Fillers play a major role in this process. The appropriate filler can restore symmetry, volume and recreate a smooth skin surface. In combination with other treatments such as chemodenervation with Botox, they may lead to more enhanced esthetic and longer lasting results.

INDICATIONS

Fillers have multiple uses, either filling pre-existing facial defects or augmenting existing facial structures. Beginning with the upper third of the face, fillers can be used to fill

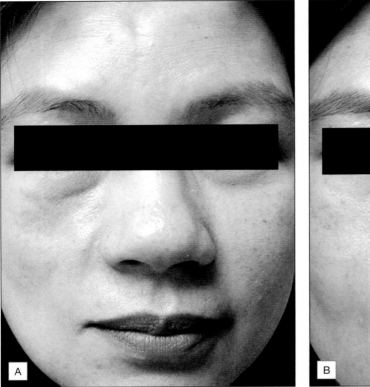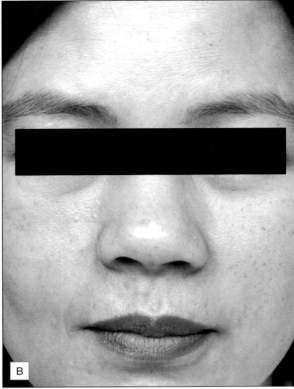

Fig. 1.1 (**A**) Patient with right-sided stable morphea. (**B**) Six months following fat transfer to the right cheek

in depressions in the forehead from acne scars and synergistically, with Botox, to treat deep resting glabellar folds. Injection under the lateral third of the brow will elevate the previously ptotic lateral brow segment. Temporal depression below the temporal fusion line, often associated with age or acquired lipodystrophy, may also be augmented. Esthetic physicians should be aware that glabellar augmentation with deep dermal hyaluronans such as Restylane appear to be safe, unlike injections of autologous fat and bovine collagen, which have caused cases of iatrogenic blindness. In the periorbital region, low viscosity fillers may be used for 'etched-in' crow's feet, particularly those that extend inferior to the inferior orbital margin, past the origin of zygomaticus major on the zygoma.

Some practitioners advocate using filler in the upper eyelid as a substitute for blepharoplasty. In the lower eyelid, restoring this subunit's volume and contour rather than ritually removing fat has become a guiding principle in restoration of the upper third of the face. The appropriate use of a filler can remove the 'double bubble' between the lower eyelid and the upper cheek as well as filling the lateral and inferior nasojugal groove as it extends into the orbitomalar groove bisecting the malar fat pad. Fillers create a more uniform smoothness in the transition

between the upper and midface by effacing the tear trough deformity; the subject promptly loses the tired appearance caused by the dark circles and is provided with a more rested, energized appearance.

In the midface, fillers can be used to fill scars from pre-existing asymmetry, and scars resulting from trauma or acne. Two common features of the aging midface are the sinking and effacing of the malar eminence and hollowing, and descent of the cheeks. Fillers can be used to augment this area. The malar region can be directly built up, often by merely adding volume to the cheeks; this will increase the malar prominence and enhance the youthful convex appearance. Similarly, cheek hollowing is often seen in subjects suffering HIV-related facial lipoatrophy. While the thinness of nasal skin may lead to a higher rate of complications or unsatisfactory results, with experience, scars, particularly on the dorsum, can be effectively filled. Occasionally, subscision of the nasal tip to relax skin adhesion to the underlying cartilage is necessary before tip contour can be improved with injected filler.

The most popular anatomic area, and the one with the most prolonged results, is the nasolabial folds (NLFs) also known as 'smile' lines. The NLFs cross the transition zone between the midface and lower face. Though initially these lines don't truly reflect the aging process, their deep-

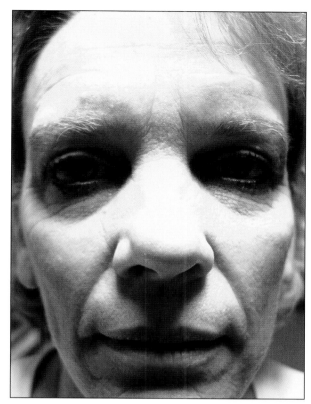

Fig. 1.2 Prominent nasolabial lines that create a sense of age, and are amenable to a filler

ening over time creates an abnormal demarcation between these two major facial regions (Fig. 1.2). The desire of even young patients to fill these lines, which initially are only a function of expression rather than senescence, reflects the esthetic aspiration for a smooth facial contour and the softening of the vertical depth of these lines, which cause a severe and angry facial expression. A variety of fillers can be used to effectively blunt these lines. A secondary effect of filling these lines will be to increase the profile of the medial cheeks, which is also esthetically desirable.

The lower face is dominated by the vermilion lips, both in contour and profile. As time passes, the vertical dimension of the vermilion lip may decrease as the vermilion display turns inside the oral cavity. Fine rhytides in the upper lip allow lipstick to 'bleed' up into the cutaneous lip, thus giving an obvious and 'smudged' appearance to the lip borders. Many types of fillers can be used in the lips to enhance and achieve a natural fullness.

Marionette or 'drool' lines are a combination of expression, aging, gravity and genetics. In many individuals, these can be not only quite pronounced, but there may be multiple perioral curvilinear depressions lateral and inferior to the oral commissures. Biomechanically, marionette lines are caused by a loss of volume and support combined with a loss of dermal elasticity. While a variety of fillers can be

used to reduce them, in older individuals or those with advanced actinic damage and sagging, filling them may create ripples lateral to the injection area. The concurrent use of neurotoxin relaxation (Botox) of the depressor anguli oris, the mentalis and the orbicularis oris will not only improve the esthetic result but also prolong the longevity of the filler in the highly mobile perioral region.

A sign of aging in the lower face is unevenness of the jawline. This is not only caused by loss of skin elasticity and gravity causing enhancement of the jowl contour, but also because of resorption of the bony mandible and subcutaneous fat. Selective injection of the appropriate filler, particularly in combination with the injection of a supporting strut of filler in the melomental fold and pre-joint sulcus, can create a smooth and robust mandibular line. Though permanent implants are the surgical procedure of choice for increasing chin projection, using injectable filler can create a more prominent chin albeit a temporary one. It may also be useful in allowing the patient to determine if he/she desires a permanent implant.

PRE-PROCEDURE PLANNING

All patients desiring cosmetic procedures should have a comprehensive medical and social evaluation. This cosmetic evaluation should first address the patient's concerns, discuss the treatment options and devise an overall treatment plan. Subjects may be helped by prioritizing their concerns and their interest in the various treatments to optimize their appearance. During this discussion, subjects can understand the components of facial aging including lines of dynamic expression, static wrinkles and folds caused by photodamage and elastosis of the skin, and loss of posterior tissue support from bone remodeling and fat atrophy. Treatments appropriate for each component should be explained and outlined. This discussion is particularly important because subjects are more accepting of treatments that they understand and have chosen themselves. Many individuals are well informed because of the Media and the Internet. Some patients may be focused on wanting only one treatment even though it may not be appropriate for their concerns. When it is determined that fillers are the appropriate therapy, several alternatives should be discussed and a choice made as to the most appropriate choice. Outlining normal postoperative sequelae such as bruising, lumpiness and swelling is important as well as the pretreatment discussion of possible adverse events. If the filler is being used in an off-label manner, then this fact should also be discussed with the patient.

A complete medical history including medications and allergies should be taken. As with any other elective surgical procedure, the patient should not take aspirin for at least 8 days, or vitamin E, or nonsteroid anti-inflammatory drugs (NSAIDs) for at least 5 days prior to treatment. If the patient is on Coumadin, the prothrombin time (PT) should be checked. Generally if the PT is under 2.0, then the risk of hematoma or excessive bruising from injection is low. It should also be ascertained whether the patient takes herbal medication such as Gingko Biloba since these can cause bleeding. Some homeopathic medications such as Arnica Montana taken preoperatively are believed to reduce bruising, but this has not been demonstrated in clinical studies.

There are very few absolute contraindications to fillers. A patient with a known allergy to a specific filler would obviously not be a candidate for the procedure. Finally, preoperative photos from the frontal, oblique and profile angles are not only important from a medico-legal standpoint, but are also an extremely important part of subsequent patient satisfaction follow up.

CHOOSING THE APPROPRIATE FILLER

The choice of filling substance to be used is perhaps the most important one after the choice that soft tissue augmentation is to be performed. A confusing array of biodegradable, nonpermanent and nonbiodegradable, permanent substances is available (Table 1.1). Traditional fillers have been biodegradable, i.e. absorbed and ultimately excreted. Though these substances can result in hypersensitivity reactions, they have a proven safety record. The disadvantage to these fillers has been their relatively short duration, in some cases necessitating injections every 3 months. Over the past decade semipermanent fillers have been used in Europe, South America and Asia. Several of these fillers are in the final stages of FDA approval. While they do have a longer effect, they may have an increased incidence of granulomas; in many cases the granulomas are of late onset (longer than 1 year after treatment). These fillers tend to have microspheres which are nonbiodegradable. Finally, there are the truly nonbiodegradable, permanent fillers. These substances may play a substantial role in patients with HIV lipoatrophy or stable morphea. Traditionally, they have resulted in a high incidence of granulomas and extrusion, but new formulations may decrease granulomas from these fillers. Ultimately, patient safety is the paramount consideration.

While autologous fat is historically the oldest available filler, bovine collagen in the form of Zyderm I, Zyderm II and Zyplast have been the most frequently used substances until 2003. They can provide excellent results for depressed acne scars, NLFs and lips. The well-known disadvantage of these fillers is the potential for allergic reaction, which necessitates two separate skin tests. Depending on the site, it is rare for collagen to have a significant effect after 6 months. In areas with increased mobility such as the lips, it is unlikely that collagen will remain for more than 3 months. Recently, human collagen has been introduced. It has the advantage of not requiring skin testing, but its duration is similar to its bovine predecessor. There have been other types of collagen derived from cadavers or from the patient. While they also don't require skin testing, their efficacy is similar to that of human collagen. Though, as mentioned earlier, these

Table 1.1 Biodegradable and nonbiodegradable fillers	
Biodegradable fillers	**Nonbiodegradable fillers**
AcHyal	Aquamid
Alloderm	Artesense (ArteFill in USA)
Autologen	Bioplastique
Biocell ultravital	Evolution
Cymetra	GoreTex
Dermal grafting	Meta-Crill
Dermaplant	Silicone oil (Adatosil & Silikone 1000)
Eleveress	Softform
Endoplast-50	
Fascian	
Fat	
Human placental collagen	
Hyal-system	
Hylaform + Hylaform Plus	**Slowly biodegradable fillers**
Isologen	Radiesse
Juvederm	Sculptra
New-Fill (Sculptra)	
Perlane	
Permacol	
Plasmagel	
Resoplast	
Restylane	
Restylane-fine/touch	
Reviderm intra	
Surgisis	
Cosmoderm & Cosmoplast	

fillers can be used in a variety of sites, because of their ease of injection and malleability, they offer superior results for lip augmentation.

Fat has been used since the late 19th century, though it has dramatically evolved in its technique, and has enjoyed a revival in its use. Fat has the advantage of volume, and the ease of using large amounts, which makes it very cost effective (Fig. 1.3). It provides excellent volume replacement. It can be used for pan-facial volume restoration. Specifically, it is an excellent substance for the NLFs, cheeks and marionette lines. Because of its volume and viscosity, fine lines and small acne scars would not be appropriate for this filler. Generally, fat is more difficult

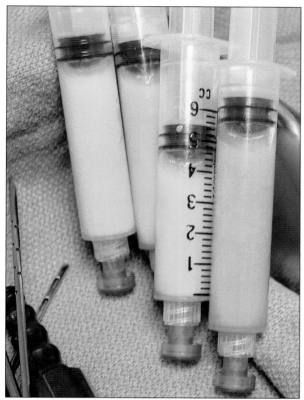

Fig. 1.3 Fat harvested by syringe for fat transfer

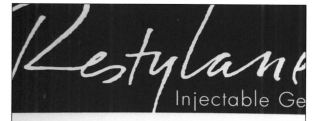

Contents:
1 Syringe (0.7 mL) containing non-animal, stabilized hyaluronic acid 20 mg/mL in physiological saline, pH 7

1 Needle 30 G x 1/2"

1 Package Insert

Indication:
Restylane is indicated for mid-to-deep dermal implantation for the correction of moderate to severe facial wrinkles and folds, such as nasolabial folds.

Fig. 1.4 Hyaluronic acid is a versatile filler for facial augmentation

to use in the lips, though in the hands of an experienced practitioner, it can provide outstanding results. The disadvantages of using fat are that the patient must have areas of fat deposits, and fat graft augmentation requires extraction and injection.

The hyaluronic acid group of fillers represents a recent breakthrough for augmentation technology (Fig. 1.4). Because this substance is completely homologous in structure between species it can be generated by both bacteria fermentation and from chicken combs so there is no need for allergy testing. It is a very versatile filler and appears to have a longer effect than earlier collagens. Initially, in Europe, there were reports that at 8 months 80% of the filler remained. However, in a multi-center double-blind, randomized study comparing hyaluronic acid to collagen in the NLFs, its effect appeared to begin to diminish at 6 months. Approved by the FDA in late 2003, it is too early to judge the exact duration of this filler. While hyaluronic acid does not quite have the ease of use of injectable collagen, it still provides excellent long lasting results for the lips, NLFs, marionette lines and acne scars. Compared to collagen, it appears that not as much hyaluronic acid is required to fill a specific defect. Longer lasting hyaluronic acid gels which have larger particles and are cross-linked are now FDA approved and tend to have a longer lasting effect than some of the previous hyaluronic acid products.

Two recent trials comparing Perlane, a hyaluronic acid gel (20 mg/mL), to Zyplast and to Hylaform for augmentation of the NLFs, demonstrated superior efficacy and less material needed.

Another recent addition to fillers has been polymethylmethacrylate microspheres. This substance has the advantage of not only remaining in the skin for an extended period of time, but also causing fibrosis around the beads leading to a longer lasting effect. It has been used successfully for the deeper lines such as NLFs and marionette lines. Because of its consistency, it can lead to lumpiness and unevenness in the lips. While it can potentially last for several years, each injection sequence is not as full as one of the biodegradable fillers. Significant granulomas have been reported with Artecoll as with other permanent fillers. However ArteFill, which has succeeded Artecoll and is now FDA approved, has been shown to have a low complication rate over a 5-year period. In the FDA-associated trials, there was a 2.2% rate of adverse effects. Less than 1% was rated as severe. Long-term efficacy at 4–5 years was also significant. In a recent retrospective series of approximately 500 patients, Carruthers and Carruthers reported only four patients who had late granulomas. These were treated successfully with triamcinolone injections. Because this filler can be less forgiving than others, the authors emphasized that thorough training and

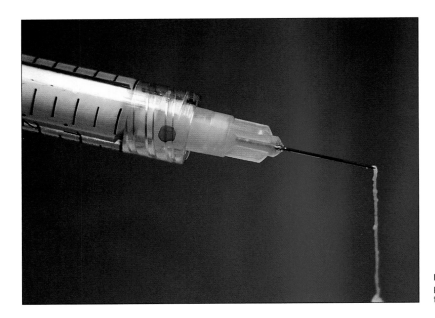

Fig. 1.5 Calcium hydroxylapatite, a semi-permanent substance, is being used off-label for facial augmentation

technique are required to produce consistently excellent results and minimal complications.

Calcium hydroxylapatite (Radiesse™), another semi-permanent substance which has been used as a radiologic marker and for vocal cord stabilization, has been used off-label for filling facial lines (it received FDA approval for cosmetic uses in late 2006) (Fig. 1.5). Based on its longevity in these other areas, it was felt that as a facial filler, it may last up to several years. That has not been the case. According to one study, it retains significant effects in NLFs for 6–9 months. In clinical experience it tends to last 10–12 months in less mobile areas of the face. Much less of this substance is needed to fill a particular defect compared to collagen. It is not difficult to inject but it should be injected in the subdermal plane. It is particularly efficacious for NLFs and marionette lines. Because of its viscosity, it is also reasonable to use for hollowing of the cheeks or substantial acne scars. In experienced hands, calcium hydroxylapatite can be very versatile. The prejowl sulcus can be augmented, which provides a smoother jawline, and there have been a number of reports of a 'nonsurgical rhinoplasty' using calcium hydroxylapatite. FDA has approved use in HIV patients for lipoatrophy as well as possible chin augmentation. Similar to Artecoll, calcium hydroxylapatite can lead to lumpiness when used in the lips and this site is not currently recommended for the current formulation of Radiesse.

Poly-l-lactic acid received FDA approval in 2004 for the treatment of HIV-related facial lipoatrophy. It is injected into the subcutis and stimulates fibroplasia. Multiple injections are necessary, but the results for cheek/malar atrophy have been impressive. In the European trials, the effect remained for 18–24 months. Cosmetic use of this product is considered off-label, but has been

used for pan facial augmentation. It is very important to inject this substance in the correct plane. Injection into the dermis will heighten the risk of granulomas.

Silicone has historically been used as a facial filler. There have been reports of granulomas, foreign-body reactions and extrusion. These adverse reactions may have been secondary to impurities. Recently, the microdroplet technique has been advocated with excellent results in selected patients using Silicone 1000. This filler is permanent, and with repeated injections can augment large defects or augment significant areas. It is currently undergoing FDA testing for cheek augmentation in subjects suffering HIV facial lipoatrophy. According to reports, it is easy to use and has had excellent cosmetic results with a minimal side-effect profile as long as the microdroplet technique is used.

TECHNIQUE

While specific techniques will be covered in the following chapters, there are several guidelines. Technique is partially dependent on the choice of filler. Positioning the patient sitting up will enable an accurate assessment of the defects or lines. Applying a topical anesthetic at least 10–30 minutes prior to the procedure will dull the pain of injection. Nerve blocks, the most common being infraorbital and submental, are often indicated. Direct injection of lidocaine with epinephrine, particularly in NLFs and marionette lines, will not only make this a much more pleasant procedure, but will reduce bleeding. Generally, waiting 15 minutes will not only allow the anesthesia to take effect, but will reduce any distortion of the target site. Massaging the site will provide a more uniform

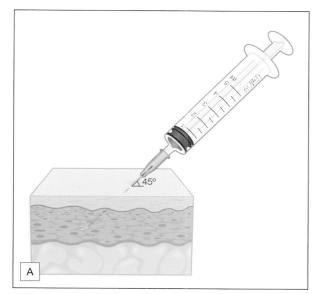

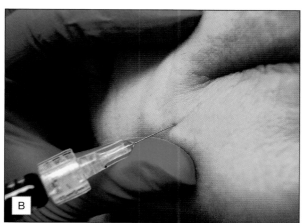

Fig. 1.6 (A) Diagram and **(B)** photograph showing correct angle for placement of filler into the deep dermis

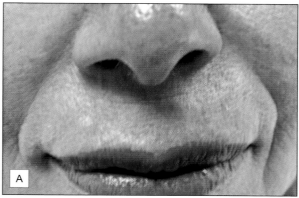

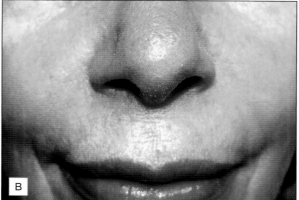

Fig. 1.7 (A) Prominent nasolabial or 'smile' lines. **(B)** Three months following injection of hyaluronic acid

distribution of lidocaine with potentially fewer needle sticks as well as reducing transient swelling.

In terms of injecting fillers such as collagen or hyaluronic acid, there are two techniques, both of which have advantages and disadvantages. For these two substances a 30 gauge needle will suffice. For thicker substances such as Artecoll or calcium hydroxylapatite, a 27 gauge needle is necessary. RJ Maxflo needles, which are also 30 gauge on the outside but 27 gauge on the inside, but permit a higher flow rate, may also be appropriate as they retain their sharpness. Fat injection requires larger gauge needles or specialized Coleman injection cannulae. Many practitioners prefer the threading technique, which injects the filler along either most or the entire length of the defect. These 'threads' are injected in toto so that they lie on top of each other. The advantage of this technique is that there are fewer needle punctures, and potentially a smoother result is obtained since it is easier to produce contiguous layering. In contrast, the multiple puncture technique requires several needle sticks. Beads of filler are injected. The advantage of this technique is more control and precise placement. With both methods, the filler is injected as the needle is retracted, thus reducing the risk of vascular injection.

The depth of injection depends on the type of filler. For Zyderm or Cosmoderm, the superficial dermis is appropriate. For Zyplast or Cosmoplast, or hyaluronic acid, the deep dermis (maintaining the needle at a 45-degree angle) provides the best results (Figs 1.6 and 1.7). Often, using Cosmoplast or hyaluronic acid in the deep dermis and then Cosmoderm more superficially will achieve very satisfying results. The dermal-subcutaneous border or subdermal plane is appropriate for both Artecoll and calcium hydroxylapatite. Fat is layered into the subcutaneous space. For these fillers, it is important not to inject too superficially as this will result in lumpiness and possibly in an increased incidence of granulomas. Of course, too deep an injection technique will result in a less than desirable augmentation. Injecting into the lips

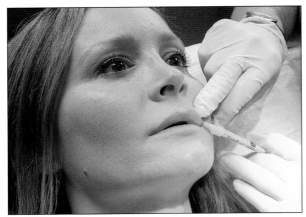

Fig. 1.8 Injecting human collagen into the upper lip. Placement of this material is at vermilion border

requires a great degree of finesse and judgment. While there are a number of different techniques, it is important to inject smoothly along the vermilion border and within the vermilion lip in order to avoid lumpiness (Fig. 1.8).

POST-PROCEDURE MANAGEMENT

It may be wise to allow the patient to rest for a few minutes following the procedure, given the needle-causing anxiety of many patients. Cold compresses or ice following the procedure will reduce some of the swelling and reduce some soreness from the multiple injections after the anesthetic wears off. Dressings are generally not needed for injectables, though the donor site for fat transfer will need to be bandaged. Though the patient may not be compliant, it is worth reminding them to try to reduce facial expressions for the first 48 hours. For some fillers such as calcium hydroxylapatite, having the patient gently pat the area injected – without a shearing motion – may help set the material. Pre- and postprocedure photographs are a necessity.

COMPLICATIONS

In addition to allergic reactions, infection and hematomas, which are rare, other adverse events may include asymmetry, granulomas, migration and extrusion. More common than the last three complications is lumpiness and dimpling, which is usually the result of placing the material in too superficial a plane. This 'bumpiness' will usually resolve over 1 or 2 weeks without therapy. Massage may expedite resolution of this problem. True granulomas are rare and can be treated initially with a low-dose steroid injection. Larger or persistent granulomas may need to be excised if treatment with intralesional steroid, topical tacrolimus or oral allopurinol is not successful.

SOFT TISSUE FILLERS ON THE HORIZON

Evolence, a collagen derivative was developed in Israel by ColBar LifeScience and introduced in Europe in 2004. This substance comes from porcine collagen, and undergoes a cross-linking process that makes it very stable and also removes its immunogenicity. Therefore pretesting is not necessary. In contrast to current collagen, Evolence is reported to last up to 12 months in less mobile facial regions such as NLFs. It has a visco-consistency similar to that of hyaluronic acid and can be injected with a 30 gauge needle. Its adverse effect profile is similar to that of commercially available collagen in the United States. Currently, it is not FDA-approved.

Polyacrylamide hydrogel is a nonabsorbable long-term filler. The gel consists of 2.5% cross-linked polyacrylamide covalently bound to 97.5% sterile water. In one animal study, it was highly bioactive inducing a tissue reaction. Yet, it has been used in Europe and Asia for the past decade with excellent results and a minimal complication rate. In a prospective study enrolling 251 patients who were injected primarily in their NLFs, lips and glabellar folds, the effect remained for up to 2 years – though only 101 patients were evaluated at 24 months. Because of its consistency and semi-permanency, hydrogel may be better for NLFs and for panfacial augmentation. Polyacrylamide hydrogel is not FDA approved, but is currently undergoing clinical safety and efficacy trials.

VALUE OF COMBINATION THERAPY

It cannot be overemphasized that the approach to facial esthetics should be a comprehensive one. No one type of procedure will achieve facial harmony in all esthetic subjects. Fillers are merely one instrument to achieve this goal. Combining fillers with other modalities will often optimize results. It has been shown for instance that the combination of hyaluronans such as Restylane and Botox will provide a superior result than either alone for the upper face. Studies have also demonstrated that it is safe and effective to combine previously injected fillers with radiofrequency skin-tightening procedures. Reports have demonstrated that Botox combined with light procedures such as intense pulsed light and laser resurfacing tend to increase the rejuvenation effect. Many practitioners have added facial fillers to this comprehensive rejuvenation philosophy, particularly when using nonablative light therapy. Similarly the combination of a rhytidectomy and fat transfer to the cheeks, or filler injection to the perioral region, will not only provide smoother lower facial contours, but will replace the volume that a face lift alone cannot achieve. This is particularly crucial in an individual with a thin, elongated face. A face lift may also reduce the amount of filler needed in the NLFs and marionette lines. The major limitation of today's fillers, and a concern of patients, is that they are very temporary in the hands of most practitioners. While this is true, permanency can present unforeseen problems when an individual's face ages, when there is deepening and subtle repositioning of lines. Perhaps in the future there will be a filler that is easy to inject, inexpensive and remains effective for 2–3 years. Until that time, appropriate education of the patient and combination therapies will result in the highest patient satisfaction.

FURTHER READING

Alam A, Levy R, Pavjani U, Ramierez JA, Guitart J, Veen H, Gladstone HB 2006 Safety of radiofrequency treatment over human skin previously injected with medium-term injectable soft tissue augmentation materials: A controlled pilot trial. Dermatologic Surgery 38:205–210

Alcalay J, Alkalay R, Gat A, Yorav S 2003 Late onset granulomatous reaction to Artecol. Dermatologic Surgery 29:859–862

Alonso D, Lazarus MC, Baumann L 2002 Effects of topical arnica gel on post laser treatment bruises. Dermatologic Surgery 28:686–688

Berman M 2000 Rejuvenation of the upper eyelid complex with autologous fat transplantation. Dermatologic Surgery 26:1113–1116

Billings E, May JW 1989 Historical review and present status of free fat graft autotransplantation in plastic and reconstructive surgery. Plastic and Reconstructive Surgery 83:368–381

Carruthers J, Carruthers A 2003 A prospective randomized parallel group study analyzing the effect of BTX-A and nonanimal sourced hyaluronic acid in combination compared with NASHA alone in severe glabellar rhytides in adult female subjects: treatment of severe glabellar rhytides with a hyaluronic acid derivative compared with the derivative and BTX-A. Dermatologic Surgery 29:802–809

Carruthers J, Carruthers A 2003 Aesthetic botulinum A toxin in the mid and lower face and neck. Dermatologic Surgery 29:468–476

Carruthers A, Carruthers JD 2005 Polymethylmethacrylate microspheres/collagen as a tissue augmenting agent: Personal experience over 5 years. Dermatologic Surgery 31:1561–1565

Carruthers A, Carey W, Lorenzi C, et al 2005 Randomized double blind comparison of the efficacy of two hyaluronic acid derivatives, Restylane perlane and hylaform, in the treatment of nasolabial folds. Dermatologic Surgery 31:1591–1598

Cohen SR, Berner CF, Bussi M, et al 2006 Artefill: A long lasting injectable wrinkle filler material-summary of the U.S. Food and Drug Adminsitration Trials and a progress report on 4- to 5-year outcomes. Plastic and Reconstructive Surgery 118:64s–76s

Conroy BF 1983 The history of facial prostheses. Clinics in Plastic Surgery 10:689–708

Danesh-Mayer HV, Savino PJ, Sergott RC 2001 Case reports and small case series: ocular and cerebral ischemia following facial injection of autologous fat. Archives of Ophthalmology 119:777–778

Donofrio L 2000 Technique of periorbital lipoaugmentation. Dermatologic Surgery 26:1129–1134

Donofrio LM 2000 Structural autologous lipoaugmentation: a panfacial technique. Dermatological Surgery 26:1129–1134

Duffy DM 1990 Silicone: a critical review. Advances in Dermatology 5:93–107

Duranti F, Salti G, Bovani B, et al 1998 Injectable hyaluronic acid gel for soft tissue augmentation. A clinical and histologic study. Dermatologic Surgery 24:1317–1325

Dzubow L 1997 The Aging Face. In: Coleman WP, Hanke CW, Alt TH (eds) Cosmetic Surgery of the Skin. Mosby, St Louis, pp 7–17

Fernandez-Cossio S, Castano-Oreja MT 2006 Biocompatibility of two novel dermal fillers: Histological evluation of implants of a hyal-

uronic acid filler and a polyacrylamide filler. Plastic and Reconstructive Surgery 117:1789–1796

Ficarra G, Mosqueda-Taylor A, Carlos R 2002 Silicone granuloma of the facial tissues: a report of seven cases. Oral Surgery, Oral Medicine, Oral Pathology, Oral Radiology and Endodontics 94:65–73

Frodel JL, Sykes JM 1996 Chin augmentation/genioplasty: chin deformities in the aging patient. Facial Plastic Surgery 12:279–283

Fulton JE, Suarez M, Silverton K, Barnes T 1998 Small volume fat transfer. Dermatological Surgery 24:857–865

Gladstone HB, Morganroth GS 2003 Evaluating calcium hydroxylapatite for facial augmentation. Presented at the Annual American Society for Dermatologic Surgery Meeting, New Orleans, LA

Goldberg RA, Edelstein C, Shorr N 1999 Fat repositioning in lower blepharoplasty to maintain infraorbital rim contour. Facial Plastic Surgery 15:225–229

Gonzalez-Ulloa M, Costillo A, Stevens E, et al 1954 Preliminary study of the total restoration of the facial skin. Plastic and Reconstructive Surgery 13:151–161

Ho TT, Chan KC, Wong KH, Lee SS 1999 Indinavir-associated facial lipodystrophy in HIV infected patients. AIDS Patient Care STDS 13:11–16

Jacovella PF, Peiretti CB, Cunille D, Salzamendi M, Schechtel SA 2006 Long lasting results with hydroxylapatite (Radiesse) facial filler. Plastic and Reconstructive Surgery 118:15s–21s

Jones DH 2003 Liquid silicone for HIV facial lipostrophy: 1 year data of 126 treated patients. Presented at the Annual American Society for Dermatologic Surgery Meeting, New Orleans, LA

Jordan DR 2003 Soft tissue fillers for wrinkles, folds and volume augmentation. Canadian Journal of Ophthalmology 2:250–253

Lam SM, Azizzadeh B, Graivier M 2006 Injectable poly-l-lactic acid (Sculptra): technical considerations in soft tissue contouring. 118:55s–63s

Klein AW 2001 Collagen substances. Facial Plastic Surgery Clinics of North America 9:205–218

Larrabee WF, Makielski KH 1993 Surgical Anatomy of the Face. Raven Press, New York, pp 3–12

Lemperle G, Romano JJ, Busso M 2003 Soft tissue augmentation with Artecoll: 10 year history, indications, techniques and complications. Dermatologic Surgery 29:573–587

Lindqvist C, Tveten S, Eriksen Bondevik B, Fagrell D 2005 A randomized evaluator-blind, multicenter comparison of the efficacy and tolerability of Perlane versus Zyplast in the correction of nasolabial folds. Plastic and Reconstructive Surgery 115:282–289

Lombardi T, Samson J, Plantier F, Husson C, Kuffer R 2004 Orofacial granulomas after injection of cosmetic fillers: Histopathologic and clinical study of 11 cases. Journal of Oral Pathological Medicine 33:115–120

Matti BA, Nicolle FV 1990 Clinical use of Zyplast in correction of age and disease-related deficiencies of the face. Aesthetic Plastic Surgery 14:227–234

Narins RS 2002 The use of tumescent anesthetic solution for fat transfer donor and recipient sites. Journal of Drugs in Dermatology 3:279–282

Narins RS, Brandt F, Leyden J, Lorenc ZP, Rubin M, Smith S 2003 A randomized, double blind, multicenter comparison of the efficacy and tolerability of Restylane versus Zyplast for the correction of nasolabial folds. Dermatologic Surgery 29:588–595

Orentreich D, Leone AS 2004 A case of HIV-associated facial lipoatrophy treated with 1000-cs liquid injectable silicone. Dermatologic Surgery 30:548–551

Peck H, Peck S 1970 A concept of facial esthetics. Angle Orthodontist 40:284–317

Reisberger EM, Landthaler M, West L, et al 2003 Foreign body granulomas caused by polymethylmethacrylate microspheres: successful treatment with allopurinol. Archives of Dermatology 139:17–20

Roy D, Sadick N, Mangat D 2006 Clinical Trial of a novel filler material for soft tissue augmentation of the face containing synthetic calcium hydroxylapatite microspheres. 32:1134–1138

Sklar JA, White SM 2004 Radiance FN: a new soft tissue filler. Dermatologic Surgery 30:764–768

Von Buelow S, Pallua N 2006 Efficacy and safety of polyacrylamide hydrogel for facial soft-tissue augmentation in a 2 year follow up: A prospective multicenter study for evaluation of safety and aesthetic results in 101 patients. Plastic and Reconstructive Surgery 118:85s–91s

Watson W, Kaye RL, Klein A, et al 1983 Injectable collagen: a clinical overview. Cutis 31:543–546

2 Fillers Esthetics

Stephen R. Tan, Richard G. Glogau

'Wrinkles should merely indicate where smiles have been'

Mark Twain, 1897

INTRODUCTION

Over recent decades, there have been major advances in the physician's ability to improve upon the signs of aging. Filler substances have abounded, and currently available products have effects which may last from a few months to many years. Filler substances are primarily utilized to restore volume to focal areas of the face, thus they are applicable to treating facial wrinkles and loss of subcutaneous volume resulting from a variety of causes. To properly use these substances to achieve the maximal cosmetic improvement while minimizing the risk of complications, the physician must have a thorough understanding of facial esthetics and the changes which occur as the patient ages.

GENDER DIFFERENCES IN ESTHETIC FACIAL APPEARANCE

The word *esthetic* is derived from the Greek word *aisthesis*, which means having a sense or love of that which is beautiful. The attractive, idealized face tends to exhibit several general characteristics, with slightly different proportions and shapes between women and men. While there are exceptions to every rule, these trends tend to be universally perceived across different cultures and across the ages. The idealized female face tends to exhibit:

❖ A larger, smooth forehead with a smaller nose
❖ Eyebrows that have an arch or gull-wing shape
❖ Eyes that are set wider apart, creating a bigger look
❖ Prominent cheekbones
❖ A heart-shaped taper to the lower face, with a smaller lower-to-upper face ratio
❖ Full, vermillion lips

The attractive masculine face tends to have:

❖ An overhanging, horizontal brow with minimal arch
❖ Deeper set eyes that appear closer together
❖ A somewhat larger nose
❖ A wider mouth
❖ A squared lower face with a more equal ratio of lower-to-upper face proportions
❖ A beard or coarser texture to the lower facial skin

Esthetics is a scientific attempt to explain a subjective concept by assigning proportions to various components of the face. Although these proportions may be used to define the 'ideal,' 'attractive,' or 'perfect' face, the real value in studying these principles lies in clarifying the range of normal relationships that exist between facial units. Harmony and balance of the face exists through a wide range of sizes, shapes, and configurations of the individual parts. The cosmetic surgeon must appreciate this in order to understand the changes that the face endures over time.

ETIOLOGY OF THE AGING FACE

The face ages in response to a number of factors, which may appear to varying degrees between individuals. Sun exposure and smoking tend to accelerate these changes:

1. **Chronic ultraviolet light damage to the skin**: Photoaging adds to the inevitable changes seen with intrinsic chronologic aging; indeed, cumulative sun exposure is the single largest factor involved in our clinical perception of aging skin, and it is responsible for a large portion of unwanted esthetic effects.
2. **Loss of subcutaneous fat**: In general, with age there is a loss of the fullness and roundness of the facial contours of youth, resulting in a flattened or sunken appearance to facial structures.
3. **Changes in the intrinsic muscles of facial expression and their influence on the skin**: The muscles of facial expression are unique in that they insert directly into the skin. Years of facial expressions constantly folding the skin result in the progressive development of hyperdynamic wrinkles, which initially appear only

with facial movement, but may ultimately remain as wrinkles at rest. Hyperdynamic wrinkles are more prominent in areas where the underlying muscles and fascia have more direct attachments to the skin, such as in the frontal, glabellar, nasolabial, perioral, and periocular areas.

4. **Gravitational changes from loss of elasticity of the tissue**: With aging, the facial soft tissues lose their inherent resiliency and ability to resist stretching; inevitably, they begin to sag under the effects of gravity.

5. **Remodeling of the underlying bony and cartilaginous structures**: Over time, bony resorption may result in a decrease in apparent facial volume, and gravitational stretch of cartilaginous structures may result in the drooping of structures such as the nasal tip. Facial asymmetry due to underlying bony or cartilaginous structural changes is difficult to correct, and pointing out these differences at the initial consultation is important in setting realistic patient expectations.

PHOTOAGING

Over the past few decades, there has been an increase in sun exposure through increased leisure time and outdoor activities. Years of people trying to acquire the 'healthy tan' have produced high rates of prematurely aged skin. Cumulative sun exposure is the greatest factor in aging skin, and is responsible for a large portion of the unwanted esthetic effects, including many of the wrinkles which may be treated with filler substances. Glogau has developed a systematic classification of patient photoaging types (Box 2.1). Depending upon the degree of sun exposure, these generalizations apply at different ages and to different degrees in patients with more pigmented skin.

Glogau type I patients have early photoaging changes, and are usually in their 20s or 30s. These patients generally have no rhytides at all, even when the face is animated during speaking or expression. Early photoaging, if present, may include mild pigmentary changes causing a disruption in the homogeneity of skin color. These patients generally wear no make-up foundation at all, as they do not require it for either rhytides or pigmentary alterations (Fig. 2.1).

Glogau type II patients are usually in their late 30s or 40s. These patients have early to moderate photoaging changes, and chronic ultraviolet damage to the elastic fibers impairs the inherent 'snap back' quality of the skin. These patients are without wrinkles while the face is at rest, but wrinkles begin to appear as expression lines when the face is in motion, appearing parallel to the melolabial fold, corners of the mouth, lateral canthal areas, and over the zygomatic arch and malar eminences. Early solar lentigines begin to appear and patients frequently utilize make-up foundation to conceal the pigmentary irregularities (Fig. 2.2) As these patients only have wrinkles while the face is in motion, they most aptly demonstrate the

Box 2.1 Glogau photoaging classification

Type I – 'No wrinkles'
- ❖ Early photoaging
  Mild pigmentary changes
  No keratoses
  Minimal wrinkles
- ❖ Younger patient – 20s or 30s
- ❖ Minimal or no make-up

Type II – 'Wrinkles in motion'
- ❖ Early to moderate photoaging
  Early senile lentigines visible
  Keratoses palpable but not visible
  Parallel smile lines beginning to appear lateral to mouth
- ❖ Patient age – late 30s or 40s
- ❖ Usually wears some foundation

Type III – 'Wrinkles at rest'
- ❖ Advanced photoaging
  Obvious dyschromia and telangiectasias
  Visible keratoses
  Wrinkles even when not moving
- ❖ Patient age – 50s or older
- ❖ Always wears heavy foundation

Type IV – 'Only wrinkles'
- ❖ Severe photoaging
  Yellow-gray color of skin
  Prior skin malignancies
  Wrinkled throughout, no normal skin
- ❖ Patient age – sixth or seventh decade
  can't wear make-up – 'cakes and cracks'

Adapted from Glogau (1994 and 1996).

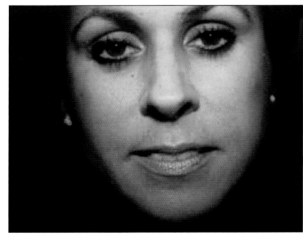

Fig. 2.1 Glogau photoaging type I. Note the absence of wrinkles and pigmentary alterations

effects of the underlying musculature on the skin, a critical consideration when contemplating the use of botulinum toxin.

Patients classified as Glogau type III have advanced photoaging changes, and are typically in their 50s or older. Damage to the cutaneous elastic fibers becomes more severe, and the wrinkles produced by facial movement

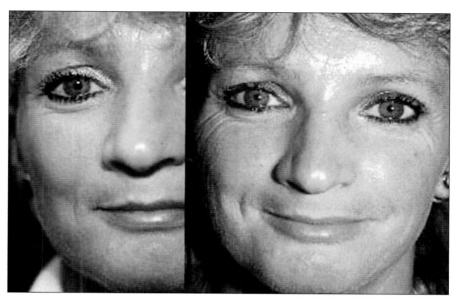

Fig. 2.2 Glogau photoaging type II. Note the absence of wrinkles while the face is at rest, and the appearance of wrinkles with facial movement

eventually persist even at rest. These may present as wrinkles radiating outwards from the lateral canthi, inferiorly from the lower eyelids onto the malar cheeks, parallel to the oral commissures, and outward from the upper and lower lips. Advanced photoaging results in obvious pigmentary dyschromias, telangiectasias, and visible keratoses. Patients commonly wear heavy make-up foundation to conceal these changes (Fig. 2.3).

Glogau type IV patients have severe photoaging changes and are usually in their 60s or 70s, but may be younger in the most severe cases. Wrinkles gradually spread to cover the majority of facial skin, and these patients may not have any unlined skin remaining on their faces. The dermis becomes engorged with thick debris, rendering a thickened, coarse quality to the skin. Pigmentary dyschromias are present as a yellow–gray sallow color of the skin, and patients have often had prior cutaneous malignancies (Fig. 2.4) Glogau type IV patients are not able to wear make-up, as the uneven facial surface often causes the make-up to have the texture of 'cracked mud.'

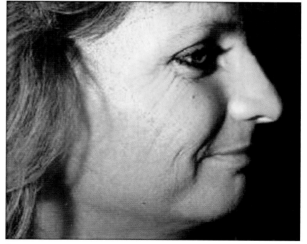

Fig. 2.3 Glogau photoaging type III. Note that wrinkles are present while the face is at rest

ANATOMIC APPROACH TO FACIAL ESTHETICS

Physicians should approach a patient seeking cosmetic improvement of the signs of aging from an anatomic standpoint. To appreciate facial symmetry and balance, one commonly used practice is to divide the face horizontally into thirds (see Fig. 2.5). The upper third ranges from the trichion to the glabella, the middle third from the glabella to the subnasale, and the lower third from the subnasale to the menton. Filler substances are mainly applicable,

either alone or in combination with other treatment modalities, to the lower two-thirds of the face.

• Upper third of the aging face

Changes in the upper third of the face are primarily related to chronic ultraviolet light damage, to the intrinsic muscles of facial expression and their influence on the skin, and to gravitational changes from loss of elasticity of

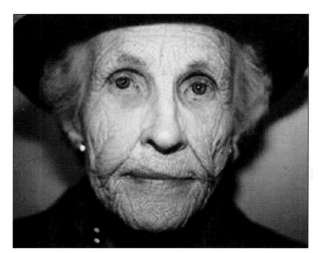

Fig. 2.4 Glogau photoaging type IV. The facial skin is entirely wrinkled, with no normal skin remaining on the face. Also note the yellow-gray, sallow color of the skin

the tissue. Occasionally filler substances may be used in conjunction with botulinum toxin to soften hyperdynamic wrinkles after the underlying causative muscles have been paralyzed. For a full description of facial esthetics and aging in the upper third of the face, please see chapter 2 entitled 'Botox esthetics' within this series.

• Middle third of the aging face

Aging of the middle third of the face affects the eyelids and periorbital regions, the cheeks, and the nose. These changes primarily result from a combination of photo-aging, loss of subcutaneous tissue, loss of cutaneous elasticity, and remodeling of underlying cartilaginous and bony structures.

Aging of the periorbital tissues results in both cosmetic and functional impairments. Dermatochalasis results from the combination of progressive cutaneous inelasticity of the eyelids and the effects of gravity. In severe cases, the upper eyelid skin may become so redundant that the visual fields are impaired. The canthal tendons and the tarsal plates provide the support structure of the eyelids, and loss of elasticity of these structures results in decreased lid tone and ability to 'snap back' after stretching of the eyelids. In severe cases, stability of eyelid position may be affected, resulting in either ectropion or entropion. The orbital septum may weaken over time, allowing for protrusions of the upper and lower lid fat compartments; however, some people may experience a loss of periorbital subcutaneous tissue, resulting in a 'sunken-in' skeletonized appearance to the orbits (Fig. 2.6).

The cheeks may be affected by volume loss of the buccal fat pad, which is positioned between the masseter muscle anteriorly and the buccinator muscle posteriorly. In childhood, an ample buccal fat pad contributes to the

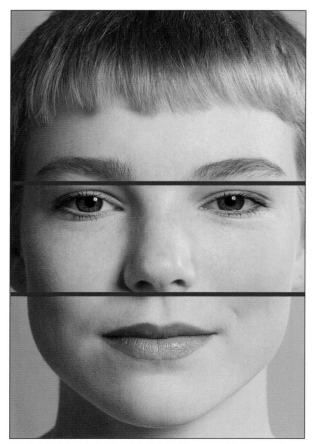

Fig. 2.5 Division of the face into thirds. The upper third ranges from the trichion to the glabella, the middle third from the glabella to the subnasale, and the lower third from the subnasale to the menton

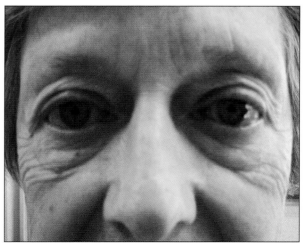

Fig. 2.6 Aging of the periorbital tissues. Note dermatochalasis and protrusion of the lower eyelid subcutaneous tissues

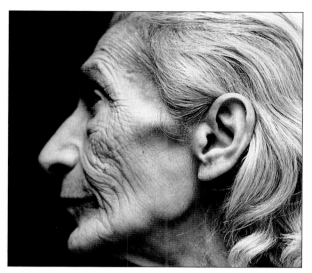

Fig. 2.7 Aging of the cheek. Note the development of a buccal depression, resulting in the appearance of a prominent malar eminence

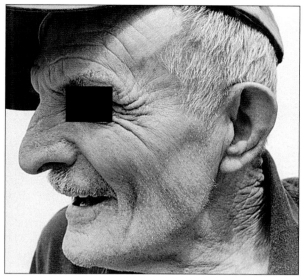

Fig. 2.9 Alterations of the proportions of the face. Note the nasal tip ptosis, which elongates the middle third of the face, while the lower third has lost height and volume with maxillary and mandibular bone resorption

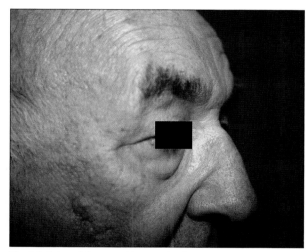

Fig. 2.8 Aging of the nose. Note ptosis of the nasal tip, with downward and posterior rotation of the nasal lobule

fullness of the cheeks; however, with age this fat pad atrophies. A buccal depression may develop, leading to the appearance of prominent malar eminences (Fig. 2.7).

Aging of the nose results in both structural and surface changes. The support mechanisms of the nasal tip may become inelastic and stretch with age, resulting in nasal tip ptosis and an apparent elongation of the middle third of the face (Fig. 2.8). The fibrous attachments between the inferior margin of the upper lateral nasal cartilage and the superior margins of the lateral crura of the alar cartilages elongate from a combination of gravity and remodeling of the underlying bony and cartilaginous

tissues. Additionally, the sling supporting the dome area weakens and there is loss of subcutaneous tissue, resulting in nasal ptosis, a downward and posterior rotation of the nasal lobule, retraction of the columella, and prominence of the nasal hump and cartilages. On the surface, enlargement of sebaceous glands may alter the skin texture, resulting in a rhinophymatous appearance.

• Lower third of the aging face

The aging changes seen in the lower third of the face affect the lips, chin, lower cheeks, and neck. Changes result from a combination of chronic ultraviolet light damage to the skin, loss of subcutaneous fat, changes due to the muscles of facial expression, gravitational changes from loss of elasticity of the tissue, and remodeling of the underlying bony and cartilaginous structures.

Changes in dentition and absorption of maxillary and mandibular bone may result in an overall loss of height and volume. The chin rotates forward and is seen to sharpen and protrude. These changes may result in the lower third of the face appearing smaller relative to the upper and middle thirds, straying from the ideal, approximately equal proportions. Aging changes from the middle third of the face may contribute to this appearance, as nasal tip ptosis may create the appearance of a shortened upper lip (Fig. 2.9). The constant effects of gravity combined with loss of elasticity in the tissue may allow for excess skin to droop off the mandible, manifesting as 'jowls' along the mandibular rim and 'wattles' in the anterior neck (Fig. 2.10).

The origin of the melolabial fold is unclear. Some authors feel that it is derived from insertions of lip

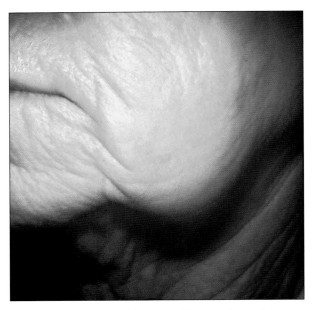

Fig. 2.10 Excess, inelastic skin drapes off the mandible as 'jowls' along the mandibular rim, and 'wattles' in the anterior neck

elevator muscles into the skin, whereas others hypothesize that it results from differences in the subcutaneous structure in the cheek and oral areas. In any case, the prominence of this fold varies with age. In childhood, the lips and cheeks contain more abundant subcutaneous tissue, such that this fold is inapparent; however, age-related loss of subcutaneous fat, combined with the loss of elasticity of the skin, results in the draping of redundant tissue over the muscular insertion point into the groove. Clinically, this results in an apparent deepening of the melolabial fold (Fig. 2.11).

Wrinkles form around the lips as a result of the constant pulling of the orbicularis oris muscle on progressively more inelastic upper- and lower-lip skin, creating angular, radial, and vertical wrinkles. Marionette lines may form as vertical wrinkles extending downwards from the oral commissures (Fig. 2.12). The effects of gravity result in drooping of the oral commissures laterally and downward, which may lead to a tired and sad appearance. Loss of elasticity may lead to lip skin redundancy, enhancing the drooping and vertical elongation (Fig. 2.13). Fullness of the lips and a strong definition of the philtrum are seen in youth; however with advancing age there is atrophy of the orbicularis oris muscle and loss of subcutaneous tissue, leading

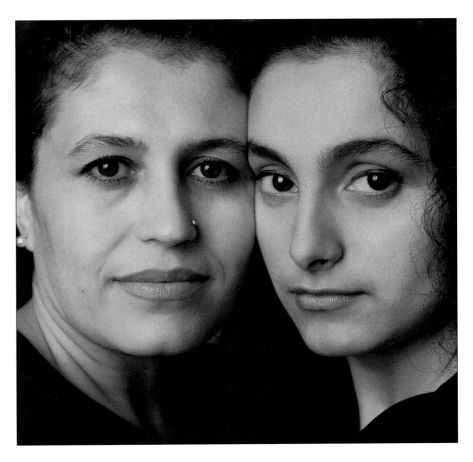

Fig. 2.11 Changes in the melolabial fold over time. Note the subtle melolabial fold in young adulthood, followed by the apparent deepening with age

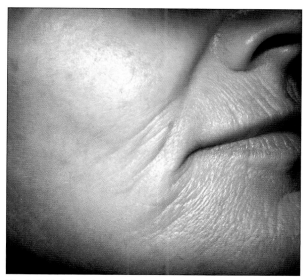

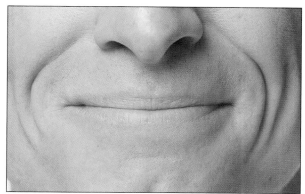

Fig. 2.14 Loss of fullness and flattening of the lips with age. Cupid's bow, the central arch of the upper lip, is flattened

Fig. 2.12 Perioral wrinkles radiating outward from the upper and lower lips. 'Marionette lines' form as vertical wrinkles extending downwards from the oral commissures

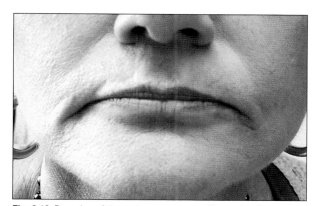

Fig. 2.13 Drooping of the oral commissures with age, leading to a tired and sad appearance

to an overall flattening and loss of fullness in the lips, with less of the vermillion showing. 'Cupid's bow', the central arch of the upper lip, may flatten (Fig. 2.14). In severe cases, there may be disruption of normal lip position. Loss of subcutaneous tissue and hypotonic lip musculature may allow the lips to invert, creating a 'sucked-in' appearance; however the occasional patient may develop a lip ectropion due to excess tissue and hypotonic lip musculature.

APPROACH TO FACIAL ESTHETICS WITH FILLER SUBSTANCES

The desire to restore the focal loss of facial volume that occurs with age has driven the development of numerous filler substances. Before embarking on a treatment plan with a patient seeking cosmetic improvement of the signs

of aging, the physician must have a thorough understanding of the realistic capabilities of the available filler substances and a systematic approach to assessing facial esthetics. The authors recommend that facial esthetics be approached from an anatomic standpoint: the determination of *what* is wrong must precede *how* it should be corrected. An anatomic approach to the aging face will allow the physician to select the optimal therapeutic tool from a wide variety of therapeutic options. Often physicians develop a preference for one or several techniques, and then apply them to all situations. Using a therapeutic technique that does not address the underlying anatomic basis for a cosmetic problem is inappropriate, and leads to mediocre results at best and disasters at worst.

During the preoperative consultation, the patient will usually indicate an area of their face that they wish to have improved. A thorough assessment of the patient's current facial structure and position of the anatomic sub-units should be made. Often patients may not be aware of subtle facial asymmetries, and using a mirror to demonstrate these may be useful in ensuring that the patient understands their own baseline condition. Underlying bony and cartilaginous causes resulting in altered facial esthetics and symmetry may not be adequately addressed with filler substances, and this should be made clear during the initial consultation. Rhytides primarily resulting from underlying facial muscle movement may be addressed with filler substances in concert with other approaches. For example, patients with deep glabellar furrows treated with filler substances may experience transient improvement; however, unless the underlying muscles causing these hyperdynamic lines are paralyzed with botulinum toxin, the wrinkles will rapidly recur.

As filler substances are applicable to restoring focal losses of subcutaneous tissue, the physician must be able to assess the quality and position of these tissues. Are the lips thin? Have they lost their shape? Are the cheekbones flattened? Is there wasting in the temporal fossae, above the eyebrows, or in the buccal fat pads? The patient's desired goals and the realistically achievable results should then be agreed upon prior to beginning treatment. With an appreciation of facial esthetics and a working knowledge of the capabilities and limitations of each filler substance, the physician will be able to use the most appropriate filler substance to achieve maximal cosmetic improvement.

REFERENCES

Dzubow L 1997 The aging face. In: Coleman WP III, Hanke CW, Alt TH, Asken S (eds) Cosmetic Surgery of the Skin: Principles and Techniques. 2nd edn. Mosby, St Louis, pp 7–17

Gliklich RE 1997 Proportions of the aesthetic face. In: Cheney ML (ed.) Facial Surgery: Plastic and Reconstructive. 1st edn. Williams & Wilkins, Baltimore, MD, pp 147–157

Glogau RG 2003 Systematic evaluation of the aging face. In: Bolognia JL, Jorizzo JL, Rapini RP (eds) Dermatology. 1st edn. Mosby, London, pp 2357–2360

Glogau RG 2002 Evaluation of the aging face. In: Kaminer MS, Dover JS, Arndt KA (eds) Atlas of Cosmetic Surgery. 1st edn. WB Saunders Company, Philadelphia, pp 29–33

McKinney P, Cunningham BL 1992 Anatomy. In: Aesthetic Facial Surgery. 1st edn. Churchill Livingstone, New York, pp 25–51

Powell N, Humphreys B 1984 Proportions of the Aesthetic Face. 1st edn. Thieme-Stratton Inc., New York

Ridley MB, VanHook SM 2002 Aesthetic facial proportions. In: Papel ID, Frodel J, Park SS, et al (eds) Facial Plastic and Reconstructive Surgery. 2nd edn. Thieme, New York, pp 96–109

Salasche SJ, Bernstein G, Senkarik M 1988 Surgical Anatomy of the Skin. 1st edn. Appleton & Lange, Norwalk, CT

3 Injectable Collagens

Seth L. Matarasso

INTRODUCTION

Injectable collagen products are temporary dermal fillers that are used to improve and reduce cutaneous defects that are the result of soft tissue loss or scarring. They are solely approved by the United States FDA for the glabrous skin of the nasolabial fold (NLF) and vermilion border of the lip. All other uses, although legal are considered off-label. The primary utility for collagen is augmentation of the central and lower third of the face; the NLF, the peri-oral area: the lips and bolstering the adjacent lateral oral commissures. Other areas that are amenable to soft tissue augmentation with collagen include the marionette lines, soft atrophic scars, and combination therapy: static rhytids that are unresponsive to chemodenervation with botulinum toxin preparations above the zygomatic arch (the forehead, glabella, peri-ocular regions), and peri-oral area (vertical 'lipstick lines', mentalis crease, and the oral commissures).

Fueled by the overwhelming success of botulinum toxin chemodenervation for dynamic rhytides, combined with patients' demand for ambulatory procedures with little time needed for recuperation, the field of soft tissue augmentation has gained significant momentum and popularity. This has been well chronicled by recent surveys by both the American Society of Dermatologic Surgery, which reported a 112% increase in the use of dermal fillers from 2001–2005, and a second poll by the American Society of Aesthetic Plastic Surgery mirrored this growth and yielded comparable statistics. Despite the development of many newer fillers, in particular the hyaluronans, injectable collagen remains an optimal minimally invasive modality. Their unparalleled historical safety profile, the admixture of anesthesia with diminished injection discomfort, and relatively reduced edema and bruising make them a treatment of choice and the cornerstone treatments for many facial 'imperfections'.

HISTORICAL PERSPECTIVE

Soft tissue fillers have been used for more than a century to improve contours, soften rhytides, blunt depressed scars, and enhance lips. The history of soft tissue augmen-

tation dates back to 1893, when Neuber first attempted to use autologous fat transfer for tissue augmentation. He utilized blocks of free fat harvested from the arms to reconstruct depressed facial defects. In 1899 Gersvny injected paraffin into the scrotum as a testicular prosthesis for a patient with advanced tuberculosis. Lexor, in 1910, used large-block grafts to treat malar depressions associated with chin recession. This was followed by Brunings, who in 1911 first described using the syringe technique to transfer free fat. In 1950, Peer reported 50% survival of transplanted fat using syringe aspiration. Baronders published a review of permanent soft tissue augmentation with liquid silicone in 1953 (Table 3.1). Although useful when injected by an experienced physician, this product has had a tumultuous history and continues to be controversial. Silicone's sole approval is for retinal tamponade in patients with retinal detachments. Fortunately, there is an ongoing multi-center study exploring the benefits of injectable microdroplet silicone for patients suffering from facial lipoatrophy due to infection with the human immunodeficiency virus (HIV). Due to the FDA Modernization Act, which allows the use of medical devices off-label, silicone (Silikon 1000, Alcon Inc., Fort Worth, Texas) has been used for off-label indications with increasing frequency for permanent soft tissue augmentation. In fact, when used appropriately by experienced physicians with the microdroplet technique, medical grade silicone has provided good results. However, when administering this product physicians must discuss its use with their medical malpractice carriers because the administration of silicone may not be covered in the event of legal action.

One of the most significant advances in soft tissue augmentation was the introduction of bovine collagen. Initial investigations began in earnest in 1958 and continued through the next 2 decades. In 1981 Zyderm I (McGhan Medical, Santa Barbara, CA) became the first FDA-approved xenogenic agent for soft tissue augmentation. Following this the two additional formulations of bovine collagen, Zyderm II and Zyplast, were granted FDA approval. Until 2003, when the injectable hyaluronic acids became available, bovine collagen remained the most commonly used dermal filler. It is perhaps the success and

Table 3.1 Historical milestones of filler substances

Year	Physician	Milestone
1893	Neuberg	First to use autologous fat for tissue augmentation
1899	Gersvny	First to use bioinjectable paraffin to correct cosmetic deformities
1910	Lexor	First to use large-block grafts to treat malar depression with chin recession
1911	Brunings	First described transfer of free fat employing the syringe technique
1959	Peer	Reported 50% survival of syringe-aspirated transplanted fat at one year
1953	Baronders	Use of liquid silicone in medicine
1976	Fischer	Cellusuctiome extraction of fat
1978	Ilouz	Liposuction as a fat source
1981		FDA approval of Zyderm I
1983		FDA approval of Zyderm II
1985		FDA approval of Zyplast
1986	Fournier	Microliposuction
2003		FDA approval of human based Collagen (CosmoDerm 1 and ComoPlast)
2004		FDA approval of hyaluronic acids (Restylane and Hylaform, Hyalaform plus, Captique)
2005		FDA approval of CosmoDerm 2
2006		FDA approval of hyaluronic acids (Juvederm)
2006		FDA approval of ArteFill (bovine collagen with polymethylmethacrylate beads) for non-resorbable soft tissue augmentation to correct smile lines.

Box 3.1 Partial list of characteristics of the ideal filler substance

Material:	Administration:
Non-allergenic (decreased risk of hypersensitivity)	Basic administration
	Painless
FDA approved	Outpatient
Non-carcinogenic/non-teratogenic	(minimal recuperation)
No migration	User-friendly
Minimal inflammation	Large amount available
No overt cutaneous change (undetectable)	Easy storage
Reproducible	
Durable	
Minimal adverse sequelae	
Stable (inert)	
Affordable	

availability of these products that ushered in a renewed quest for the ideal formulation for soft tissue augmentation (Box 3.1). In 2006, following the acquisition of Inamed Corporation (Santa Barbara, CA), all of the commercially available collagen products became available from the sole distributor, Allergan (Irvine, CA).

No two wrinkles are created equal as each has a different derivation, and they vary in shape and size. As such there is no one filler agent that is suitable for all defects.

Therefore treatment should be predicated based on the defect and individualized to each patient's needs. The selection of the appropriate implant; whether dermal or subcutaneous, temporary or permanent; liquid or solid, requires knowledge of all of the available materials as well as their characteristics. Furthermore filler substances may be used as monotherapy or combined with other dermal implants or other procedures such as resurfacing, botulinum toxin, or surgery.

FILLER MATERIALS

There is an ever-expanding menu of materials and devices for soft tissue augmentation and they can be classified, based on either derivation or site of cutaneous placement. Autologous materials (adipose, collagen) are harvested from the same patient and hence have no risk of immunologic reaction. However they require an initial harvesting procedure and are limited by a potentially limited donor reservoir. Xenografts are semi-synthetic formulations harvested from a different species (bovine and porcine collagen, avain hyaluronic acid derivatives). These are readily available and carry a low risk of infection and rejection. Allograft materials are harvested from human cadaveric tissue, have a minimal risk of hypersensitivity reaction but pose a theoretical risk of infection from the donor tissue. While synthetic substances (expanded polytetrafluoroethylene) may provide longer lasting results and have an unlimited supply, they frequently require surgical insertion, as opposed to injection, and they may cause site-specific mechanical difficulties. The injectable collagen products meet many of the criteria of the ideal product for soft tissue augmentation as they are ambulatory, reproducible, predictable in their effect and FDA-approved, and they have an extensive safety profile.

• Collagen products

In the late 1980s, research began on extracting intact human collagen fibers and acellular dermal matrix from cadavers for human dermal implants. There are three human cadaveric collagens: Alloderm and Cymetra, both of which are manufactured by Lifecell Corporation (Branchburg, NJ) and Dermalogen (Collagenesis Inc., Beverly, MA). They are allograft materials that are derived from American tissue banks that are subject to FDA screening for all infectious processes. They primarily contain the acellular dermal layer of cadaver tissue consisting of intact collagen and elastin fibers. Alloderm is processed into sheets and widely used in the treatment of full-thickness burns, blistering disorders as well as in soft tissue augmentation procedures. Alloderm requires surgical implantation under local or general anesthesia. Cymetra is the micronized form of Alloderm and is reconstituted in the physician's office with lidocaine. Like Alloderm, no known hypersensitivity has been reported and therefore no allergy testing is required. Cymetra is injected deep in the dermis – above the dermal/subcutaneous junction and is used to treat scars and for lip augmentation. Although the manufacturer addressed the original difficulties in reconstituting this product, it nevertheless remains a viscous material that generally requires a larger bore needle (23 or 26 gauge) for injection. Therefore local or regional anesthesia is required for placement. According to the manufacturer the results lasted between 3–6 months. Although theoretically nonimmunogenic and incapable of producing allergic reactions, with the introduction of newer fillers, all three of these cadaveric agents seem to have lost much of their initial appeal, and the two injectable forms, Cymetra and Dermalogen are no longer commercially available.

The advent of human-derived collagen from fibroblast cultures further increased the popularity of injectable products. More recently, cultured autologous collagen and several other formulations of collagen have been undergoing clinical trials or are available outside of the United States. These advances in collagen technology may deliver products that are more persistent in duration and comfortable to administer than the materials that are presently in use.

Some of the injectable products presently used outside of the United States or that are in clinical trials include: Evolence, Permacol, Atelocollagen, Isolagen, Resoplast, Endoplast-50 and ArteFill.

Evolence (ColBar LifeScience, Herzliya, Israel) a xenographic product derived from porcine (pig) tendons, is the most recent addition to the injectable dermal collagens. It is produced in vitro by polymerization of porcine collagen followed by 'Glymatrix technology', a cross-linking technology that uses a sugar (ribose) moiety rather than chemicals. Porcine collagen is supposedly less immunogenic than its bovine counterpart. Furthermore, an additional potential advantage is that during the production of this product, there is removal of the allergenic telopeptides, thus ensuring compatibility with human collagen. No allergic responses have been reported in the clinical trials or in postmarketing surveillance follow up and, theoretically allergy testing is unnecessary. Each syringe contains 30 mg/mL of product without anesthetic. As it is a collagen, it may have the added benefit that it stimulates the clotting cascade, resulting in less bleeding and bruising upon injection. The longevity of implantable material is purportedly equivalent to that of Zyplast collagen, and may in fact be longer and last up to 12 months. The product was made available for sale in Europe, Canada and Israel in 2005 and has received US FDA approval for clinical investigation (Fig. 3.1 A and B).

Permacol (Tissue Science Laboratories, Aldershot, Hampshire, UK) is a porcine dermal collagen matrix graft and is primarily manufactured as a firm sheet of material that is used for reconstructing human dermal tissue defects. Permacol injection is the cross-linked micronized formulation of the sheet form. It is in a saline vehicle with a 60% wet weight per volume and in Europe is available in 2.5 cc syringes. It is intended for urinary bulking for patients with urinary incontinence; however some have used it off-label as a dermal filler.

Atelocollagen (Koken Co. Ltd., Tokyo, Japan) is obtained from Australian-bred calves no older than 6 months old to decrease the transmission of bovine spongiform encephalopathy (BSE). It is supplied in 1 cc/mg cartridges and injected with dental syringes. It is commercially available outside of the United States and comes in three solutions containing 2%, 3.5% and 6.5% monomolecular solutions without anesthesia. It contains approximately 95% type I collagen, but as it is of bovine derivation, allergy testing is recommended. There is limited information available regarding its duration and biologic cosmetic response.

Isolagen (Isolagen Inc., Houston, TX) is significantly different from other collagens because it uses intact fibroblasts, collagen, and elastic fibers harvested from each patient. This unique method of creating autologous collagen requires a small (3 mm) skin biopsy typically obtained from the patient's postauricular sulcus. The tissue is shipped to a central facility, which cultures the specimen and generates a syringe (approximately 1.2 mL) of the patient's own collagen, which can then be administered to the original donor for soft tissue augmentation. Phase III clinical trials to determine the efficacy of this technique are presently underway.

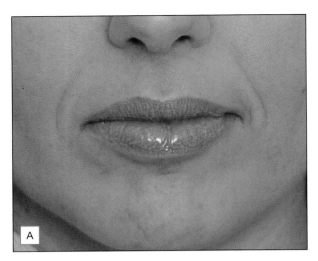

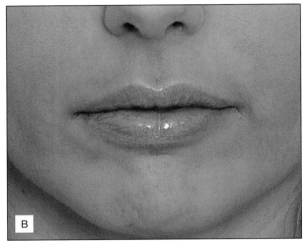

Fig. 3.1 (**A** and **B**) Frontal photograph before and after 1.0 cc on Evolence was injected into the NLFs

Resoplast is collagen extracted from the skins of calves that were raised within closed herds in Germany (Rofil Medical International, Breda, Holland). It is a monomolecular bovine collagen product suspended in saline solution at 3.5% and 6.5% concentrations. It is available in 1.0, 1.5 and 2.0 cc syringes. As it has similar antigenicity to Zyderm collagen, a skin test is required.

Endoplast-50 (Filorgra Laboratories, Moscow, Russia) consists of solubilized elastin peptides with bovine collagen. Injected intradermally, the material influences the proliferation of fibroblasts to produce collagen. As it is bovine, two negative skin tests are required prior to treatment and augmentation is reported to last as long as 12 months. Currently this product is only available in Europe and is not FDA-approved in the United States.

ArteFill (Artes Inc., San Diego, CA) is a bi-phasic product that combines bovine collagen with a suspension of polymethylmethacrylate (PMMA) beads. The collagen serves both as a temporary vehicle to introduce the PMMA beads into the dermis as well as an initial filling agent. Autologous collagen is subsequently created by fibroplasia as the PMMA beads become encapsulated in a dermal fibrous network. ArteFill initially received a conditional approval letter from the FDA pending collection of data of 1000 treatment sessions and a commitment to use bovine collagen obtained from a closed herd of cattle. In October 2006, this product received final FDA clearance and marked the sanctioning and availability of the first non-resorbable injectable wrinkle filler to correct smile lines.

FDA-APPROVED COLLAGEN PRODUCTS

There are many forms of injectable collagen but the two that have maintained the widest appeal and diversity are the bovine-derived Zyderm family of products, and the human bioengineered form; the CosmoDerm family (Table 3.2). Both are now manufactured by Allergan (Irvine, CA) and are subdivided into three categories based upon the viscosity of the material and their corresponding indications. Each is available in boxes of six preloaded single-use syringes containing white-opaque collagen suspended in phosphate-buffered physiologic saline with 0.3% lidocaine, and are stable up to 1 year when stored in a refrigerator (4°C). The manufacturer recommends that following a treatment any unused collagen should be disposed of and not be stored in between patient visits. If there is any separation of the microfibrils of the product or if there is no uniform consistency of the material, the syringe should not be used and should be returned to the manufacturer. The single-use syringes are accompanied by labels with a lot number and expiration date that can be affixed to the patient's chart for tracking purposes. Also in the box are 30 gauge 0.5 in or adjustable-depth gauge (ADG) needles. The latter may be manually adjusted to alter the distance between the distal end of the needle and the skin surface of the patient.

• Bovine collagen

The bovine-derived collagen products are Zyderm I, Zyderm II and Zyplast. These collagen products have been used safely and effectively as biomaterials since 1982 due to their unique physical properties and weak immunogenicity. To date well over 1 million patients have been treated with highly purified reconstituted bovine collagen. All three Zyderm collagen implants are 95–98% type I collagen, with the remainder being type III. Zyderm I is the least concentrated and contains 35 mg/mL of collagen. It is generally used for very superficial rhytides or to layer on top of another filling agent. Placement of Zyderm I should be in the superficial papillary dermis. Because a significant portion of Zyderm I is saline, which is rapidly reabsorbed, the defect should be overcorrected by 150–200% imparting a white blanch or peau d'orange appearance to the epidermis. Zyderm II is a more concentrated

Table 3.2 FDA-approved collagens					
Type of Collagen	Concentration of collagen	Indications	Size of syringe available	Placement	Degree of overcorrection
Zyderm I	35 mg/ml Bovine	Fine lines: perioral periocular glabellar	0.5; 1.0; 1.5 cc	Superficial papillary dermis	150–200×
Zyderm II	65 mg/ml Bovine	Mild-moderate rhytids: scars perioral	0.5; 1.0 cc	Mid dermis	100–150×
Zyplast	35 mg/ml Cross-linked with glutaraldehyde Bovine	Deeper rhytids and folds: nasolabial vermilion border marionette lines	1 cc; 1.5; 2 cc; 2.5 cc	Deep dermis	No overcorrection
CosmoDerm 1	35 mg/ml Human derived	Fine lines: perioral periocular glabellar	1 cc	Superficial papillary dermis	150–200×
CosmoDerm 2	65 mg/ml Bovine	Mild-moderate rhytids: scars perioral	0.5; 1.0 cc	Mid Dermis	100–150×
CosmoPlast	35 mg/ml Cross-linked with gluteraldehyde Human derived	Deeper rhytids and folds: nasolabial vermilion border marionette lines	1 cc	Deep Dermis	No overcorrection

and viscous form of Zyderm I and contains 65 mg/mL of collagen. It is intermediate in durability between Zyderm I and the more robust Zyplast. Zyderm II is appropriate for deeper lines and wrinkles and is placed deeper in the papillary dermis with about 100–150% overcorrection. Zyplast has a concentration of 35 mg/mL but it has the longest duration because it is cross-linked by the addition of 0.0075% glutaraldehyde. This characteristic decreases proteolytic degradation by collagenase and enhances its in vivo stability lasting longer than the 3 months generally anticipated for the other Zyderm products. Typically Zyplast is placed deeper in the dermis and is recommended for deep rhytides and folds. There should be no overcorrection upon injection of this material.

Prior to therapy with any of the three bovine products, potential allergic response to the products must be excluded. Hypersensitivity can be reduced with double skin testing. A skin test is available in 1.0 cc tuberculin syringes that contain 0.3 ml of Zyderm I, which screens for all three forms of bovine collagen. Approximately 0.1 cc is injected subcutaneously in an inconspicuous area, such as the volar aspect of the forearm. Hypersensitivity is characterized by swelling, induration, tenderness, pruritis and/or erythema at the injection site and resolves with time as the implant is absorbed. This has been found in approximately 3% of patients and indicates a pre-existing allergy to bovine collagen. Despite a negative preliminary test, an additional 1–2% of patients will develop allergic reactions to the products at subsequent treatments. Therefore, it is the standard of practice to perform a second challenge 2 weeks after the initial skin test. This test, using a similar volume, can be injected on the contralateral arm or the periphery of the face (pretragal area, anterior hairline), and should be monitored for two additional weeks. A positive reaction occurring with either of the tests is an absolute contraindication. Conversely negative skin testing allows the patient to proceed with treatment 4 weeks after the initial test or 2 weeks after the second test. An amended protocol is recommended for patients who have previously been successfully treated with bovine collagen, but have not had soft tissue augmentation for 1 year or longer. If these patients do not wish to switch to the newer form of human-derived collagen or an alternative class of agents and elect to continue with bovine products, to reduce the risk of bovine hypersensitivity, a single re-test with a 2-week observation period is suggested prior to commencing treatment.

• Synthetic human collagen

The development of human-derived collagen was prompted by the need for a product that would eliminate hypersensitivity reactions and the mandated skin testing. Based on the safety profile following their use in burns and wounds, the first of the CosmoDerm family of products was granted approval by the FDA for soft tissue augmentation in March of 2003. There are currently three formulations: CosmoDerm 1 and 2, and CosmoPlast. They have the same consistency and injection properties as Zyderm and Zyplast but are grown from a single human fibroblast cell culture and unlike other human-derived products are not cadaveric in nature. They are the result of tissue-engineered technology and have undergone extensive pathogen screening for viral and bacterial contamination to avoid the possibility of disease transmission. As these products are nonanimal based they have the significant advantage that they do not require initial skin testing to exclude the risk of hypersensitivity prior to administration and hence can be injected on the same day as the initial consultation. Similar to its bovine counterpart Zyderm I, CosmoDerm 1 has a concentration of 35 mg/mL and is placed into the superficial papillary dermis with a comparable degree of blanching and overcorrection. It is also primarily indicated for superficial lines and defects. CosmoDerm 2 has 65 mg/mL of human-derived collagen and is analogous to Zyderm II in its indications and technical aspects. CosmoPlast, like Zyplast, is the more robust of the three and contains 35 mg/mL of human-derived collagen cross-linked with glutaraldehyde, which not only increases its durability but also makes it less immunogenic. It is a deeper dermal implant; appropriate for injections to a depth of approximately 2 mm. CosmoPlast does not require overcorrection to improve deep folds and wrinkles. Although the two collagen families, CosmoDerm and Zyderm, are remarkably similar there is anecdotal evidence that the CosmoDerm products have better rheology (flow characteristics) but perhaps briefer clinical duration than the Zyderm collagens.

PATIENT SELECTION

Patients seeking treatment with soft tissue augmentation often do not adequately appreciate the nature of their defect and hence should be educated about the underlying 'anatomy of a wrinkle'. The distinction must be made between dynamic versus static lines, and those secondary to chronology and gravitational pull. Although these defects are not mutually exclusive and, in fact, often appear in combination, their treatment mandates individual evaluation.

While the type of defect is clearly important, so too, is its size, depth, and location, as well as the appearance and integrity of the adjacent surrounding tissue (Box 3.2). The patient must therefore also be informed of the many different means for improving them. A discussion regarding therapeutic options should include the alternatives of

---

Box 3.2 Soft tissue augmentation preinjection considerattions	
Defect Parameters: Medications (anticoagulants) History of hypersensitivity reaction History of herpes labialis Volume required Location Alternative/simultaneous treatments Medical history Pregnancy/lactation Autoimmune disease	Patient Goals: Expectations (longevity) Degree of improvement (what is of concern to the patient?) Morbidity patient is willing to sustain Risk/benefit ratio

---

surgery (rhytidectomy or excision), resurfacing and chemodenerervating agents (botulinum toxin), as well as the option of no intervention at all. Although not often comprehensive, patients should have a fundamental understanding of all of the different dermal filler options appropriate to their specific anatomy, any preferences and their budgetary restrictions. They should have an adequate comprehension of the indications and technique, advantages and disadvantages, and inherent risks of each procedure, with an estimate of the time needed for full recuperation. As with any treatment, the success is largely proportional to the extent of realistic and appropriate goals and expectations set by both the physician and the patient. Patients undergoing soft tissue augmentation must be especially aware of the temporary nature of the procedure as well as its primary purpose of replacing lost or atrophic subcutaneous tissue. It is the physician's responsibility to critically evaluate the defect, determine its etiology, and provide treatment parameters.

TREATMENT GUIDELINES

Prior to any form of soft tissue augmentation it is recommended that for approximately 10–14 days before their appointment that patients abstain from medications that can inhibit platelet aggregation and potentiate ecchymosis. After an informed consent form that is specific to the specific filler is signed, the area should be photographed and corroborated by the patient with a hand-held mirror. The areas should then be cleansed of all debris and make-up with an antiseptic solution. When necessary, the area to be addressed can be delineated with a marker and a topical anesthesia may be applied. Percutaneous injections can be painful and this is especially true in the central face and perioral areas and anesthesia should be offered to patients. Adequate cutaneous anesthesia may be obtained with topical preparations and injected local anesthesia and nerve blocks are often not necessary. For adequate pain management the topical anesthetics should be applied liberally and left intact for 15–30 minutes. Enhanced penetration of the topical anesthetic may be achieved with occlusive dressings. Although not mandatory, to aid in diminishing patient discomfort and anxiety, it is also helpful to have auditory (music and interesting conversation) and tactile (a soft rubber ball placed in their hand) diversions available during the procedure.

Patients should be situated in a dependent or seated position with their heads upright so that their lines and folds are accentuated. Reclining positions, which can diminish or obliterate the rhytides, should be avoided. To further appreciate the defects, overhead lighting and magnification are helpful.

Before penetrating the skin surface all topical preparations inclusive of anesthetics should be removed in a non-abrasive manner with gauze and then the filler can be injected. For easier access, it may be preferable to bend the needle to a 45-degree angle and insert it with the bevel up gently through a pilosebaceous opening. The material can then be placed in the proper dermal location with the serial puncture technique, linear threading or a combination of the two. The former, serial puncture, is preformed by inserting small discrete amounts of material at the leading edge of the previously injected deposit. The latter, threading, is one continuous uninterrupted injection. Massage and ice applied to the treated area can reduce erythema and edema. Unlike many other facial procedures the results are immediate with few post-procedural restrictions and patients can reapply make-up and promptly resume their normal daily activities.

• Indications

Areas that are amenable to treatment with Zyderm I or CosmoDerm I include the superficial periorbital and peri-oral lines that radiate from the eye and lips (lipstick lines). Lines in the glabella and forehead may be treated with Zyderm I or II or CosmoDerm 1 or 2. The oral commissures, vermilion borders and nasolabial creases are best suited to the thicker products – Zyplast or CosmoPlast – as the noncross-linked products do not provide sufficient long-term augmentation. Shallow soft distensible scars due to trauma, surgery or infection such as varicella or acne vulgaris respond well to any of the forms of collagen. While there are few absolutes with respect to selection of collagen, and there can be a great deal of personal physician preference, the one irrefutable contraindication is the use of the thicker fillers, Zyplast and CosmoPlast, in the glabellar complex. The deeper placement required of these products has been associated with vascular compromise and sloughing of the skin (Fig. 3.2).

• Scars

Patients who are good candidates for scar correction with collagen include those who acknowledge that the results are temporary and will need multiple visits for optimal outcomes. Anatomically the indications are for non-ice pick, shallow and distensible scars (approximately 1–2 mm in depth) and are not prominent (2–4 mm).

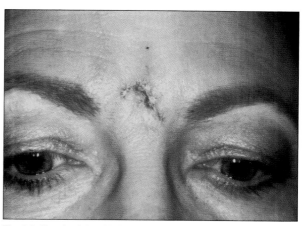

Fig. 3.2 Slough of the skin following vascular embarrassment from deep placement of Zyplast into the glabellar region. The use of any cross-linked products is an absolute contraindication in this area

It is important to appreciate the thickness and amount of sebaceous glands of a patient's skin prior to selecting the collagen to be used. For patients with thin skin (underlying blood vessels can be seen), a noncross-linked collagen such as Zyderm or CosmoDerm is adequate. Men, and in general patients with thicker skin, with a greater density of glands should be treated with a cross-linked collagen such as Zyplast or CosmoPlast.

Prior to injecting collagen into a scar some have advocated 'subcising' the area. Under local anesthesia using an 18 gauge Nokor needle and a windshield-like action, a dermal pocket can be created where the collagen material can be deposited. This serves to trap and immobilize the implanted material and eliminates mechanical forces that could lead to early degradation. The collagen injection should begin at the junction between the scar and adjacent uninvolved skin. Several injections from different angles may help to release any remaining subcutaneous fibrous attachments and assist in uniform and homogenous placement. Correction of small annular scars should be directed towards the center, and with linear scars, injections should be oriented at about 45 degrees with the long axis of the scar.

• Lip augmentation

Lip augmentation and peri-oral rejuvenation is one of the most frequently requested regions for enhancement. Patients often present with atrophy of the lips secondary to age, vertical rhytides emanating from the vermilion ('smokers lines') and depressed oral commissures. Unlike other areas, the lips are the central focus of the face and patients express very strong feelings about their size and shape. It is wise to have a frank discussion of what can reasonably be achieved. While patients often will provide photographs from lay publications of what they may consider their 'ideal lip' it is prudent to maintain appropriate goals when augmenting the lips. The most significant contraindication to this procedure is patients with unrealistic expectations. A relative contraindication is patients with recurrent herpes labialis. These patients may be treated but they require prophylaxis with oral antiviral medications.

The basic parameters of lip augmentation are: definition of the vermilion border, oral commisure elevation, volume replacement and vertical rhytid correction. The vermilion is the only FDA-sanctioned indication and the thickest forms of collagen; Zyplast and CosmoPlast are used here and in the angles of the mouth. For volume and perioral rhytides the noncross-linked formulations such as Zyderm I and II and CosmoDerm 1 and 2 are recommended.

Understanding lip anatomy and the esthetics and ratios of the lower face are essential to optimum lip augmentation. Lip rejuvenation should not be perceived in terms of treating a single homogenous, linear structure, but rather as a complicated augmentation of a structure that has different contours, volumes and inflection points. The proportions of the lip change with time and in a youthful lip the ideal ratio of the upper lip to the lower lip is 1 : 1.6 and it is important to attempt to restore the lower lip to a more youthful dominant proportion. The two constants of lip augmentation are that the lip should have transition points and there should be no downward slope, but rather an elevation of the lateral commissures.

Prior to injection, any pre-existing asymmetries should be identified and pointed out to the patient. In combination with the lidocaine already mixed in with the collagen the discomfort can be adequately managed with various topical preparations. Regional nerve blocks (infraorbital, mental) are effective in completely eliminating pain but are generally not needed as they can distort the oral anatomy and impart a false sense of fullness to the patient.

To accentuate the vermilion border and define the lip, Zyplast or CosmoPlast is injected in a threading manner into the potential space that runs continuously along the lip edge. This thin channel runs the entire length of the lip and allows collagen to flow uniformly with minimal pressure on the syringe plunger. By itself this creates a demarcation that defines the lip margin, stops lipstick from 'bleeding' from their lips and restores some volume. However, when one of the goals is to further increase the volume of the lip, it is recommended to place small (0.1 cc) aliquots of Zyderm I or CosmoDerm 1 with the serial puncture technique along the 'wet/dry' (epidermal–mucosal) junction. This however is an area where the Fordyce glands are typically located. Showing these glands to the patient prior to injection avoids confusion and concerns that the collagen caused them. Although not an FDA-approved location for collagen implantation, when a patient requests greater volume, the physician may evert the lips slightly with a nondominant hand and inject directly to the labial mucosa. This technique will produce a slight eversion and give the appearance of a fuller lip.

Upon injection it is important to monitor both the amount being used to maintain symmetry and to avoid deep placement that would interfere with the labial artery. The 'cupid's bow' may better be defined by additional Zyplast or CosmoPlast in that midline curvilinear structure as well as injecting directly into the philtral columns (the 'Paris Lip'.) Patients who require treatment of the radiating perioral rhytides tend to be women whose genetics, musculature, smoking habits or photodamage have resulted in moderate vertical lines. Patients with profound perioral rhytides should be informed that they may have a better and longer lasting result with resurfacing procedures rather than with soft tissue augmentation. In order to correct these superficial lines a noncross-linked material such as Zyderm I or CosmoDerm 1 is used. The cross-linked products have a tendency to produce contour irregularities with superficial deposits of material. The needle is placed at the vermilion border pointing away from the mouth and is inserted under the entire length of the rhytid and the collagen is injected in a retrograde manner as the needle is slowly withdrawn. This allows for an even distribution. Alternatively the collagen can be injected in a serial puncture manner. However, using this technique, careful control of the plunger must be exercised to ensure that very small amounts are placed with each injection or beading will occur. Following either injection technique, gentle massage is performed.

Ptosis correction at the angle of the mouth, the lateral commissure, is an ideal indication for collagen as it bolsters up the lower lip and acts like a buttress, restoring the 'drool area' to a more neutral position. Since the goal is volume replacement and not line reduction the material selected for this region should be one of the cross-linked products. Adding volume is done with serial injections of Zypast or CosmoPlast. Beginning inferiorly just above the edge of the mandible these injections address the marionette lines that extend down from the lateral oral commissure. For an adequate cosmetic improvement, some filling agent should also be placed in the lateral third of the lower lip – this raises the corner of the lip (Figs 3.3 A and B and 3.4 A and B).

In many cases, the lip position, texture and volume can be softened with collagen but the patient continues to have deep perioral rhytides or malposition of the angles of the mouth. This is often secondary to hypertrophy or hyperkinetic movement of the perioral musculature. A technique that can help to improve the appearance of the senescent mouth is the adjunctive use of botulinum toxin (Botox Aesthetic, Allergan Inc., Irvine, CA). Upon completion of soft tissue augmentation of the lips, reconstituted Botox (2.0 cc preserved normal saline/100 u vial; 5 u/0.1 cc) can be injected into the orbicularis oris muscle of both the upper and lower lips. The patient is instructed to purse their lips to visualize maximum muscle mass and 1–2 u of reconstituted Botox is injected superficially into each quadrant of the lips. Injecting toxin into the midline of the upper lip is contraindicated as it can result in blunting of the Cupid's bow. Reducing the mimetic perioral

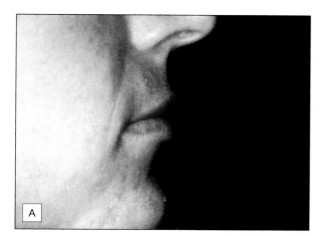

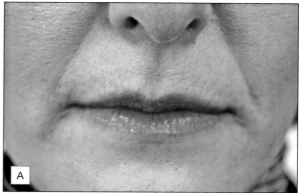

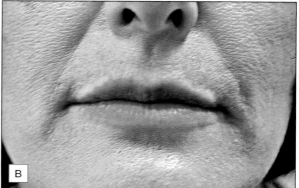

Fig. 3.4 (**A** and **B**) Before and after frontal photographs of vermilion augmentation with CosmoPlast

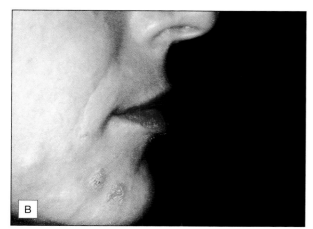

Fig. 3.3 (**A** and **B**) Profile before and after lip augmentation with Zyplast collagen into the vermilion border and oral commissures

lines with Botox has the added benefit of simultaneously weakening the sphincter activity of the orbiclaris oris muscle, which further everts the lip and gives the appearance of a fuller lip (pseudoaugmentation) (Fig. 3.5 A and B). Similarly inducing paresis of the lower lip depressor, relaxing the depressor anguli oris muscle, with 2–3 u of Botox eliminates its downward pull and aids in elevation of the lateral commissure. This small muscle can be located just anterior to the masseter muscle as it crosses the mandible.

An additional modification for those wishing to combine different filler products, is to flow one of the collagens along the vermilion border. The lidocaine in the collagen will provide some degree of anesthesia so that a second agent such as one of the recently approved hyaluronic acids that does not contain lidocaine can be injected with less patient discomfort. The patient must be forewarned that this technique provides further fullness to the lip.

• Nasolabial fold

'Smile lines', wrinkles that extend from the angle of the nose to the corner of the upper lip are a frequent site for soft tissue replacement. Treatment of nasolabial creases is performed in order to correct volume defects in the deep dermis and the amount required should be predicated on the depth of the fold. To insure patient satisfaction, placement of adequate volume is important. There is no perfect filler for all defects and when very large volumes are necessary for adequate volumetric correction and collagen is not sufficient an alternative should be discussed with the patient (Table 3.2.)

Effacing the nasolabial creases involves injections with a needle at a depth of about 1.0–2.0 mm. The material, Zyplast or CosmoPlast, should be placed medial to the crease to avoid lateral extravasation. Beginning at the distal portion of the crease, collagen is injected in a cephalad direction. It is wise to evaluate the symmetry and predict the total quantity that will be needed and divide half of the allotted material for the contralateral fold. One area that often is neglected when correcting nasolabial creases is the triangle at the nasal sill immediately adjacent

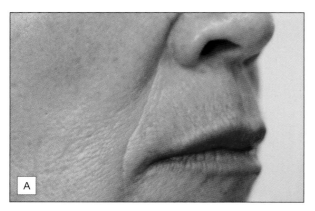

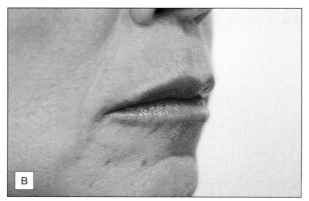

Fig. 3.5 (**A** and **B**) Combination therapy: before and after three-quarters view using CosmoPlast into the vermilion border and CosmoDerm1 and Botox for the perioral rhytids

to the ala. If this is not treated adequately, the entire cosmetic unit will appear undercorrected. Injection should involve injecting the entire expanse of the nasolabial crease to its termination at the nasal ala. Care must be taken as the angular vein and artery are located in this triangle and deep injections can eventuate into profound bruising and intravascular placement can result in tissue necrosis and slough. Following treatment of the NLF with collagen, one gloved finger can be inserted inside the patient's mouth and another finger placed on the outside; gentle massage with the two opposing digits may reduce bumps and locate any areas that have been skipped.

• Periorbital rhytides

Treatment of periocular rhytides, those radiating from the lareral ocular canthus (crow's feet) and in the infraocular sulcus, is one of the more challenging uses of collagen. The periorbital skin is very thin with a rich superficial vascular plexus and treating this region with fillers is unforgiving, often resulting in visible beading and significant eccyhmosis. It is routinely considered as an ancillary treatment to Botox, resurfacing procedures and blapharoplasty surgery.

Since many of these lines are dynamic, due to activity of the underlying orbicularis oculi muscle, Botox is considered the primary treatment of choice. The subsequent addition of fillers primarily addresses any of the remaining static and photodynamic lines. Selectively inactivating fibers of the large annular orbicularis oculi muscle that encircles the eye sustains and preserves the benefits of collagen in this area. Botox (10–15 u) placed lateral to the ocular rim eliminates many of the dynamic horizontal crow's feet lines. An additional 2–4 u: 1–2 at the lateral canthus and 1–2 approximately 3 mm below the ciliary margin at the midpupillary line, will greatly improve the appearance of the lower eyelid rhytides. Any of the remaining fine lines can be treated with collagen. The collagen used for periocular rhytides should be a thin product such as Zyderm I or CosmoDerm 1. When placing collagen around the eyes, the technique is similar to that used for the vertical perioral rhytides. The needle should be very superficial and with minimal force on the plunger serial injections of about 0.05 cc should be used to gradually fill the rhytides. Treating the deep infraorbital sulcus and the lateral superior brow should be done with a hyaluronic acid. Deep placement with one of these fillers not only reduces the sunken 'hollowed' appearance of the infraorbital area but also helps to raise the lateral brow. When injecting collagen and hyaluronic acids around the eyes, patients should be told that swelling may be significant; in addition bruising can be significant and may last many days. Both ecchymosis and edema can be minimized with cool compresses and massage. Patients should be instructed in the use of green-based make-up, which aids in camouflaging bruising.

• Glabellar complex

The etiology of glabellar wrinkles is primarily due to hypertrophy of the bilateral corrugator supercilii and midline procerus muscles. Paralysis of these muscles with 20–35 u of Botox eliminates much of the muscular movement and eliminates the folds in this region. However despite adequate muscular immobility, often due to both chronic photodamage and repetitive movement, there often remains a pair of superimposed deeply etched parallel lines in the skin. Zyderm I or CosmoDerm 1, the non-cross-linked products, can be used to soften these residual static lines. Zyplast and CosmoPlast are absolutely contraindicated for this area due to their deep placement and the risk of vascular embarrassment and subsequent skin necrosis. Injecting glabellar lines is analogous to those in the periocualar and perioral regions.

• Complications

A common source of frustration for patients receiving collagen injections is the temporary nature of the correction. Duration of implanted dermal filling substances are dependant on the volume used, the type of defect, and the mechanical stresses at the implantation site. Patient satisfaction is a combination not only of anatomic defect and physician expertise, but also managing expectations. This can be tempered if patients are provided with a range of how long augmentation can be sustained. In general, patients can anticipate 3–6 months of improvement with gradual diminution of results; however patients can receive additional treatment or maintenance therapy at any time.

The adverse treatment responses for both classes of injectable collagen can be nonhypersensitive, and additionally for bovine collagen, hypersensitive reaction patterns may occur (Box 3.3). Many of the former are technique dependent, and include injection site ecchymosis, superficial placement with apparent beading and deep placement with intravascular injury. Vascular occlusion following dermal placement of collagen presents as an immediate cutaneous blanch associated with pain. Immediate vasodilation with warm compresses and topical nitroglycerin paste can reduce the vasospasm. Ultimately, if tissue necrosis and slough occur, sustained emotional support and appropriate wound care are essential to expedite resolution.

With bovine collagen there are two forms of true classic type IV hypersensitivity to the implants. They develop in about 1% of those whose two skin tests were negative and who subsequently received treatment. Due primarily to Zyderm I and occurring at approximately 2 weeks after treatment the more common reaction is manifested by swollen, indurated granulomas at both the treatment and test sites. Although they resolve spontaneously and without permanent scarring, they can take up to 1 year to completely dissipate. In addition to reassurance, treatment has included nonsteroidal anti-inflammatory drugs and intralesional injections of dilute corticosteroids such as Triamcinolone. There has been anecdotal evidence that oral cyclosporine and topical immune modulators (tacrolimus) have expedited resolution. Sterile abscesses are the second form of delayed hypersensitivity that has been associated with bovine collagen. The incidence is low, approximately 1–4 in 10,000 treatments, and is due in large part to Zyplast. Adverse reactions are characterized by the sudden onset of pain, usually a few weeks after injection, followed by tense edema and erythema with fluctuant nodules. The lesions can be treated by incision and drainage, intralesional steroids, and oral antibiotics, however scarring can occur. The circulating anti-bovine-collagen antibodies that occur in these reactions do not cross-react with human collagen products, and there has not been any statistical association between bovine collagen and autoimmune connective tissue disease. It should also be noted that all bovine collagens are derived from the hides of a closed herd of American cattle, and therefore do not come in contact with animals exposed to the prions that cause bovine spongiform encephalopathy (BSE).

CONCLUSION

Facial soft tissue deformities and age-related cutaneous changes have a great impact on psychosocial interactions. There are many causes for these defects, and in the practitioner's quest to enhance the appearance of facial skin there is a correspondingly wide range of techniques for improving them. The vast array of available filler products and those on the horizon provide a safe and effective means to provide volume and improve contour irregularities associated with aging and trauma. The injectable collagens, whether bovine, porcine or synthetically human based, will continue to be a mainstay in the treatment of the 'aging face' as they are predictable and have a long history of safety and efficacy.

FURTHER READING

Aschinoff R 2000 Overview: Soft tissue augmentation. Clinics in Plastic Surgery 274:479–487

Bauman L, Kerdel F 1999 The treatment of bovine collagen allergy with cyclosporine. Dermatologic Surgery 25:247–249

Cosmetic Surgery National Data Bank Statistics 2004. New York, The American Society for Aesthetic Plastic Surgery

Drake L, Dinehart S, Farmer E, et al 1996 Guidelines of care for soft tissue augmentation. Journal of the American Academy of Dermatology 34:695–697

Elson ML 1989 The role of skin testing in the use of collagen-injectable materials. Journal of Dermatologic Surgery and Oncology 15:301–303

Kaminer MS, Kraus MC 1998 Filler substances in the treatment of facial aging. Medical and Surgical Dermatology 15:215–221

Lemperle G, Romanon JJ, Busson M 2003 Soft tissue augmentation with Artecoll: 10 year history, indications, techniques, and complications. Dermatologic Surgery 29:573–587

Matarasso SL, Matarasso A 2001 Treatment guidelines for botulinum toxin type A for the periocular region and a report on partial upper lip ptosis following injections to the lateral canthal rhytides. Plastic and Reconstructive Surgery 108:208–214

Matarasso SL, Sadick NS 2003 Soft tissue augmentation. In: Bolognia J, Jorizzo JL, Rapini RV, Horn T (eds) Dermatology. Mosby, Harcourt Health Sciences, London, pp 2439–2449

Matarasso SL, Carruthers JD, Jewell ML 2006 Consensus recommendations for soft-tissue augmentation with nonanimal stabilized hyaluronic acid (Restylane). Plastic and Reconstructive Surgery 117:3–43

Matarasso SL 2006 The use of injectable collagen for aesthetic rejuvenation. Seminars in Cutaneous Medicine and Surgery 25:151–157

Matarasso SL 2007 Injectable collagen: Lost but not forgotten: A review of products, indications, and injection techniques. Plastic and Reconstructive Surgery Plas Recons Surg 120 (Suppl) 15–105

Orentreich DS, Orentreich NO 1989 Injectable fluid silicone. In: Roenigk RK, Renigk HH (eds) Principles of Dermatologic Surgery. Marcel-Dekker, pp 1349–1395

Moody BR, Sengelmann RD 2001 Topical tacrolimus in the treatment of bovine hypersensitivity. Dermatologic Surgery 27:789–791

Rohrer TE 2001 Soft tissue filler substances. Current Problems in Dermatology 13:54–60

Stegman SJ, Chu S, Armstrong RC 1988 Adverse reactions to bovine collagen implant: Clinical and histologic features. Journal of Dermatologic Surgery and Oncology 79:39

Toman DP, Egbart BE, Thomas JA, DeLustro FA 2004 Development of a novel nonantigenic dermal implant composed of human placental collagen. Plastic and Reconstructive Surgery 113:1015–1023

Yoshiko M, Fumitaka T, Nobuyoshi K, et al 2004 Atelocollagen mediated synthetic small interfering RNA delivery for effective gene silencing in vitro and in vivo. Nucleic Acids Research 32:109

4 Hylans and Soft Tissue Augmentation

Rhoda S. Narins, Jason Michaels, Joel L. Cohen

INTRODUCTION

Hyaluronic acid fillers have rapidly become the new 'gold standard' in soft tissue augmentation, and are the fastest growing noninvasive esthetic procedure in the United States today according to the American Society for Aesthetic Plastic Surgery. From 2003–2004 alone they have experienced a nearly 700% increase in use. Baby boomers and older retirement ages, along with a projected 2010 US population of 81 million people aged 44–64 years old are driving demand for minimally invasive procedures. Collagen once commanded the market, but hyaluronic acids have demonstrated distinct advantages that have made them more popular. These include higher biocompatibility, the ability to volumize and longer residence times in the skin (Table 4.1). There are several forms in clinical use as soft tissue fillers (Box 4.1). This chapter will review the most commonly used agents, their indications (Box 4.2), safety, efficacy, uses, and advantages compared to other fillers.

Hylans are ideal for patients who like the results of temporary tissue fillers, but desire something longer lasting than collagen. As with other fillers, the folds and wrinkles that are most readily distensible will respond the best. Deep, nondistensible, and 'ice-pick'-type scars that do not easily efface with gentle, manual stretching of adjacent skin will not respond well (Box 4.3). Rejuvenation of age-related facial changes, such as static rhytids, deepened nasolabial folds (NLFs), and atrophy of the lips and oral commissures can also be addressed well with hylans. Other uses include facial (re)contouring of atrophic, volume-depleted changes in the face. Contraindications are similar to other soft tissue fillers (Box 4.4). Patients allergic to bovine collagen, as well as first-time patients who want treatment 'today' (no skin test required) are able to benefit from these derivatives of hyaluronic acid.

Discovered in 1934 by Karl Meyer and John Palmer, hyaluronic acid (hyaluronan, sodium hyaluronate [HA]) is found in all vertebrate animals as a naturally occurring linear polysaccharide composed of alternating residues of the monosaccharides D-glucuronic acid and N-acetyl-D-glucosamine (Fig. 4.1). It is widely distributed in the extracellular matrix of connective tissues, synovial fluid, the aqueous and vitreous humor of the eye, and other tissues. In the skin, it forms the elastoviscous fluid matrix in which collagen fibers, elastic fibers, and other intercellular structures are embedded. Synthesized on cell membranes and then extruded into the extracellular space, HA is the largest (mass of 50 kDa) and most plentiful glycosaminoglycan (GAG) in the extracellular matrix of the dermis with an average adult concentration of 200 mg/kg (0.02%). Unlike other GAGs (chondroitin sulfate, heparin sulfate), it is not sulfated or bound to a core protein. It is negatively charged and binds enormous amounts of water (up to 1000 times its volume). Unlike collagen, it exhibits no species or tissue specificity; its chemical structure is uniform throughout nature, and it thus has no potential for immunogenicity in its pure form. With age, the amount of hyaluronic acid decreases in the skin, resulting in reduced dermal hydration and increased wrinkling.

Medically useful HA was first isolated and purified in 1962 and licensed by the Food and Drug Administration (FDA) to Pharmacea as Healon for ophthalmic use. It then evolved into use as an intra-articular injection for the treatment of osteoarthritis. Because of its stabilizing, hydrating, and cushioning properties with high biocompatibility, it seemed to be a logical alternative as a soft tissue filler material. However, in contrast to the earlier mentioned medical applications, cutaneous soft tissue augmentation requires a sustained presence at the site of deposition. Since the half-life of natural unmodified HA in tissue is only 1–2 days (exogenous HA is rapidly cleared from the dermis and degraded in the liver to form carbon dioxide and water), it is a poor candidate for soft tissue augmentation in its pure natural form.

In the 1980s, cross-linking was established to address this concern and increase tissue residence time. By chemically cross-linking molecules of HA, more stable macromolecules are formed that have the same biocompatibility as native HA, but are water-insoluble and thus have

Table 4.1 Hylans compared to collagen as soft tissue fillers

	Collagen	Hyaluronic acid
Compatibility	Species and tissue specific	Identical in all species and tissues
Duration in tissue	Lasts 3–5 months	Lasts 6–12 months[a]
Origin	Bovine or human	Animal or bacterial
Pattern of loss	Steady volume loss	Isovolemic degradation[a]
Viscosity	Constant viscosity	Dynamic (shear-thinning) viscosity
Anesthesia	0.3% lidocaine included	No lidocaine included
Discomfort	Slightly less injection pain	Slightly more injection pain
Target correction	50–100% overcorrection	No overcorrection
Pre-op skin test?	Double skin test required[b]	No skin test required
Allergy prevalence	3% population allergic[b]	<0.4% population allergic[c]
Shipping and storage	Refrigerated	Room temperature

[a]When in HA gel (hylan) form, [b]for bovine collagen, [c](Lowe 2001).

Box 4.1 Hyaluronic acid preparations in clinical use as soft tissue fillers

Hylaform	Restylane	Restylane Fine Lines	Perlane	Contura	DermaDeep
Hyacel	Esthelis	Hylan Rofilan,	Matredar	Dermalive	
Viscontour	Captique	Juvederm, Hydrafill	Macrolane	Synvisc	
Surgiderm	Achyal (Hyal 2000)	Beletero	Elevesse		

Box 4.2 Conditions treated with hylans

Static facial rhytids
Forehead ('worry' lines)
Periorbital lines ('crow's feet')
Perioral (upper lip and smile) lines
Glabellar lines
Nasolabial folds
hollowsLabiomental folds (marionettes)
Horizontal neck bands

Lip sculpture
Volume enhancement
Vermilion border definition
Philtral crest definition
Oral commissure effacement

Facial contouring
Cheek augmentation
Chin augmentation
Temporal augmentation
Infraorbital augmentation

Other
Distensible scars
Earlobe enhancement
Hand rejuvenation
Brow augmentation
Perimental
Nasal contouring

increased durability and prolonged tissue residence times after injection. In addition, cross-linked HA molecules retain their affinity for water (hygroscopic) and swell to form a three-dimensional network known as a gel. Hyaluronic acid gels (hylans) are classified as both chemical gels (connected by covalent bonds) and hydrogels (swollen with water rather than an organic solvent).

Hylans have several other physicochemical attributes that make them especially attractive as soft tissue fillers. First, hylans have the unique attribute of **dynamic viscosity**, where viscosity decreases with increasing shearing forces (Fig. 4.2). Under the pressures of injection (high

shear rate) the gel can pass through a relatively small-gauge needle. Upon removal of the shearing forces the viscosity increases and forms a thick gel at the site of tissue implantation. Viscosity also decreases with increasing temperature. Their molecular weight, concentration, and degree of cross-linking determine their rheological (flow) properties, which vary among different hylans.

Second, their disappearance from tissue is anecdotally said to show some degree of **isovolemic degradation**; that is, as individual molecules of HA are degraded, those remaining are able to bind more water. In other words, the concentration of the gel decreases during reabsorption while some of the volume is maintained due to more water binding being available even though less overall HA remains in the skin. Clinically, this translates into an implant that maintains some space-filling volume until the last of the material is completely resorbed (Fig. 4.3).

HYLAFORM

The first preparation widely used for soft tissue augmentation was hylan B gel (Hylaform Gel, Biomatrix Inc., Ridgefield, NJ). Developed in the mid-1980s, it was first made available in Europe in 1996. It uses HA derived from the dermis of nongender chicken combs, which is then purified and chemically cross-linked with divinyl sulfone. It has a concentration of 5.5 mg/mL and a duration of effect of 3–6 months. It is currently used in the treatment of soft tissue defects and facial augmentation throughout most of the world (Canada, Europe, Australia, South America, Asia, etc.). It became available in the USA in April 2004 (Hylaform, Hylaform Plus, Inamed, Santa

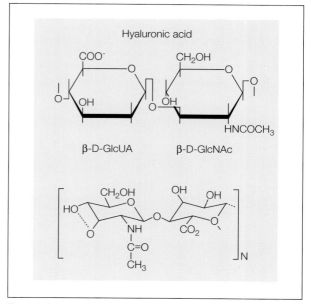

Fig. 4.1 Chemical structure of hyaluronic acid

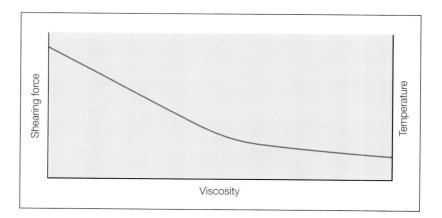

Fig. 4.2 Dynamic viscosity of hylans

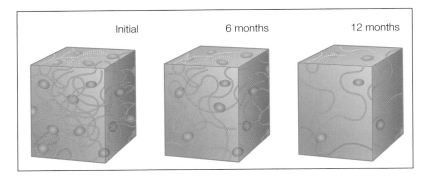

Initial   6 months   12 months

Fig. 4.3 Isovolemic degradation of hylans

Barbara, CA) and is distributed in 0.75 cc syringes. It is also known as Hyladerm in Europe.

Preclinical animal studies demonstrate that hylan B gel implants do not elicit clinically significant immunogenic, inflammatory, or foreign-body reactions, and remain stable in tissue over time. In a study by Piacquadio et al in 1997 comparing intradermal injection of collagen and hylan B gel implants in guinea pigs, most of the injected collagen was resorbed after 26 weeks, while 75% of hylan B gel injection sites still showed histologic evidence of residual material up to 52 weeks.

To determine the safety and efficacy of Hylaform Gel for facial scars and wrinkles, Pollack conducted a six-center, open-label, 12-month study of 216 patients. Treatment success, defined as 60% of all sites showing at least a 33% degree of correction, was noted in both wrinkles/folds and scars at 18 weeks. Treatment reactions included mild erythema, itching, swelling and pain. Less than 2% of all treatments were associated with persistent erythema, acne, or ecchymoses, and all resolved without long-term sequelae.

Clinically, in the FDA US clinical study, Hylaform lasted the same as collagen, about 3 months.

CAPTIQUE

Captique (Allergan-Inamed, Santa Barbara, CA) was FDA approved in December 2004 for use in mid-to-deep dermal injections for the correction of moderate to severe facial wrinkles and folds, such as nasolabial folds (NLFs). It is very similar to Hylaform: 5.5 mg/mol, 500 μ particle size and cross-linked by divinyl sulfone. The main difference lies in its source of production, that is, bacterial fermentation rather than animal derived rooster combs. The FDA approval process for Captique considered it an extension of Hylaform with a new manufacturing source (*Streptococcus* bacteria) rather than a new product. In fact, the only studies referred to in the Captique package insert are based on the Hylaform studies. It has a concentration of 5.5 mg/mL, and is sold in 0.75 cc syringes, also just like Hylaform. Matarasso et al recently reported a case of a

hypersensitivity reaction to Captique 2 weeks after injecting the NLFs. This apparent Captique HA reaction presented as 'small bumps,' and was presumed secondary to a protein contaminant introduced during the fermentation process.

RESTYLANE

Restylane (Medicis Scottsdale, AZ) was the first hyaluronic acid product to be FDA approved in the United States (December 2003). It is a stabilized, partially cross-linked HA produced by bacterial fermentation of *Streptococcus equi*, a Non-Animal Stabilized Hyaluronic Acid (NASHA) formulation and cross-linked with epoxides (butane-diol-diglycidyl ether). The material is heat sterilized in its final container and has a shelf life of 1.5 years from the date of manufacture.

Restylane is distributed in several forms worldwide: Restylane, Restylane Fine Line, Perlane, and Restylane SubQ. All Restylane products have a concentration of 20 mg/mL. In the United States is Restylane, which is distributed in 0.4 cc and 1.0 cc syringes with a duration of effect of 6–12 months, Perlane has been approved recently by the FDA.

There are several key differences between the most commonly used hylans (Table 4.2). Prior to Restylane's release in the United States, early comparisons of Restylane and Hylaform by Manna et al and Micheels found Hylaform to be 'rheologically superior', behaving as a stronger (more elastic) hydrogel. Further, Olenius detected low levels of impurities in both products: avian proteins in Hylaform and fermentation byproducts and additives (to enable cross-linking) in Restylane. Restylane was also found to contain small, undetermined amounts of phosphate, calcium, and other ions. For these reasons, Restylane was reformulated in 1999 to decrease its foreign protein content. The protein contaminant levels in Hylaform and Restylane products are now reportedly similar.

Table 4.2 Comparison of FDA-approved hyaluronic acids				
	Hylaform	**Captique**	**Restylane**	**Juvéderm**
Cross-linking	Divinyl sulfone	Divinyl sulfone	Epoxides	Epoxides
HA source	Rooster combs	*Strep. equi*	*Strep. equi*	*Strep. equi*
HA concentration	5.5 mg/mL	5.5 mg/mL	20 mg/mL	24 mg/mL
Particle size	500 μ	500 μ	250–400 μ	Nonparticulate
Supplied in	0.75 mL	0.75 mL	0.4, 1.0 mL	0.8 mL
Degree cross-linked	20%	20%	<1%	6–8%

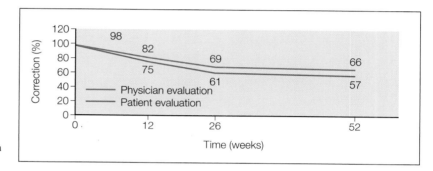

Fig. 4.4 Physician and patient evaluations of correction after Restylane injection. (Data from Olenius 1998)

In 1998, a Swedish study by Olenius of the clinical safety and efficacy of Restylane revealed that the physician-evaluated treatment sites maintained an average of 82% and 69% of correction at 12 and 26 weeks, respectively, while subjects self-reported 75% and 61% improvement at these same time points (Fig. 4.4). An Italian study by Duranti et al of Restylane's clinical efficacy and tolerability also showed favorable results: 78% of patients had moderate to marked improvement at 8 months with the NLFs and lips maintaining the most improvement (Fig. 4.5). In addition, the Duranti group demonstrated Restylane implants histologically apparent at 12 months. More recent reports by both Bennett and Soparkar, demonstrate the remains of Restylane implants up to 23 months and 5 years, respectively.

In 2003, Narins et al compared the treatment of NLFs with Restylane to Zyplast. In this six-center, randomized, double-blinded study of 138 patients with moderate to severe NLFs, investigators found Restylane to be superior to Zyplast at maintaining correction at all post-baseline time points (Fig. 4.6). Although the number of treatment sessions required to reach the initial baseline of an 'optimal cosmetic result' did not differ between the two fillers (mean 1.4, range 1–3), the total injection volume needed to produce this effect was lower for Restylane (mean 1.0 mL, range 0.3–2.8 mL) than for Zyplast (mean 1.6 mL, range 0.1–5.0 mL).

Jaggi conducted a randomized study of 80 patients in a report in November 2005 comparing Restylane and Hylaform in the treatment of NLFs. The blinded, independent reviewer panel attributed an average improvement score of 2.86 of 5 for Hylaform and 3.78 of 5 for Restylane, even at lower volumes of injected material for Restylane (1.0 ml versus 0.7 mL, respectively). At a similar time, Carruthers conducted a randomized, double-blind comparison of Perlane and Hylaform in the treatment of nasolabial folds. Perlane was also considered superior in 64% of patients, though treatment-related adverse events tended to be more frequent with Perlane.

Restylane may exhibit mild and transient side effects including redness, swelling, darkening of the treatment site, bruising, and slight pain, most of which resolve within 3 days. Red spots, bumps, and hematomas are infrequent and seem to be associated with injection technique. In some cases, swelling is stimulated by exercise, sun exposure and menstruation and was judged to be due to the hydrophilic properties of the implant. Duranti, Olenius and Narins have all reported varying degrees of adverse events from 12.5% to 93.5% (Table 4.3), with intermittent swelling and erythema the most reported. Narins et al report a much higher incidence of adverse events probably because patients were required to keep a daily diary of any adverse events for 2 weeks after each injection session

Soft Tissue Augmentation

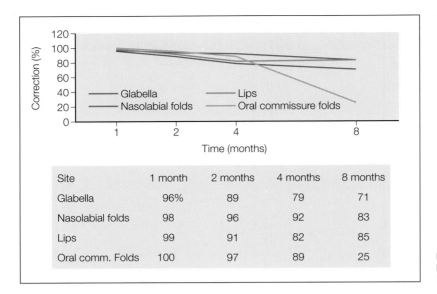

Fig. 4.5 Persistence of Restylane correction by implantation site. (Data from Duranti et al 1998)

Site	1 month	2 months	4 months	8 months
Glabella	96%	89	79	71
Nasolabial folds	98	96	92	83
Lips	99	91	82	85
Oral comm. Folds	100	97	89	25

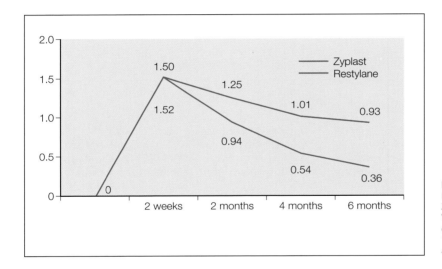

Fig. 4.6 Maintenance of improvement in NLFs after treatment with Restylane vs Zyplast. Mean change from pretreatment in WSRS over 6 months. WSRS is a method of quantifying facial folds, in which 1 = absent, 2 = mild, 3 = moderate, 4 = severe and 5 = extreme

(i.e. possibly recorder bias with patients feeling that they had to report 'something' in their diary). They also found injection site pain to be slightly higher for Restylane than Zyplast (57.2% compared to 42.0% in patient diaries), perhaps due to the absence of lidocaine and its more viscous character.

Hypersensitivity or other allergic reactions to hylans have also been reported. Prior to 1999, Lowe et al reported delayed implant site reactions in three of 709 patients (0.42%) treated with hylan implants in London between 1996 and 2000 (438 Hylaform, 271 Restylane). Positive skin testing to both agents implies causes other than avian protein reactivity, which would be expected only with Hylaform. Micheels treated 219 patients with Hylaform

(106) or Restylane (133) between 1997 and 2001. In that time, eight patients (3.7%) developed delayed inflammatory reactions of redness, pruritus, painful swelling, or 'nettle-like rash' reactions. Biopsies in four of these patients revealed strong granulomatous foreign-body reactions with giant cells, including reactions to both agents. Lowe's study determined the overall incidence of granulomatous reactions to be low (0.4%). Examining the worldwide adverse events database of Q-Med Esthetics, Friedman performed a retrospective review of reactions to Restylane in 1999 and found that 1 of every 1400 (0.07%) patients get 'swelling, erythema and induration at the implant site, sometimes with edema in the surrounding tissue with a median duration of 15 days'

Table 4.3 Implant-related adverse events (AEs) associated[a] with Restylane[a]

Event	Duranti (% sites)	Olenius (% sites)	Narins (% patients)
Intermittent swelling	4.8%		87.0%
Erythema	2.6	6.6%[b]	84.8
Edema	1.8		NR
Discomfort	1.8	NR	NR
Tenderness	1.1	NR	77.5
Bruising/dark area	1.1	3.2[d]	52.2
Itching	0.4	NR	30.4
Pain	0.4	0.4	57.2
Other[c]	NR	NR	24.6
Overall AE rate	12.5%	13.4%	93.5%[e]

NR = not reported. [a]In Duranti & Olenius studies AEs were directly observed by investigators; in Narins' study they were recorded from daily patient diaries. [b]Includes erythema, swelling, and edema. [c]'Other' includes injection site stiffness, nodules, and pimples. [d](1.4% injection related, 1.8% technique related). [e]In comparison, local injection site reactions to Zyplast during the same time period were reported in 90.6% of diaries. Most were mild or moderate in intensity such that at the investigator evaluation at 2 weeks, less than 15% of all reactions were still clinically apparent, similar to the other two studies.

Table 4.4 Reports of incidence of delayed hypersensitivity from hylan implants

Implant	Incidence (No. of cases/total)	Time period	Source
H or R	0.42% (3/709)	1996–2000	Lowe[a]
H or R	3.7% (8/219)	1997–2001	Micheels[a]
R	0.07% (104/144 000)	1999	Friedman[b]
R	0.02% (52/262 000)	2000	Friedman[b]

H = Hylaform, R = Restylane. [a]From personal observation. [b]From retrospective review of adverse event database of Q Med Esthetics.

(0.07%). Most reactions resolved spontaneously in 4 days. The exact incidence of delayed hypersensitivity reactions has varied among reports (Table 4.4). In 2000, Friedman found that of the estimated 262,000 patients treated, one out of every 5000 developed a localized cutaneous hypersensitivity appearing an average of 22 days after injection and lasting 15 days. Studies suggest that most reactions are a response to protein contaminants rather than to the hyaluronic acid itself, supporting the convictions of several key opinion leaders (including Arnold Klein, M.D. *Dermatologic Surgery* editorial) that allergy to hyaluronic acid is not the chief cause of these reactions.

Other incidental reports of cutaneous hypersensitivity have also been reported. Lupton and Alster described a case of delayed hypersensitivity in a 54-year-old Caucasian woman after having three injections of Restylane over a 14-month period. Two weeks after the last injection into the melolabial folds, she developed multiple acute tender red nodules in the treatment area that eventually resolved with treatment. This was before 1999 with the original and not the upgraded product that is the only one that has been used in the United States. In 2005, Leonhardt reported an angioedema acute hypersensitivity reaction of the upper lip and nose within 1 hour after injection, which significantly improved after 4 days. Again, in 2006, Matarraso described a case of delayed hypersensitivity to Captique that spontaneously resolved at 4 months after multiple ineffective attempts at therapy.

Case reports of other reactions have also occurred, including abscess-like swellings, tender nodules, arterial embolization, venous occlusion, and granulomatous reactions. Two cases of injection site necrosis were recorded, both in the glabella area. Narins and Cohen et al describe a protocol to manage focal necrosis and 'angry red bumps', as does Glaich and Cohen et al for glabellar necrosis. Hirsch, Cohen and Carruthers have reported a case of delayed impending necrosis beginning several hours after HA treatment. Voy and Andrea also reported several cases of facial atrophy similar to that of HIV patients under highly active antiretroviral therapy. A list of reported side effects from hylans appears in Box 4.5.

Lastly, early indications from both animal and human clinical studies show that using popular ablative and non-ablative energy sources before or after injection of Restylane does not adversely affect either the efficacy or persistence of the filler. Alam shows that radiofrequency

Box 4.5 Side effects reported from use of hylans

Common
Erythema
Swelling/edema
Pain
Tenderness at injection site
Bruising
Itching

Rare
Angioedema acute hypersensitivity reaction
Delayed local hypersensitivity
Granulomatous reaction
Abscess-like swelling
Arterial embolization
Venous occlusion resulting in lip varix
Acneiform eruption
Facial atrophy similar to HIV lipoatrophy
Superficial blue nodules (Tyndall effect)

treatment over skin previously injected with Restylane does not appear to cause gross morphological changes in the filler material or the surrounding skin. However, a recent report by Hirsch and Narurkar showed that superficial injections with hyaluronic acids (Tyndall effect) could be improved with Q switched 1064 nm lasers.

JUVÉDERM

The newest hyaluronic acid product to reach the United States market is Juvéderm (Allergan, Irvine CA). Approved for use in the European market in 2001 (aka Hydrafill), it was FDA-approved in the United States in June 2006 for mid to deep dermis correction of moderate to severe facial wrinkles and folds.

Developed by bacterial fermentation and cross-linked with butane-diol-diglycidyl ether (BDDE, like Restylane), Juvéderm differs from the other HA products as it is a homogeneous gel with the highest concentration of cross-linked hyaluronic acid (>90%) of any dermal filler currently available. There has never been a head-to-head comparison of Restylane versus Juvéderm and it is not known which one, if any, lasts longer or provides more volume per unit. The Juvéderm products inject very smoothly. Some speculate that the impurities involved in the higher degree of cross-linking process may raise the chance for hypersensitivity reactions.

In Europe, Juvéderm is available in five formulations: Juvéderm 18, 24, 24 HV, 30, and 30 HV. HV indicates higher viscosity or a greater degree of cross-linking for that product. Though Juvéderm 30 has also been FDA-approved, the first products released in the US are Juvéderm Ultra (24 HV 24 mg/cc) and Juvéderm Ultra Plus (30 HV, also 24 mg/cc with more cross-linking) and are prepackaged with 30 and 27 gauge needles for mid to upper dermal and mid to deep dermal injection, respec-

tively. They all have a concentration of 24 mg/mL and are differentiated by their degree of cross-linking; that is, higher numbers equate to a higher degree of cross-linking. Both Juvéderm Ultra and Juvéderm Ultra Plus are distributed in 0.8 ml syringes.

OVERVIEW OF TREATMENT STRATEGY

• Evaluate defect to be treated/patient interview

The first step in performing any sort of soft tissue augmentation is having a detailed discussion about what the patient wants to change, soften or improve. Does a fold, wrinkle, or scar exist that is particularly bothersome? Having the patient hold a hand mirror so both physician and patient can see and discuss individual lines or lesions is helpful. Make sure you and the patient are talking about the same thing, and fully understand the goals of the patient. Consider using a pointer (wooden end of a cotton-tipped applicator, etc.) to precisely indicate the area(s) of concern. Many of the changes the patient requests may be better served by other treatment approaches (Box 4.3). Dynamic rhytids (present only when the patient furrows brow, smiles, purses lips, etc.) are the best example, and are best addressed with botulinum toxin. In general, botulinum toxin is the most useful agent for prominent/hyperdynamic musculature in the upper face which is beginning to cause etched-in lines in specific areas (glabella, forehead, crow's feet), while fillers are most useful for lines and folds in the lower face (NLFs, oral commissures). Often these treatments can be combined. Carruthers demonstrated the synergy of these types of products in a report that showed moderate to severe glabellar rhytides were treated more effectively by botulinum toxin A combined with HA injections than by HA alone. Lips and NLFs respond best to fillers, and hylans in particular. Use manual stretching of skin to estimate how well a certain wrinkle, fold or scar will or will not respond is often helpful, often demonstrating this to the patient as they look into the mirror.

Ask questions to confirm the patient's understanding of the filler and its potential, as well as what it can and cannot do (Box 4.6). Discuss that hylans are temporary (although longer lasting than collagen) fillers. Determine if the patient is at increased risk for scarring (history of hypertrophic scars, keloids, etc.) Have they had soft-tissue augmentation in the past, and if so, were they pleased with the results? Do they have a history of herpes simplex in the area to be treated (especially the lips) that could be reactivated with the trauma of an injection? Injections should also be deferred until any active inflammation in the area (acne, rash, etc.) has resolved.

Injection-related hematomas, which result from the entrapment of hemoglobin from small bleeders during injection, can leave dark spots that may remain for a time if they become entrapped in the implant. Consider having the patient discontinue the use of aspirin, nonsteroidal anti-inflammatory medications (NSAIDs), St John's Wort, some vitamin supplements (including vitamin E) and other nonmedically necessary blood thinners for 7–10 days prior to the procedure. To minimize the effects of bruising, anecdotal evidence has led some physicians to advocate applying 1% vitamin K cream twice daily or ingesting homeopathic arnica before or after treatment.

Hyaluronic acid fillers currently available in the USA today are only indicated for the treatment of moderate to severe facial wrinkles and folds, such as the NLFs. All other uses are currently considered off-label. Also, HA implants have not been studied in patients who are pregnant, breastfeeding, under 18 years of age or on immunosuppressive therapy.

Box 4.6 Patient interview questions

Does the patient have:

❖ Experience with soft tissue fillers in the past?
❖ History of hypertrophic scars or keloids?
❖ History of herpes simplex infection?
❖ History of easy bruising/bleeding?
❖ History of pigmentary disorders?
❖ History of autoimmune conditions?
❖ A current pregnancy or breastfeeding?
❖ Dermatologic condition that exhibits pathergy (pyoderma gangrenosum, Sweet's syndrome)?
❖ Any active inflammation (acne, rash, etc.) in area to be treated?
❖ High pain tolerance (need for anesthesia)?
❖ Important social plans in next 3–7 days?
❖ Realistic expectations?

• Choosing an implant agent

As more hylans become available, there will be a greater opportunity to match specific HA preparations to certain types of treatment areas and defects. In general, fine, superficial wrinkles and distensible scars respond best to thin fillers placed at the upper to mid-dermal level. Deeper, more substantial wrinkles, such as the nasolabial folds, require a thicker filler to be placed more deeply in the dermis. Areas requiring true volume augmentation, such as the cheeks or temples, need a more robust filler with placement at the dermal-subcutaneous interface or deeper. Some wrinkles may have both a superficial and a deep component, and require both to be addressed to achieve optimal results.

The Restylane family of products is a good example of different hylan formulations which are designed for use at different dermal depths: Restylane, Restylane FineLine, Perlane and Restylane SubQ (Table 4.5). The concentration of hyaluronic acid is identical in all four preparations (20 mg/mL). They differ in the size of their HA particles (expressed in number of gel particles per mL) as well as the depth of their implantation (Fig. 4.7). Restylane Fine-Line has the smallest particles (200,000/mL), and is therefore the least viscous. It is injected through a 31 gauge needle and is designed for use in the most superficial dermis to correct fine lines and superficial, easily distensible defects. Restylane has larger particles (100,000/mL), is injected through a 30 gauge needle and is placed in the mid dermis to correct moderate NLFs and provide lip augmentation. Perlane has an even larger particle size (10,000/mL) and requires a 27 gauge needle for injection. It is designed for implantation into the deep dermis and superficial subcutaneous tissue to treat deep folds and provide facial contouring (cheek and chin augmentation, etc.) Lastly, Restylane SubQ has the largest particle size (1000/mL) and is therefore the most viscous. It is injected

---

Table 4.5 Comparison of four forms of Restylane

	Restylane	Restylane FineLine	Perlane	Restylane SubQ
HA concentration	20 mg/mL	20 mg/mL	20 mg/mL stabilized HA	20 mg/mL
No. of gel particles/mL	100 000	200 000	10 000	1000
Indications	Wrinkles, lips	Thin superficial lines	Deep folds e.g. NLFs), lip augmentation, facial contouring	Facial contouring
Target depth	Mid-dermis	Upper dermis	Deep dermis/upper subcutis	Subcutis, supraperiosteum
Degree correction	100%	100%	100%	100%
Syringe volume	0.4, 1.0 mL	0.5 mL	1.0 mL	2.0 mL
Needle size	30 gauge	31 gauge	27 gauge	18 gauge
Perlane	Restylane SubQ		Coleman cannula	

Soft Tissue Augmentation

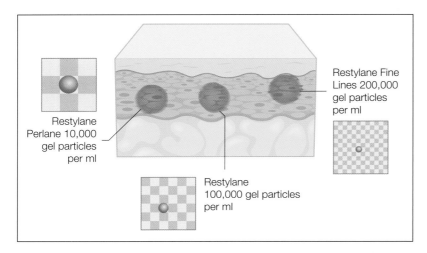

Fig. 4.7 Comparative gel particle sizes and suggested sites of implantation for Restylane Fine Lines, Restylane and Restylane Perlane

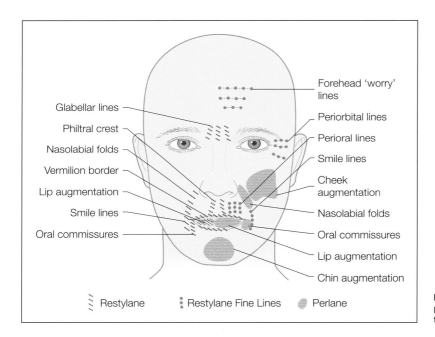

Fig. 4.8 Suggested uses for Restylane preparations based on site and defect to be treated

with a 16 gauge or 19 gauge Coleman cannula into the subcutaneous tissue and periosteal areas for facial contouring. The four different products can be used in concert, layering one over another for optimal clinical results. Only Restylane is FDA-approved for use in the United States. Currently, Perlane is in the final phases of getting FDA approval for use in this country and will likely be the next Restylane product available in the United States. The currently available Hylaform and Juvederm products can be layered as well, with Hylaform Plus and Juvéderm Ultra Plus being placed in the deep dermis, while Hylaform and Juvéderm Ultra are injected more superficially in the mid-dermis overlying the respective deeper filler.

As these and other hylans become available in the United States, more tailored agents can be matched to individual defects (Fig. 4.8).

TREATMENT TECHNIQUES

• General implantation technique

After removing any make-up, the area to be treated should be cleansed with an alcohol prep pad or some other antiseptic (such as chlorhexidine). It is useful for the patient to sit upright during treatment, as the contour of some facial folds and tissues change when the patient is reclining. For this reason, it seems intuitive that general anesthetic procedures (such as face lifts) are not the most appropriate times to inject fillers. The use of a motorized surgical table though can be very helpful for physician comfort and appropriate patient positioning.

None of the currently available hylan preparations include lidocaine and in most patients, some type of anesthesia is needed prior to treatment. Topical anesthetics (EMLA, LMX, or compounded betacaine/lidocaine/tetracaine etc.) can be useful, but must be thickly applied for 20–30 minutes before injection. For other patients, injecting small amounts of local anesthetic around the area to be treated in a 'field block' fashion may be preferable (such as a mini-dental or 'sulcus block' prior to lip augmentation). If this is performed, care must be taken not to alter the defect itself with the tumescence of the anesthetic causing distortion. Peripheral nerve blocks (infra-orbital and mental nerve blocks) can also be performed, which provide the deepest anesthesia but often some degree of distortion of the area being treated. Nerve blocks are also technique dependent and require 10–20 minutes to achieve a complete effect. Some patients can tolerate treatment of NLFs, oral commissures, or the glabella area without any anesthesia. For injections of the lips, however, peripheral nerve and/or field blocks are usually needed (Fig. 4.9, Fig. 4.10). In any area, the thicker the filler, the deeper the implantation depth, the larger the needle required, and the more likely some type of anesthesia is required. Vibration anesthesia, described in an article by Smith, can also make injections much more tolerable through the Gates principle of afferent stimulation.

Hylans are thicker and more viscous than collagen, and take more injection pressure to be pushed out of the syringe and through a needle. Their viscosity slightly decreases with mild increases in temperature. Duranti found that mildly warming the syringe in the hand prior to injection might help to improve product flow. Also, before injecting the patient, push the plunger forward to feel the intrinsic resistance of the filler moving through the needle until a small droplet appears at the needle tip. This should then be wiped off prior to the injections beginning.

Four different implantation techniques have been suggested: linear threading, serial puncture, fanning, and cross-hatching (Fig. 4.11). The serial puncture technique is technically easiest (since the needle tip doesn't move during injection), and is often preferred by beginners. Here the needle enters the skin to the desired depth and a small aliquot of filler is deposited. The needle is then withdrawn. Individual injections of this type work well to fill distensible acne scars, while successive injections can be used to efface a wrinkle.

The linear threading technique is probably the most commonly used. Holding the syringe parallel to the length of the wrinkle or fold to be treated, pierce the skin and advance the needle to the mid to deep dermal level. Then, while slowly withdrawing the needle, apply even pressure on the plunger to dispense material into dermis. To avoid

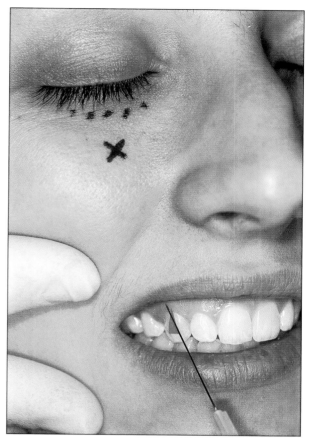

Fig. 4.9 Infraorbital block, intraoral approach (infraorbital foramen indicated by purple 'X'. canine indicated by red triangle

waste and at the same time prevent superficial placement of product, make sure to discontinue the pressure as the needle is almost at the surface. For very fine lines and superficial wrinkles, the extrusion of material from the needle tip can to some extent push the needle backwards. Short, superficial lines and wrinkles can often be softened with a single injection, while several successive 'threads' below, above, or beside previous injections may be required to fill larger folds, lines, or wrinkles. Deeper defects may require layering with thicker preparations (Perlane or Juvéderm Ultra Plus).

Some practitioners enter the skin with a needle angle of 30 degrees or 45 degrees, while others prefer it more parallel to the skin; it is really a matter of personal preference. Some even bend the needle in order to keep it more parallel during their injections. Most authors recommend keeping the needle bevel up, but this is not essential. Studies have shown that the direction of the bevel does not influence the direction of the flow of the material, which follows the course of least resistance.

The most difficult part of the technique for beginners is developing a feel for needle depth. It is better to err on

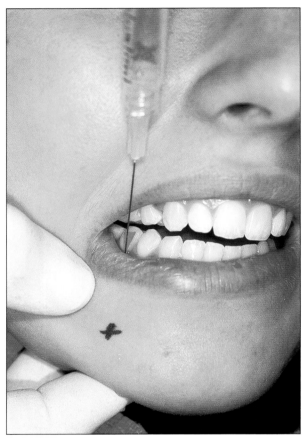

Fig. 4.10 Mental block, intraoral approach (mental foramen indicated by purple 'X', second premolar indicated by red triangle

the side of injecting too deeply, which will simply not give as much benefit. In contrast, injecting too superficially can overcorrect defects and leave surface irregularities. In addition, superficial placement of the clear hylan gels can cause the epidermis to become transparent, which leads to 'bluish spots' (Tyndall effect) on the skin.

Keep the tip of the needle at constant depth during implantation, depositing all filler material within the same plane to get even results. The depth of needle placement (and thus filler implantation) should be high dermis for superficial lines, mid-dermis for more substantial wrinkles, and deep dermis/subcutaneous border for heavy folds. When injecting in the mid-dermal plane, the needle's contour should be visible, but not its color. When injecting thinner materials placed high in the dermis (Restylane Fine Lines) guide treatment by visual response, and when injecting thicker substances (Perlane) guide treatment by tactile response. Resistance should be felt placing thicker substances into deep dermis; a sudden drop in such resistance may indicate injection into the subcutaneous plane.

Hylans should be used to correct to the desired volume. If overcorrection is seen, massage firmly to roll out and spread some of the product. Approximately 20% overcorrection can be massaged out; more will usually lead to a persistent undesirable cosmetic result while the implant is present. Hyaluronidase (Vitrase, Amphadase) has been used to remove unwanted or overcorrected hyaluronic acid, as described by Brody. In addition, hyaluronidase has recently been described by Hirsh, Cohen and Carruthers to decompress 'impending necrosis' after HA injections.

After HA injections, patients can return to normal activities almost immediately after treatment. The authors recommend avoiding exercise and use of make-up until 8–10 hours after the injection visit. Use an ice pack or other cold compress to help minimize swelling (on lips especially); some patients also feel it alleviates post injection discomfort. The duration of correction depends on the character of the defect being treated, implant depth, injection technique, tissue stress at the implant site (i.e. frequency of muscular activity) as well as seemingly the amount of previous filler still present in the skin (i.e. many physicians and patients alike have anecdotally indicated HA products lasting longer on the second and successive treatment sessions).

APPROACH TO SELECTED ANATOMIC AREAS

• Lips

PATIENTS/INDICATIONS

Lip enhancement is one of the most popular procedures in soft tissue augmentation. There are two main aspects to lip enhancement. The first is improvement of lip line definition, achieved by injecting along the cutaneous/vermilion border. The second is augmentation, produced by direct injection into the bulk of the mucosa of the lip to produce enlargement of one or both lips. The former is useful for patients who complain that lipstick bleeds into vertical wrinkles of the upper lip, or who simply need more lip definition, while the latter is used for patients who want bigger, more robust lips. Atrophy of the lips is a natural change as we age, and (re)enlargement can provide a rejuvenating effect. Finally, enhancement of the natural philtrum of the upper cutaneous lip can provide esthetic improvement. One such approach, popular several years ago called the Paris Lip, creates a 'pouting' look.

EQUIPMENT (RESTYLANE, PERLANE, HYLAFORM, CAPTIQUE, JUVÉDERM ULTRA)

One syringe is usually adequate for the initial treatment of the lips. Depending on the product used, enhancement can last 4–6 months, although occasionally patients maintain improvement for 6–9 months.

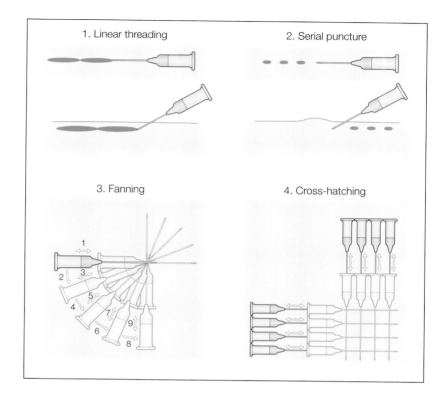

Fig. 4.11 Hylan implantation techniques

TREATMENT ALGORITHM (LINEAR THREADING, SERIAL PUNCTURE)

The lips are one of the most sensitive areas of the entire face; unlike other areas, most patients will require a nerve block for all but the most minimal treatments. Some practitioners prefer to replace these blocks by injecting anesthetic under the mucosa in the sulcus of the posterior (mucosal) aspect of the upper and lower lips. Niamtu describes the 'mucosal lip block' as a method to limit the profound level and extent of anesthesia from nerve blocks. For the needle-phobic patient, Smith describes a 'needle-less,' painless form of anesthesia using topical 5% lidocaine cream simultaneously applied to the skin, vermilion and mucosa of the lips (the latter with the use of a barrier film, such as a Telfa pad) for 20–30 minutes prior to injection.

To improve lip line definition, inject into the potential space between the lip mucosa and the skin along the vermilion border (Fig. 4.12). Any sequence of lip injection can be used; the specific approach is one of personal preference (Fig. 4.13). Holding the syringe parallel to the lip with the noninjecting hand, pierce the vermilion just anterior to the oral commissure and advance it medially along the vermilion border. Using a retrograde flow (pulling back the needle upon placing pressure on the plunger) threading technique, inject the implant into the potential space between the lip mucosa and skin. Continue with successive threads onward toward the center of the lip.

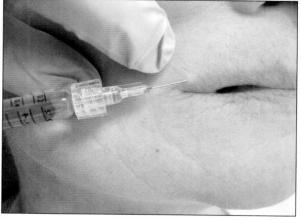

Fig. 4.12 Syringe is held parallel to the long axis of the lip for injection of vermilion border

Then repeat the process for the other three quadrants. An 0.5 in needle will reach 20–25% of the lip line in most patients, so four or five threading injections should cover the entire lip. Placing filler in the lateral aspects of the lower lip will also serve to lift the corners of the mouth and provide a 'happier' rejuvenating look. Holding the syringe vertically, perpendicular to the upper lip, the philtrum of the lip can also be made more defined by implanting threads of filler below each philtral crest (with care to

44

Soft Tissue Augmentation

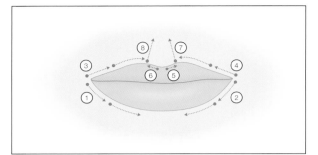

Fig. 4.13 Schematic of injection sequence for lip line enhancement

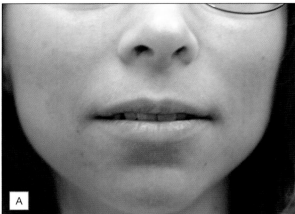

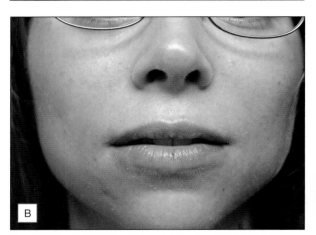

Fig. 4.14 (**A** and **B**) A 37-year-old woman who received Juvéderm Ultra 0.8 cc into the body of her lips (0.3 cc upper lip, 0.5 cc lower lip)

stay very superficial to avoid placement into the superior labial artery).

If volume augmentation of the lip is also desired, outlining the vermilion border is followed by injection into the mucosa itself, above the orbicularis oris muscle. Roughly equal amounts of material are normally used for lip margin enhancement and volume expansion (for example, half a syringe for each). Inject along the 'wet line' where the dry outer mucosa meets the moist inner mucosa. Use either a linear threading or serial puncture technique. Be sure to cease injection just prior to needle withdrawal in order to avoid too superficial placement of the gel. Massage gently throughout the treatment to ensure a smooth final contour (Fig. 4.14).

TROUBLESHOOTING

Owing to the thin, distensible tissue of the lips, patients may develop localized swelling during treatment. This can make it difficult to judge lip symmetry and the overall degree of augmentation that is appropriate or desired by the patient. It is best to invite the patient to return for a touch-up in 1–2 weeks, rather than risk overcorrection by continually trying to 'equalize' the two sides. Each patient will have a different idea of what is 'too much' lip enhancement, and most will not appreciate over-augmentation. Another helpful tip is to inject the entire upper or lower lip first, rather than injecting the right half of the upper and the right half of the lower (i.e. asymmetry is more likely if the injector waits for swelling to set in prior to treating the other side of the lip).

SIDE EFFECTS, COMPLICATIONS, AND ALTERNATIVE APPROACHES

Significant post injection swelling and bruising are the most common side effects of lip injection. Immediate postoperative ice packs can help minimize the swelling ('kiss the ice'), as can keeping the head elevated after injection. The swelling will decrease in 1–2 days, but bruising can last 7–10 days. A short course of systemic steroids can also be used if needed.

A rare complication is reactivation of labial herpes infection, which should respond to an appropriate course

of systemic antiviral therapy. Many injectors will pre-treat known herpes carriers, or more often those who suffer from more frequent outbreaks, with antiviral prophylactic therapy.

The lips are very vascular structures. The most concerning complication of lip augmentation is inadvertent injection into or near a vessel to the point of occlusion with resultant localized necrosis. While this can occur with any injectable filler, it is more likely with thicker substances (Zyplast, Perlane). Since blood cannot be easily drawn back through a 30 gauge needle to ensure a vessel has not been entered, the best insurance is to stay superficial and to keep the needle moving during injection to minimize implantation in any single perivascular location. Also, watch for signs of occlusion (pain, blanching) during implantation so injection can be quickly discontinued if needed.

• Upper lip rhytids

PATIENTS/INDICATIONS

Many patients have vertical rhytids of the upper cutaneous lip that can be improved with hylan fillers. If a patient is also interested in lip enhancement, however, we recommend augmenting the lips first as many of the radial lines may soften as they are effaced by the increased volume of the adjacent vermilion alone.

EQUIPMENT (RESTYLANE, RESTYLANE FINE LINE, JUVÉDERM ULTRA)

Most of the lines of the upper cutaneous lip are superficial and are best treated with thinner fillers such as Restylane, Restylane Fine Line or.Juvéderm Ultra. Smaller needles are generally employed (such as a 32 gauge), especially when the injector is trying to tuck into more shallow etched-in lines. Typically, however, the human-derived collagen product CosmoDerm can be most useful for these types of shallow finer lines. Few patients will require more than 0.3 mL of a filler product in a single treatment session.

TREATMENT ALGORITHM (LINEAR THREADING, SERIAL PUNCTURE)

Unlike the vermilion of the lips, patients often can tolerate injection of the cutaneous portion of the upper lip vertical lines with topical anesthesia alone. Be sure to allow an adequate amount of time for the topical anesthetic to take effect before injection. The patient can also use an ice pack ('kiss the ice') before and in between injections to supplement anesthesia. Treatment is easily performed by standing in front of the patient and holding the syringe upright to inject into the vertical rhytids (Fig. 4.15).

TROUBLESHOOTING

In this area, the most important issues are ensuring adequate anesthesia so the patient can remain still during implant placement, and not injecting the filler too superficially, which can lead to unsightly beading. The latter can be evident as 'bluish' nodules in the skin (Tyndall effect). If this does occur, massage the implant firmly between two fingers (one inside and one outside the lip) or against the underlying bone to try to salvage an acceptable result.

SIDE EFFECTS, COMPLICATIONS, AND ALTERNATIVE APPROACHES

Necrosis is a possibility with any filler material, but is much less likely here as the plane of injection should be very superficial, and the orientation of the needle is perpendicular to the underlying vessels. Hirsch has shown that hyaluronidase or QS 1064 nm lasers can be effective should the Tyndall effect be induced.

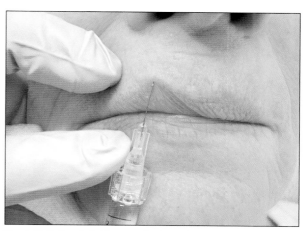

Fig. 4.15 Syringe is held perpendicular to the long axis of the lip (parallel to rhytid being filled) for injection of static upper lip rhytids

Reactivation of a herpes infection may also be of concern in this area, so prophylactic antivirals should at least be considered in patients with a history of frequent cold sores.

• Nasolabial and labiomental folds (marionette lines)

PATIENTS/INDICATIONS

Patients who would like to diminish these prominent folds can attain significant improvement with hylan fillers. Layering of several fillers in these areas can allow the practitioner to achieve a more ideal result and likely a greater longevity to their treatments. Injecting the NLFs allows for a volume improvement to a saggy midface, while injecting the labiomental folds creates a happier disposition to the saddened look of inferiorly directed mouth corners.

EQUIPMENT (RESTYLANE, PERLANE, CAPTIQUE, JUVÉDERM ULTRA, JUVÉDERM ULTRA PLUS)

Hyaluronic acids work well for these areas. If the fold is shallow, Restylane or Juvéderm Ultra alone may do well. If it is more pronounced, a thicker agent (Perlane, Juvéderm Ultra Plus) may be required for deeper filling, followed by layering Restylane or Juvéderm Ultra on top. The volume injected will depend on the severity of the folds. Generally, larger volumes tend to be needed in these areas to adequately efface the 'triangles' of the upper NLFs as well as to create the buttresses of the labiomental folds. Appropriate treatments to these sites go beyond just 'filling' a line.

TREATMENT ALGORITHM (LINEAR THREADING, SERIAL PUNCTURE, FANNING, CROSS-HATCHING)

Many patients do not require more than topical anesthesia, though some may prefer injection of anesthetic around the area to include the infra-orbital nerve. The linear threading technique is most easily used to deposit the filler beneath the fold and efface it. The peri-alar sulcus, a triangular-shaped concavity at the upper end of the fold, may be more effectively filled with the fanning technique or cross-hatching to 'bridge' cosmetic subunits more adequately. Wide portions of the fold may require several threads placed side by side. When treating the marionette lines, the practitioner must build a buttress under the oral commissures to support the lateral portion of the lip (Fig. 4.16). Also, injecting a small amount into the modeolus of the lip can help to raise the corners of the mouth. In treating this area, Carruthers showed that esthetic satisfaction was greatest in the first 3 months post-hylan treatment, with 40% of subjects still noting improvement at the 6-month follow-up visit and those getting optimum volume in studies had results lasting up to 12 months (Figs 4.17 and 4.18).

TROUBLESHOOTING

Treatment of this area is generally easy and straightforward, and satisfying for patients and practitioners. It is important to stay medial to the folds to fill them; injecting lateral to the folds can accentuate them. Be careful not to overfill these areas in order to prevent the look of a 'sausage' vertically thickening the cheek.

SIDE EFFECTS, COMPLICATIONS, AND ALTERNATIVE APPROACHES

Bruising is the most common side effect in this area and usually resolves in 5–7 days. Necrosis is possible, though rare via injections either compressing the facial artery or its branches or more likely a small nidus of frank intravascular injection of filler. A case of delayed 'impending' necrosis has been reported by Hirsch, Cohen and Carruthers and was effectively treated with multiple small aliquot injection stabs of hyaluronidase along the course of the facial and angular arteries. Lastly, it is important to focus on trying to achieve some degree of symmetry for both folds.

• Glabellar lines

PATIENTS/INDICATIONS

Patients with static glabella lines can have a good response to hylan fillers. Many practitioners will first maximize treatment with botulinum toxin to improve these 'frown' lines, dispelling dynamic rhytids and softening static ones. Then, the etched-in residual lines can be softened with fillers.

EQUIPMENT (RESTYLANE, RESTYLANE FINE LINES, JUVÉDERM ULTRA)

Depending on the severity of the rhytid, Restylane, Restylane FineLine, or Juvéderm Ultra can be used to

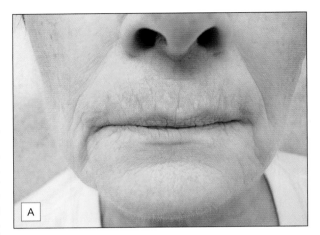

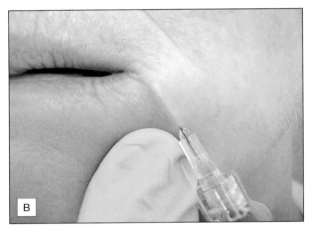

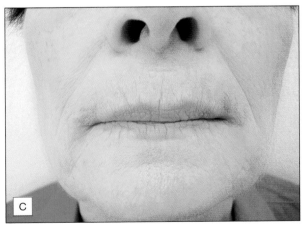

Fig. 4.16 (A) Before treatment of bilateral melolabial folds with 0.7 ml Restylane gel **(B)** Technique used. **(C)** 2 weeks after treatment

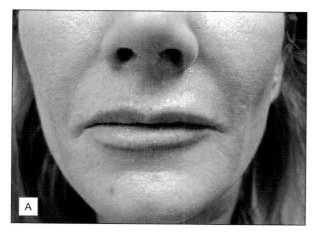

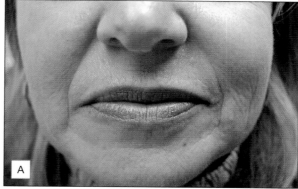

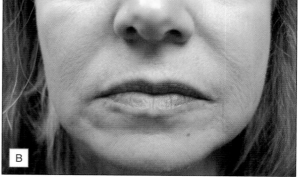

Fig. 4.18 A 52-year-old woman who received Restylane 2.00 cc into her NLFs (1.2 cc right side, 0.8 cc left side)

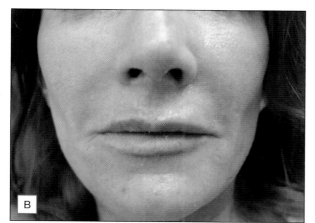

Fig. 4.17 A 54-year old woman who received Restylane 2.00 cc into her NLFs (0.4 cc each side) and then Juvéderm Ultra (0.4 cc each side)

treat fine to moderate wrinkles in this area. Thicker preparations such as Perlane or Juvéderm Ultra Plus should be used with caution, due to the rare but concerning risk of vascular occlusion in this area of the supra-trochlear artery arborizations (thicker, cross-linked collagen preparations such as Zyplast are contraindicated in the glabella area for this reason). However the thinner very superficially placed collagen products, Zyderm and Cosmoderm, are often the treatment of choice in this area, though longevity is less than with most HA products.

TREATMENT ALGORITHM (LINEAR THREADING, SERIAL PUNCTURE)

Most patients do well with only topical anesthetic in the glabellar area. With the patient seated, immobilize the area to be treated with the noninjecting hand. Since most lines in this area are in a vertical orientation, it is easy to stand directly in front of the patient, holding the syringe upright injecting at a 45-degree angle to the skin surface (Fig. 4.19). Linear threading and/or serial puncture techniques can produce good results. To help stay superficial in this higher risk area for necrosis, the injector can pinch the skin to 'tent' upward during injections. In addition, using low volumes and possibly spacing the treatment over 2–3 sessions may also be helpful in avoiding necrosis due to compression in this area of watershed vasculature. Remember to inject slowly intradermally in this area and don't use the thicker fillers like Perlane or Juvéderm Ultra Plus.

TROUBLESHOOTING

Using the thinnest possible filler substance to place most superficially will help to minimize concerns of vascular occlusion (such as the collagens Zyderm or Cosmoderm or the Restylane Fine Line formulation).

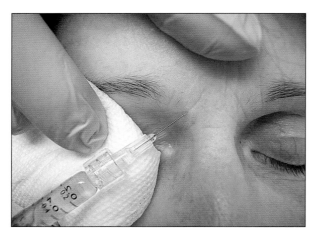

Fig. 4.19 Injection of glabellar lines

SIDE EFFECTS, COMPLICATIONS, AND ALTERNATIVE APPROACHES

The most concerning side effect of treatment of the glabella is localized necrosis from partial or total occlusion of a vessel. Owing to the limited collateral circulation in this area, 56% of all necrotic events from collagen injection (mostly Zyplast) occur here. If symptoms of vascular occlusion (pain, blanching) occur during treatment, stop the injection immediately. Glaich and Cohen have written a definitive protocol for the prevention and treatment of glabella necrosis.

• Facial (re)contouring

PATIENTS/INDICATIONS

Patients who desire filling of 'sunken' areas of the midface, as from HIV lipodystrophy or other atrophic losses, or those who desire true augmentation as in the chin, cheekbones and eyebrows, are also appropriate candidates for hylan implantation. Other innovative uses include 'revolumizing' the nasojugal folds ('tear trough'/'infra-orbital hollow'), perimental hollows, and earlobes. There are also reports of nasal recontouring with HA products. HA products can also be very helpful in the treatment of postsurgical depressed scars, especially of the cheek, nose and helical rim. Results should last at least 6 months with most HA products.

EQUIPMENT (RESTYLANE, PERLANE, RESTYLANE SUBQ, JUVÉDERM ULTRA PLUS)

Contouring of larger areas (cheeks, chin) generally requires deeper augmentation with more robust fillers such as Perlane or Juvéderm Ultra Plus. Still, it is surprising how much improvement can be obtained through careful mid- to deep dermal placement of Restylane or Juvéderm Ultra.

TREATMENT ALGORITHM (LINEAR THREADING, FANNING, CROSS-HATCHING)

Highlight the area to be treated with a surgical marking pen prior to anesthesia as both topical and injected formulations alter the contour through swelling or volume, respectively.

Fanning and cross-hatching implantation techniques are useful when depositing the larger volumes of filler needed for facial contouring (i.e. cheek bones). Fanning, however, has been shown to cause more bruising. The correct target depth of implantation is the deep dermis and dermal-subcutaneous planes. Carruthers suggests that the subdermal rather than the intradermal injection plane is an important advance in this technique to replace the lost volume of the atrophic subdermal fat and age-related remodeling of the maxillary and mandibular areas. In phase 4 clinical trials in press, it has been shown that Restylane lasts in every layer of the skin. Supraperiosteal bolus injections can also be helpful (i.e. perimental hollows and tear troughs). Supraperiosteal injections can also be performed by the linear threading technique in certain areas, such as the nasojugal folds ('tear troughs'). When treating here, most injectors layer along the bone of the orbital rim, making sure not to penetrate the orbital septum. Conversely, a minority of injectors such as Kane have had great success in this area with meticulous supramuscular placement using a 31–32 gauge needle, though this technique is only for skilled injectors with substantial product knowledge to understand the filler's behaviors extremely well. It is much easier to develop persistent, visible nodule formation in the thin lower eyelid skin with superficial injections.

Restylane SubQ must always be placed into the subcutaneous tissue and PRE periosteal planes. De Lorenzi demonstrated that Restylane SubQ maintained esthetic correction of the cheeks and chin for at least 3 months after subcutaneous and/or supraperiosteal placement.

TROUBLESHOOTING

The most difficult aspect of facial contouring is having an artistic eye. Symmetry is critical, as is an understanding of the bony landmarks and esthetics of the face. For example, use of fillers in the lateral brow can create a 'Cro-Magnon' look if not injected with caution and low volumes, just as recontouring the zygomatic arch too medially will create an ill-placed 'ball' in the middle of the cheek. Also, with deeper injections there is a greater risk of vessel and nerve damage as well as parotid duct trauma. Facial contouring with fillers is best reserved for seasoned injectors with a thorough understanding of facial anatomy.

SIDE EFFECTS, COMPLICATIONS, AND ALTERNATIVE APPROACHES

Most patients do well after use of hylans for facial contouring. If they are pleased with the results using temporary fillers and want to avoid repeated injections, they may want to consider treatment with more permanent fillers instead (ArteFill, silicone, etc.) The current authors truly feel that only very experienced injectors should use these types of permanent fillers.

• The question of skin testing

One of the major advantages of hylans over collagen is the decreased incidence of delayed hypersensitivity reactions. However, while this incidence is very low, there have been very sporadic case reports of hypersensitivity reactions with HA derivatives. Since it should be impossible to react to pure hyaluronic acid, which is identical in all species and tissue types, any such reactions are thought to be due to impurities in hylan production: residual avian proteins (Hylaform) or byproducts of bacterial fermentation (Restylane, Juvéderm, Captique. Skin testing prior to hylans would still not prevent all reactions, as some patients do not react until after their third treatment session. In addition, the incidence of such reactions seems to be dropping significantly as the manufacturing process of hylans becomes more refined, resulting in purer products (for example, Restylane reformulation in 1999).

• Other fillers containing hyaluronic acid or its derivatives

Many other fillers now contain hyaluronic acid as a major or minor constituent. The hyaluronic acid may or may not be cross-linked, and may or may not be the substance responsible for volume augmentation. Following is a list of the some of the more common fillers worldwide containing hyaluronic acid in current use.

Beletero (Esthelis) is another HA that is cross-linked by BDDE. Phase 3 FDA Cosmetic Clinical Trials were begun in the United States in December 2006. Beletero is a cohesive, monophasic HA gel with zones of greater and lesser density called Cohesive Polydensified Matrix (CPM) technology. It is distributed by Merz Pharmaceuticals.

Achyal (Hyal2000, Hylan SES) is a 1% solution of the sodium salt of hyaluronic acid. Since it is not cross-linked, it is not considered a hylan (it does not form a gel). It is distributed in 2.5 mL pre-filled syringes with 30 gauge needles, and can be stored at room temperature for up to 3 years. Similar to the hylans, it is used for wrinkles, scars, lip and contour deformities. It is manufactured by Tedec Meiji Farma, S.A., Madrid, Spain, and is not available in the United States.

DermaLive (see also Chapter 7) is a semi-permanent nonanimal filler composed of hyaluronic acid and acrylic hydrogel fragments. Here the hyaluronic acid is merely the delivery system (which accounts for 60% of the volume); the acrylic hydrogel filler is a copolymer of hydroxyethylmethacrylate (HEMA) and ethylmethacrylate (EMA), a nonbiodegradable material belonging to the acrylate family that has demonstrated a good level of tolerance for many years in eye surgery (same acrylic hydrogel as used in intraocular lens implants in cataract surgery). The smooth-walled 45–65 µ hydrogel particles are intentionally irregular (nonspherical), which is thought to help integrate them into newly formed collagen fibers and prevent concentric fibrosis. It is supplied in 0.8 mL syringes and delivered through a 27.5 gauge needle. Produced by Dermatech, the product was first marketed in France in 1998 and has now become very popular throughout Europe. The manufacturer suggests several treatment sessions, each separated by a minimum of 3 months. There have been reports of granulomatous reactions from the acrylic particles, manifesting as palpable nodules appearing about 6 months after injection. As with other HA products, no pre-operative skin tests are required.

DermaDeep (see also Chapter 7) is similar to DermaLive, except that the acrylic particle sizes are larger, from 80–110 µm. It is provided in 1.2 mL syringes and delivered through a 26.5 gauge needle. One study describing the use of DermaLive and DermaDeep in 455 patients (859 syringes) over 3 years reports that patients were satisfied in 88% of cases, with 20% developing transient redness or edema at the injection site.

Hyacell is an HA derivative which is widely used in India and Latin America. In addition to hyaluronic acid, it contains zinc, selenium, vanadium, and unspecified 'embryonic extracts'. Its illicit use by a nonphysician was suspected to have caused nine cases of *Mycobacterium abscessus* infection in New York City in 2002 (Toy et al), although it is unknown whether the material was contaminated during manufacture or from the individual posing as a physician who injected it with unclean technique.

Hylan Rofilan Gel (Matredur) is a hyaluronic acid gel cross-linked with a natural acid instead of a chemical compound. It has not been FDA-approved for use in the United States. It is manufactured and distributed by Rofil Medical International B.V., Breda, The Netherlands.

Viscontour is a sodium hyaluronic acid product which has been developed in three forms to address wrinkles, contour defects, wound healing, and tissue hydration. A noncross-linked injectable version has been marketed in Europe since 2002, and Aventis Dermatology is developing a cross-linked injectable version.

FURTHER READING

Alam M, Levy R, Pavjani U, et al 2006 Safety of radiofrequency treatment over human skin previously injected with medium-term injectable soft-tissue augmentation materials: a controlled pilot trial. Lasers Surg Med 38:205–210

Andre P, Wechsler J, Revuz J 2002 Facial lipoatrophy: report of five cases after injection of synthetic filler into nasolabial folds. Journal of Cosmetic Dermatology 1:19

American Society for Aesthetic Plastic Surgery. February 24, 2006

Bennett R, Muba T 2005 Restylane persistent for 23 months found during Mohs micrographic surgery: a source of confusion with hyaluronic acid surrounding basal cell carcinoma. Dermatologic Surgery 31:1366–1369

Brody HJ 2005 Use of hyaluronidase in the treatment of granulomatous hyaluronic acid reactions or unwanted hyaluronic acid misplacement. Dermatologic Surgery 31:893–898

Carruthers J, Klein AW, Carruthers A, et al 2005 Safety and efficacy of nonanimal stabilized hyaluronic acid for improvement of mouth corners. Dermatologic Surgery 31:276–281

Carruthers J, Carruthers A 2005 Facial sculpting and tissue augmentation. Dermatologic Surgery 31:1604–1609

Carruthers A, Wayne C, de Lorenzi C, et al 2005 Randomized, double-blind comparison of the efficacy of two hyluronic acid derivatives, Restylane Perlane and Hylaform, in the treatment of nasolabial folds. Dermatologic Surgery 31:1591–1600

Carruthers J, Carruthers A, Maberley D 2003 Deep resting glabellar rhytids respond to BTX-A and Hylan B. Dermatologic Surgery 29:539–544

DeLorenzi C, Weinberg M, Solish N 2006 A multicenter study of the efficacy and safety of subcutaneous nonanimal stabilized hyaluronic acid in aesthetic facial contouring: interim report. Dermatologic Surgery 32:205–211

Duranti F, Salti G, Bovani B, Calandra M, Rosati ML 1998 Injectable hyaluronic acid gel for soft-tissue augmentation. A clinical and histological study. Dermatologic Surgery 24:1317–1325

Fernandez-Acenero MJ, Zamora E, Borbujo J 2003 Granulomatous foreign body reaction against hyaluronic acid: Report of a case after lip augmentation. Dermatologic Surgery 29:1225–1226

Friedman PM, Mafong EA, Kauvar AN, Geronemus RG 2002 Safety data of injectable nonanimal stabilized hyaluronic acid gel for soft tissue augmentation. Dermatologic Surgery 28:491–494

Glaich A, Cohen J, Goldberg L 2006 Injection necrosis of the glabella: protocol for prevention and treatment after use of dermal fillers. Dermatologic Surgery 32:276–279

Gooderham M, Solish N 2005 Use of hyaluronic acid for soft tissue augmentation of HIV-associated facial lipodystrophy. Dermatologic Surgery 31:104–109

Hallen L, Johansson C, Laurent C 1999 Cross-linked hyaluronan (hylan B gel): a new injectable remedy for treatment of vocal cord insufficiency – an animal study. Acta Oto-laryngologica (Stockh) 119:107–111

Hirsch RJ, Narurkar V, Carruthers J 2006 Management of injected hyaluronic acid induced Tyndall effects. Lasers Surg Med 38:202–204

Hirsch R, Cohen J, Carruthers J Treatment of impending necrosis after soft tissue augmentation. Dermatologic Surgery (in press)

Jaggi R, Chi G, Goldman M 2005 Clinical comparison between two hyluronic acid-derived fillers in the treatment of nasolabial folds: Hylaform versus Restylane. Dermatologic Surgery 31:1587–1591

Kane MA 2005 Treatment of tear trough deformity and lower lid bowing with injectable hyaluronic acid. Aesthetic Plastic Surgery 29:363

Klein AW 2004 Granulomatous foreign body reactions against hyaluronic acid. Dermatologic Surgery 30:1070–1071

Klein AW 2001 Skin filling: Collagen and other injectables of the skin. Dermatology Clinics 19:491–508

Leonhardt J, Naomi L, Narins R 2005 Angioedema acute hypersensitivity reaction to injectable hyaluronic acid. Dermatologic Surgery 31:577–580

Lowe NJ 2003 Arterial embolization caused by injection of hyaluronic acid (Restylane). British Journal of Dermatology 148:379

Lowe NJ, Maxwell A, Lowe P, Duick MG, Shah K 2001 Hyaluronic acid fillers: Adverse reactions and skin testing. Journal of the American Academy of Dermatologists 45:930–933

Lupton JR, Alster TS 2000 Cutaneous hypersensitivity reaction to injectable hyaluronic acid gel. Dermatologic Surgery 26:135–137

Manna F, Dentini M, Desideri P, DePita O, Mortilla E, Maras B 1999 Comparative chemical evaluation of two commercially available derivatives of hyaluronic acid (Hylaform from rooster combs and Restylane from *Streptococcus*) used for soft tissue augmentation. Journal of the European Academy of Dermatological Venereologists 13:183–192

Matarasso SL, Herwick R 2006 Hypersensitivity reaction to nonanimal stabilized hyluronic acid. Journal of the American Academy of Dermatology 55:128–131

Micheels P 2001 Human anti-hyaluronic acid antibodies: Is it possible? Dermatologic Surgery 27:185–191

Narins R, Jewell M, Rubin M, Cohen J, et al 2006 Clinical conference: management of rare events following dermal fillers-focal necrosis and angry red bumps. Dermatologic Surgery 32:426–434

Narins RS, Brandt F, Leyden J, Lorenc ZP, Rubin M, Smith S 2003 A randomized, double-blind, multicenter comparison of the efficacy and tolerability of Restylane versus Zyplast for the correction of nasolabial folds. Dermatologic Surgery 29:588–595

Olenius M 1998 The first clinical study using a new biodegradable implant for the treatment of lips, wrinkles, and folds. Aesthetic Plastic Surgery 22:97–101

Piacquadio D, Jarcho M, Goltz R 1997 Evaluation of hylan B gel as a soft-tissue augmentation implant material. Journal of the American Academy of Dermatologists 36:544–549

Pollack SV 1999 Some new injectable dermal filler materials: Hylaform, Restylane, and Artecoll. Journal of Cutaneous Medical Surgery 3(suppl 4):27–35

Ramelet AA 2000 Homeopathic arnica in postoperative haematomas: a double-blind study. Dermatology 201:347–348

Schanz S, Schippert W, Ulmer A, et al 2002 Arterial embolization caused by injection of hyaluronic acid (Restylane). British Journal of Dermatology 146:928

Smith KC, Melnychuk M 2005 Five percent lidocaine cream applied simultaneously to the skin and mucosa of the lips creates excellent anesthesia for filler injections. Dermatologic Surgery 31:1635–1638

Smith KC, Comite SL, Balasubramanian S, et al 2004 Vibration anesthesia: a noninvasive method of reducing discomfort prior to dermatologic procedures. Dermatology Online Journal 10:22

Soparkar CN, Patrinely JR, Tschen J 2004 Erasing Restylane. Ophthalmic Plastic Reconstructive Surgery 20:317–318

Toy BR, Frank PJ 2003 Outbreak of *Mycobacterium abscessus* infection after soft tissue augmentation. *Dermatol Surg* 29:971–973

Voy ED, Mohasseb J 2002 Lipoatrophie als seltene komplikation nach auffullung der nasolabialfalten mit injizierbaren implantaten. Magazin Aesth Chir 3:36

5 Management of the Lips and Mouth Corners

Jean Carruthers, Vic A. Narurkar

INTRODUCTION

The perioral region is an extremely important area for esthetic enhancement. With the passage of time, hereditary factors, photodamage, and smoking contribute to the development of the typical features of perioral rhytides, decrease in vermilion lip fullness, and prominence of melolabial and melomental folds in the context of gravitational ptosis of the lower face (Fig. 5.1).

Successful rejuvenation of the perioral region requires sophistication in the application of multiple technologies. Injectable biodegradable biologic fillers include collagen implants (Zyderm/Zyplast, CosmoDerm/CosmoPlast, Evolence), nonanimal stabilized hyaluronic acids (Restylane/Perlane, Juvéderm), animal-derived hyaluronic acids (Hylaform Plus), polylactic acid (Sculptra/Newfill), and autologous fat. More permanent fillers such as Artecoll and perhaps Radiesse, ablative, fractional, nonablative resurfacing and BTX-A injections are also important components of the therapeutic armamentarium for perioral rejuvenation.

The Glogau photoaging classification offers a rational approach to perioral rejuvenation. In general, the more advanced staging on the classification, the more common it will be to incorporate a plurality of treatments.

THE PROBLEMS BEING TREATED

The deflating vermilion lip is the most common concern for perioral rejuvenation. Photoaging, smoking and repetitive muscular pursing of the orbicularis oris combine with intrinsic aging to produce reduced show of the vermilion with superficial and deep lip rhytides (so called 'smokers lines' or 'lipstick lines').

Atrophic changes in the chin produce the 'apple dumpling' effect. Resorption of maxillary and mandibular bone as well as subcutaneous fat allows the mouth corner complex to descend, resulting in the 'mouth frown' and deep melomental folds, and hollowing of the chin behind the mentum and anterior to the jowls.

PATIENT SELECTION

The selection of the appropriate patient for perioral rejuvenation is based on the extent of damage as described by the Glogau photoaging classification, the Fitzpatrick skin type of the patient, and the extent of associated bone and fat resorption. Semipermanent fillers that do not require skin testing are usually suitable in all patients. In addition, subjects must disclose any tendency for herpes labialis and whether there are any other general health-related issues, including allergy.

Depending on the composition of the desired filler, skin testing may be necessary. Fillers containing bovine collagen such as Zyderm and Zyplast and Artecoll (Artefill) require skin testing, and approximately 3% of candidates have shown an allergic reaction to Zyderm. Evolence is a new porcine derived atelomeric cross-linked collagen that does not appear to require a skin test. In addition, patients with known connective tissue disorders such as systemic lupus erythematosus are not suitable candidates for these implants. Nonanimal stabilized hyaluronic acid fillers do not require skin testing and show less than 1/10,000 incidence of delayed-type hypersensitivity reactions.

Semipermanent fillers such as ArteFill show overall complication rates of 3%. Patients with a known history of recurrent oral herpes simplex should be premedicated with systemic antiviral therapy such as valacyclovir prior to injection, particularly with deeper placed implants, as herpetic reactivation can produce epidermal compromise and atrophic and hypertrophic scarring. Individuals who are professional musicians or singers may need to consider the treatment and the initial effect it may have on oral expressive tone. There is no absolute contraindication for BTX-A injections for the perioral area but proper technique and conservative dosing is necessary to avoid asymmetry and unwanted facial paralysis.

Lasers and light sources for photorejuvenation are highly dependent on Fitzpatrick skin type. Visible lasers and intense pulsed light with low cut-off filters (500–

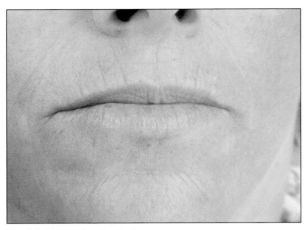

Fig. 5.1 Advanced perioral aging

Table 5.1 Approaches to perioral rejuvenation	
Entity	**Approach**
Superficial rhytides	Botulinum A toxin injection
	Nonablative treatments
	Nonablative fractional resurfacing
	Superficial fillers
Moderate rhytides	Medium and deep placed fillers
	Nonablative fractional resurfacing aggressive settings
Deep rhytides	Ablative laser resurfacing and fillers
Lip augmentation – architecture	Medium placed fillers
Lip augmentation – volume	Superficial placed fillers

600 nm) should be used with caution in those with darker skin types for nonablative rejuvenation as there is significant overlap with melanin and this can lead to hypopigmentation and hyperpigmentation in darker skin types. Near infra-red lasers (1064, 1320, and 1540 nm) are the safest wavelengths for nonablative rejuvenation in darker skin but inadequate cooling may result in unwanted thermal injury leading to atrophic scars. Nonablative fractional laser resurfacing (NFSR) in the mid-infrared region offers an innovative approach to produce more consistent results than nonablative devices with reduced risks and recovery compared to ablative devices. The most widely studied wavelength is the 1550 nm device (Fraxel laser) for this indication. Zones of microthermal damage up to 1000 μ are created with extrusion of microscopic epidermal necrotic debris. The effect is twofold – with semi-ablative effects that produce more immediate results and nonablative effects producing neocollagensis which ensues at several months following the procedure. Treatment densities can be varied to tailor the degree of damage from 5–45%, resulting in the majority of the epidermis remaining intact, thereby producing a more rapid recovery. A 1540 nm fractional laser also employs the principles of fractional photothermolysis in the mid infra-red region and prototype devices using the 10,600 nm wavelength (fractional ablative resurfacing [FAR]). Skin types I to VI can be safely treated with NFSR. Ablative laser resurfacing of perioral rhytides is not recommended in darker skin types and segmental ablative laser resurfacing carries the risk of post-treatment unmatched pigmentation, even in lighter skin types, as the resurfaced region shows a difference in pigmentation (typically hypopigmentation) from the untreated skin.

EXPECTED BENEFITS

Table 5.1 summarizes expected benefits of the various approaches to perioral rejuvenation. Superficial rhytides are best addressed with BTX-A injections, nonablative

rejuvenation, and superficially placed semipermanent fillers. The duration of these treatments is typically 3–4 months. These are ideally suitable in younger patients with limited damage. Moderate and deep perioral rhytides are best addressed with layering techniques of medium- and deep-placed longlasting fillers. NFSR offers a viable solution to mild to moderate rhytides as monotherapy but requires a series of three to five treatments. Skin types I to VI can be safely treated with fractional resurfacing and segmental treatments can be performed safely without obvious lines of demarcation.

Ablative laser resurfacing, manual dermabrasion/dermasanding, and chemical peeling are also viable options but carry the risk of post-treatment segmental pigmentary changes. Combination nonablative and fractional laser/light therapy and medium and deep fillers may be synergistic. The duration of these treatments is typically 4–9 months. One of the authors (VN) is conducting a study on the duration of fillers with fractional resurfacing and preliminary results indicate that nonablative resurfacing can be performed safely over most semi-permanent fillers. The best approach to lip augmentation depends on the nature of the defect and the subject's esthetic desires. For genetically thin lips, structural augmentation with a deeper placed filler followed by volume correction with a superficial filler is ideal. For pure cosmetic enhancement of lips, a superficially placed filler with emphasis on the white roll and expansion of the vermilion is ideal.

The onset of benefits varies depending on the conditions being treated. Placement of fillers often produces an immediate result, although edema and bruising can temporarily mask the true correction. The onset of effect of botulinum toxin (Botox) injections typically is evident at 2–10 days post injection. Nonablative laser and light source rejuvenation shows a highly variable clinical outcome and multiple and repeated treatments may show clinical effects at varying intervals. NFSR produces con-

Glogau type	Nonablative technique	NFSR	Botulinum toxin A injections	Superficial filler	Medium filler	Deep filler	Ablative resurfacing
			Table 5.2 Algorithm for perioral rejuvenation				
1	+	+	+	+/–	–	–	–
2	+	+	+	+	+	–	–
3	+/–	+	+	+/–	+	+	+/–
4	–	+/–	+/–	+/–	+	+	+

sistent results and three to five treatments spaced 4–6 weeks apart is recommended. Ablative resurfacing results in immediate epidermal and dermal injury, which can take 4–6 weeks to resolve. The final results of ablative resurfacing may not be evident for up to 6 months following resurfacing.

Topical anesthesia (Ela-Max, Betacaine) is typically sufficient for most BTX-A injections, nonablative lasers and light sources, and selected fillers for lower melolabial fold augmentation. Infraorbital and mental nerve blocks and topical anesthetic are essential for most peroral fillers except collagen implants as there is no anesthetic in the injectable material. For lip augmentation and lip rhytides, nerve blocks are essential. Fractional resurfacing requires stronger topical anesthetics such as a mixture of 7% lidocaine and 7% tetracaine and regional blocks are often beneficial. Ablative segmental resurfacing often requires sedation and/or general anesthesia if the entire face is also being treated.

Biologic fillers and BTX-A are the most gratifying in-office procedures as they produce consistent and reproducible results with little risk. The main disadvantage that patients express is the need for repeated treatments. Nonablative light and laser treatments are usually very safe and comfortable but in the perioral area have a lower patient satisfaction rate and are best performed as an adjunct to fillers and BTX-A. NFSR produces more consistent and predictable results than nonablative treatments, is safe in skin types I–VI but does require multiple treatments for optimal results. Postoperative recovery usually consists of edema and erythema, as re-epithelialization is usually complete in less than 24 hours. Ablative resurfacing produces more definitive and longer lasting results but the exaggerated healing time and risks make these procedures less popular.

The art of perioral rejuvenation involves careful patient selection, the use of the appropriate technology for the appropriate indication, and the use of combination therapies for a complete result. Often, combination of resurfacing, BTX-A and semipermanent fillers produces a more complete result. Thorough patient education with emphasis on realistic outcomes is essential for patient satisfaction.

OVERVIEW OF TREATMENT STRATEGY

• Treatment approach

An algorithm for perioral rejuvenation is presented in Table 5.2. Glogau photoaging classifications provide an excellent guideline to treatment strategies. Patients with Glogau type I photoaging typically have minimal damage in the perioral area. True rhytides are just discernible. Nonablative laser and pulsed light resurfacing may have some benefits for these patients, with the possible addition of BTX-A for very superficial vertical lip rhytides.

Patients with Glogau type II photoaging have mild to moderate vertical lip rhytides, early signs of vermilion atrophy, and some lower melolabial ptosis. Superficial and mid-dermal filler placements are appropriate for these patients with adjuvant laser and pulsed light nonablative and fractional laser treatments and BTX-A injections.

Patients with Glogau type III photoaging have more prominent vertical lip rhytides, further vermilion atrophy, and prominent melolabial ptosis. Mid-dermal and deep-dermal filler placements, lip and chin BTX-A injections are essential with the possibility of lip augmentation with fillers. There is limited use of nonablative resurfacing. Fractional resurfacing at aggressive settings produces consistent results in this subgroup and can be done segmentally without risks of lines of demarcation.

Patients with Glogau type IV photoaging have severe perioral rhytides, extreme lip atrophy, deep melolabial folds, and drooping and significant photodamage. The role of fillers and BTX-A are purely adjunctive in these patients. Ablative resurfacing, typically for the full face, is often warranted and surgical procedures are indicated prior to placement of fillers and BTX-A. These patients often require large volumes of fillers for complete correction of defects and therefore may not be suitable candidates for nonsurgical/ablative treatments as the primary modality for correction. A face lift may also be required.

• Patient interviews

Careful patient selection and a detailed consultation are key factors for successful outcomes in any esthetic procedure. What the patient may desire may not be realistically possible and it is crucial to educate the patient about the realistic outcomes of perioral rejuvenation. Box 5.1 is a summary of a patient checklist and is a useful guide for consultation. An excellent approach during the patient screening process is to provide a mirror for the patient and elicit the patient's perspective of esthetic goals. This is particularly critical as the physician's perception of the esthetic goal may be different from the patient's perception. Once the therapeutic goals are established, a thorough explanation of treatment options is performed, with emphasis on the repetitive nature of these procedures. These include the onset of action of the various technologies, the duration of effect, and the appropriate intervals for treatments (Table 5.3). An atlas and diary of before and after pictures may be helpful but can often be misleading as they may convey only the optimal results. Patients seeking more 'permanent' options should be educated about the duration of these procedures, as surgical and ablative options for perioral rejuvenation also have their limits. The current authors avoid using the word 'permanent' for any procedure. When there is hesitation about maintenance treatments, they emphasize how main-

tenance is part of any therapeutic goal, the same as for diet, exercise, and overall physical wellness. Once the consultation is complete, a patient care coordinator can discuss the costs and the patient signs a form which states they have been informed of the fees. A copy is given to the patient and the original form is placed in the chart. If the patient elects to schedule a procedure, an appropriate deposit is collected at the time of booking. It is critical for the physician to be removed from discussion of the fees and their collection and this entire process should be performed in a private and discrete setting with a patient care coordinator.

TREATMENT TECHNIQUES

We have outlined treatment techniques based on Glogau photoaging, which provides a useful guide to address the sequence and modalities of treatment. Table 5.4 outlines the Glogau photoaging classification and the treatment techniques suitable for the appropriate patient.

• Glogau photoaging I

This patient will typically present for cosmetic lip augmentation. The patient is advised to take Arnica Montana 2–3 days prior to the procedure to reduce ecchymoses and valaciclovir 2 g twice daily the day before the procedure if they have a history of recurrent oral herpes simplex. Anesthesia is first administered with a topical anesthetic such as Elamax over the vermilion area. An infraorbital and mental block is then performed with 1% lidocaine (plain or with epinephrine) (lidocaine) through the intraoral approach and a small amount is injected at the junction of the gum line and lip mucosa. It is critical not to distort the lip. The current authors' approach is to utilize a medium-depth filler such as Restylane for lip architecture. A 30 gauge needle bent at 45 degrees is utilized and a serial puncture technique is utilized (Fig. 5.2) inferior to the white roll in the vermilion border. For patients desiring additional volume, a more superficially placed filler such as Restylane fine lines or Cosmo-Derm is placed in the white roll with a 30 gauge needle

---

Box 5.1 Patient checklist for perioral rejuvenation

1. Synchronization of patient expectations and physician expectations
2. Detailed discussion of realistic outcomes of various modalities used in perioral rejuvenation
3. Detailed discussion of therapeutic options and their limitations
4. Detailed discussion of the time of onset, time of maximum benefit, and duration of treatments
5. Emphasis on repetitive nature of these procedures
6. Avoidance of the word 'permanent' correction
7. Education of ablative and surgical procedures when indicated
8. Discussion about maintenance treatments
9. Discussion of costs of procedures by a patient care coordinator in a discrete and private setting without the presence of the physician

---

Table 5.3 Perioral rejuvenation summary

Approach	Onset of effects	Duration of effects	Potential risks
Botulinum toxin A	2–10 days	3–4 months	Asymmetry of lip
Nonablative treatments	6 weeks	Variable	Superficial blistering and potential for scars
Fractional resurfacing	4–6 weeks	3–5 years	Superficial blistering, petechiae
Biodegradable fillers	Immediate	3–9 months	Edema, ecchymoses, allergic reaction, migration
Semipermanent fillers	Immediate	12–60 months	Similar to biodegradable fillers, granuloma formation
Ablative resurfacing	6 weeks to several months	3–5 years	Pigmentation change, erythema, infections, atrophic and hypertrophic scars

Glogau photoaging type	Defect(s)	Treatment
Any	Cosmetic lip enhancement	Superficial/medium depth fillers
I	Superficial vertical lip rhytides	Nonablative laser and pulsed light
		Fractional resurfacing
		Botulinum toxin A
II	Superficial lip rhytides	As above
	Lip atrophy	Medium depth fillers
	Melomental folds	Medium depth fillers
III	Superficial lip rhytides	As above
	Dyschromia/telangiectasias	Nonablative laser and pulsed light
	Moderate vertical lip rhytides	Medium depth fillers +/− NFSR
	Corner of mouth droop	Medium depth fillers
	Advanced melolabial and melomental folds	Deep fillers
IV	Deep rhytides	− As above and ablative laser resurfacing (sequential and combination therapy)

Table 5.4 Glogau photoaging classification for perioral rejuvenation

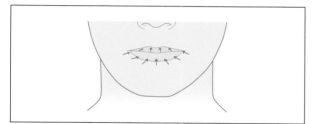

Fig. 5.2 Technique for lip augmentation for lip architecture. Placement of filler in the body of the lip using a serial threading technique

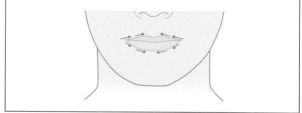

Fig. 5.3 Technique for lip augmentation for volume. Injection of filler in white roll (natural tunnel) at the junction of the vermilion border and the body of the lip

bent at 45 degrees (Fig. 5.3). The philtrum and the angle recently identified as the Glogau–Klein point can be peaked for fullness. An ice pack is applied postoperatively. The patient is advised the volume of the lips may increase significantly and may not return to the expected size for 1 week. For patients who have an important event or social function and desire immediate lip augmentation, the authors limit the treatments to superficially placed fillers such as CosmoDerm and advise against placement of medium-depth fillers. Prednisone 30 mg as a single dose after the injection, or possibly repeated once or twice, may be necessary in some individuals to reduce the swelling for the first few days.

Lip augmentation with fillers produces immediate results and has an outstanding patient satisfaction rate. It is critical to educate the patient about the degree of volume achieved by these procedures, as the immediate results are often disguised by edema. Some patients may experience anxiety over the nature of the edema and need to be informed that this will subside in 24–48 hours. The current authors' approach for lip augmentation is to be initially conservative and typically administer a single syringe of fillers for new patients and then reassess in 1 week if the patient desires additional augmentation. For patients with thinner lips, the layering technique is preferable, even in new patients, using vermilion placement of medium-depth fillers and white roll placement of superficial fillers (Fig. 5.4).

Expected postoperative results of lip augmentation include edema and ecchymoses. Complications are

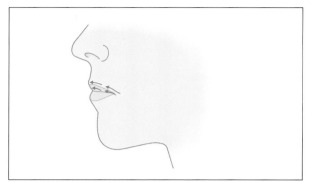

Fig. 5.4 Layering technique for lip augmentation. Superficial filler placed in white roll. Medium-depth filler serial threading into body of lip

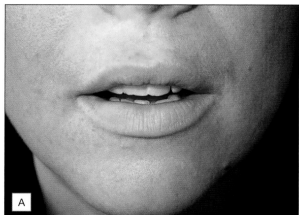

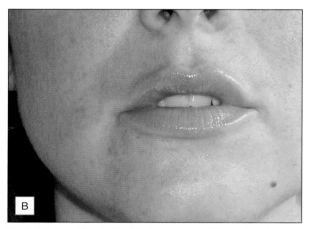

Fig. 5.5 Before (**A**) and after (**B**) photographs of Glogau type 1 photoaging for perioral rejuvenation

exceedingly rare and include inadvertent intravascular injection resulting in immediate blanching of the site, exaggerated edema, hypersensitivity reaction to the filler, and herpetic reactivation. Careful technique can avoid intravascular injection, and if it does occur the lip, with its superb collateral circulation, is highly forgiving. Warm compresses, the use of Wydase for hyaluronic acid fillers, and close follow up is critical for favorable patient outcomes. Hypersensitivity reactions are also exceedingly rare and can be treated with intralesional steroids and pulsed dye/intense pulsed light treatments. Exaggerated edema can be prevented by postoperative ice, head elevation, and anti-inflammatory agents such as Celebrex or Naprosyn. Herpetic reactivation can be prevented by preoperative treatment with valaciclovir.

• Glogau photoaging II

This patient typically presents with superficial vertical lip rhytides, some lip atrophy, and the appearance of lower melolabial fold drooping and superficial melolabial folds. The approach to lip augmentation is identical to Glogau photoaging type I. In addition the vertical lip rhytides are more prominent. BTX-A injections will address early superficial lip rhytides. Topical anesthetic is administered with Elamax and 4–6 units of BTX-A are placed in the shoulders of the lip rhytides (Fig. 5.5) with a tuberculin or diabetic syringe. Often these patients may be undergoing nonablative photorejuvenation. BTX-A injections can be performed on the same day as nonablative rejuvenation and fractional resurfacing. For more advanced vertical lip rhytides, placement of a filler is indicated and superficially placed fillers are ideal. Regional anesthesia is performed along with topical anesthesia and the fillers are placed with a bent 30 gauge needle directly into the groove of the rhytide (Fig. 5.6). Overcorrection is not indicated. Simultaneous white roll enhancement and/or vermilion augmentation result in a more complete effect, as lip atrophy is often evident with the presence of vertical lip rhytides. Combinations of BTX-A injections, direct filler injections

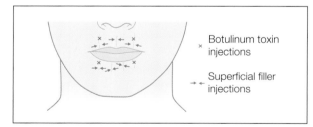

Botulinum toxin injections

Superficial filler injections

Fig. 5.6 Technique for vertical lip rhytides

into rhytides, and vermilion augmentation produce the most complete effect in these patients. The true efficacy of nonablative laser and pulsed light rejuvenation in this region remains controversial but may have synergistic effects when combined with the aforementioned techniques. NFSR is a good device option for this subgroup as consistent results are seen with monotherapy and can be augmented with combination therapy. The lower melolabial folds and chin drooping is addressed by injection of

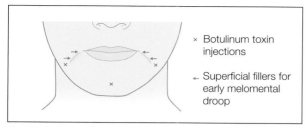

Fig. 5.7 Technique for superficial melomental folds and chin droop

× Botulinum toxin injections

← Superficial fillers for early melomental droop

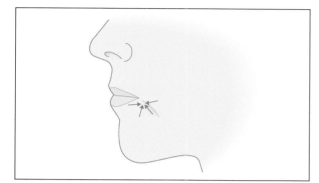

Fig. 5.8 Fanning technique for corners of mouth

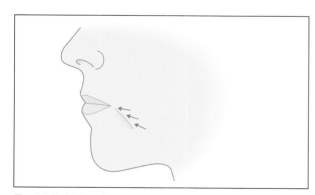

Fig. 5.9 Serial threading technique for melomental folds. Medial injection of filler towards melomental folds serial threading

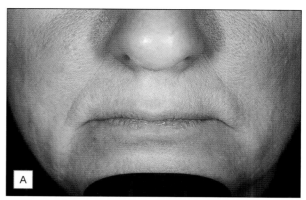

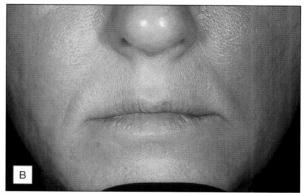

Fig. 5.10 Before (**A**) and after (**B**) photographs of Glogau type II photoaging patient for perioral rejuvenation

medium-depth fillers and BTX-A into the depressor anguli oris (Fig. 5.7). Hyaluronic acid derivatives such as Restylane and Juvederm are ideal and the technique of fanning (Fig. 5.8) is performed to the corners of the mouth while a serial threading technique (Fig. 5.9) is ideal for placement of the filler in the lower melolabial folds. Both procedures utilize a bent 30 gauge needle which is directed medially. Gentle massaging of the material immediately after injection with a Q-tip for proper placement may be necessary for perfect results, but in general the current authors aim to place the material in its final position rather than injecting and then massaging. Full correction of the region

(Fig. 5.10) is an ideal postoperative result. The postoperative sequelae and care are identical to the treatment of lip augmentation.

The most common pitfall encountered in these patients is incomplete correction, thereby stressing the importance of combination therapies. If vertical rhytides are approached by direct injection of fillers alone, the results are generally unsatisfactory. Overcorrection of the rhytides results in patients complaining of lumps in the upper and lower cutaneous lip, exaggerating the problem instead of correcting it. The use of lip augmentation and vertical rhytide correction produce a more cosmetically enhanced perioral region, with the placement of the fillers in the white roll further enhancing the effects of vertical rhytide improvement. The addition of BTX-A completes the effect. If the sole concern is superficial vertical rhytides, the current authors prefer BTX-A as the sole modality, as even the most superficial filler placement is difficult and may result in a worse cosmetic outcome. Treatment of melolabial folds and corner of the mouth droops have limited complications. Placement and correction of the filler are critical as many materials may migrate. Medially directed injections directly to the rhytide avoids lateral migration of the filler and gentle massage with a Q-tip to position the filler assures adequate placement. Inadvertent vascular injection of filler can be avoided with proper technique and is particularly critical in the lower melolabial folds to avoid intra-arteriolar injection. Use of small volumes, withdrawal prior to injection, and monitoring for tissue blanching prevents these outcomes. As placement is more superficial, inadvertent vascular injury is exceedingly uncommon in this region. Nonablative laser and pulsed light treatment of this region as a single modality is generally unsatisfactory. Typically, if photorejuvenation is being performed on the entire face, the perioral region can be treated on the same day with fillers. If fractional resurfacing is being perfomed, the authors do not recommend same-day treatment with fillers, as the potential for epidermal compromise as well as the masking of true filler volume by the edema from this procedure can compromise the final outcome. The authors typically recommend waiting 1 week after these procedures to perform fillers in this region.

• Glogau photoaging III

These patients are ideal candidates for perioral rejuvenation with combination therapies. The chief concern in these patients is moderate vertical lip rhytides, significant vermilion atrophy, corner of mouth drooping, and prominent lower melolabial folds. It is critical to inform these patients that a multimodal approach is essential for complete correction and that adequate amounts of filler materials are necessary. These patients often have moderate photodamage and will also benefit from full-face nonablative photorejuvenation and/or NFSR. A blended technique is often utilized, where segmental fractional resurfacing is performed to address rhytids and textural concerns and photorejuvenation to address telangiectasias and lentigines. Simultaneous NFSR and pulsed light delivery is being investigated at the moment.

A step-wise approach to perioral rejuvenation in these patients is aggressive fractional resurfacing (Fig. 5.11) photorejuvenation (Fig. 5.12) to correct dyschromia and telangiectasias, aggressive NFSR for mild to moderate rhytids and photodamage, BTX-A injections for hyperdynamic perioral rhytides, lip and lip rhytide augmentation with medium depth and superficial fillers, and lower melolabial folds and corner of mouth drooping with deep- and medium-depth fillers. The authors usually separate the photorejuvenation/NFSR component and BTX-A injections from fillers, as these multiple procedures may be too time and cost prohibitive in a single session. At times, photorejuvenation is not indicated, as the primary focus is the perioral region where NFSR, fillers and BTX-A may suffice alone. The interval between photorejuvenation/NFSR and fillers is typically 1 week (Fig. 5.12).

In addition to the treatments for Glogau photoaging types I and II, these patients have more exaggerated lip rhytides, further lip atrophy, very prominent lower melolabial folds, and chin drooping. Topical anesthetic and regional anesthesia are first administered followed by ice

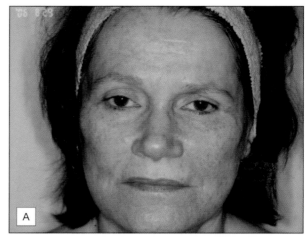

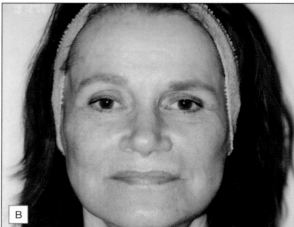

Fig. 5.11 Before (**A**) and after (**B**) photographs of Glogau type III photoaging with NFSR (non ablative fractional laser resurfacing with 1550 nm laser)

pack application. The BTX-A injections are performed first for the lip rhytides (4–6 u) and the chin (2–4 u). The melolabial folds are then addressed. Placement of the deeper filler such as Perlane is performed with a 27 gauge bent needle aimed medially, followed by layering with a superficial or medium-depth filler. Typically two syringes of filler material are the absolute minimum requirement in these patients. The corner of the mouth is then treated with the identical fanning technique using a medium-depth filler such as Restylane. The lip rhytides and lip augmentation is performed last, allowing the regional anesthetic to take its maximum effect. Some patients may not desire multiple regions within the perioral area to be treated at the same time. For these patients, the authors treat the areas that are most visible to them, typically the lower meloabial folds and chin drooping during the first visit, and then treat the lip rhytides and vermilion on a subsequent visit. This is particularly evident in new

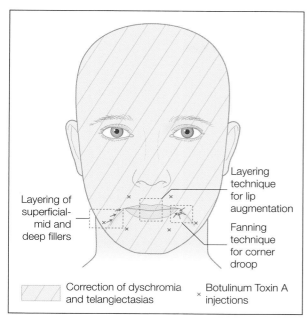

Fig. 5.12 Technique for perioral rejuvenation in more advanced Glogau photoaging type III stepwise approach

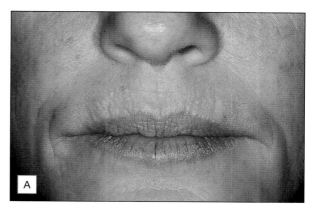

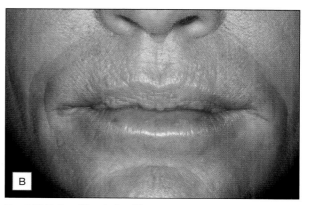

Fig. 5.13 Before (**A**) and after (**B**) photographs of Glogau type III photoaging for perioral rejuvenation

patients who have never been treated with any fillers. A conservative approach is best in these patients to familiarize them with fillers but it is critical to address all of their concerns.

While this category of patients is the ideal group for perioral rejuvenation (Fig. 5.13), it is often the group of patients where undertreatment can result in patient dissatisfaction. The degree of rhytides is significant and therefore it is important to educate the patient on the synergistic approach of combination therapy. Often undercorrection is a pitfall in these patients, resulting in a high incidence of dissatisfaction. The authors often compare this with BTX-A injections in the male glabella, where inadequate dosing results in an incomplete result. However, if the patient is focused on one particular concern (e.g. vertical lip rhytides), it is not unreasonable to address that defect initially and schedule a return appointment to assess the esthetic outcome and then address additional areas. The patient's expectations and the physician's expectations need to be synchronized.

The complications in these patients, in addition to those already discussed in the previous photoaging group, primarily deal with placement of the filler material. Layering of fillers is most critical in these patients, as the lower melolabial folds are quite deep and require the placement of a deep and superficial filler for complete correction. In addition, if the entire face shows photodamage and dynamic rhytides and the only area addressed is the perioral region, the results are generally unsatisfactory. These patients are ideally suited for a series of photorejuvenation and/or fractional resurfacing procedures and BTX-A injections for the upper third of the face. Timing of perioral

rejuvenation depends on patient expectations. Fillers can be performed after the first NFSR/photorejuvenation as their duration is compatible with the duration of the series of NFSR/photorejuvenation procedures, which usually consists of five treatments spaced 4–6 weeks apart. A more conservative approach is to introduce fillers after the final NFSR/photorejuvenation procedure. With aggressive settings of fractional resurfacing, spacing of fillers is particularly important as edema often masks the placement and quantity of filler material. This enables the patient to appreciate the dramatic effects of NFSR and photorejuvenation, and establishes a relationship between the physician and patient to address the introduction of semipermanent biologic fillers as part of global esthetic enhancement.

• Glogau photoaging IV

These patients are the least favorable candidates for non-invasive perioral rejuvenation as a single modality. They are best approached after definitive surgical and/or ablative procedures. A prototype fractional carbon dioxide laser is being investigated for these indications, which may reduce the risks and recovery time for traditional ablative resurfacing procedures. However, they will often present

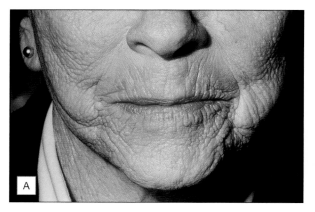

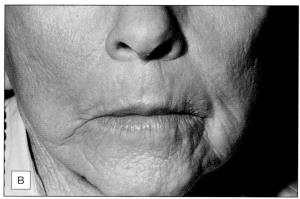

Fig. 5.14 Before (**A**) and after (**B**) photographs of Glogau type IV photoaging of perioral areas for ablative resurfacing

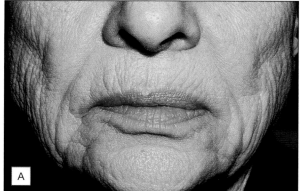

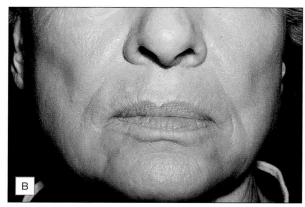

Fig. 5.15 Before (**A**) and after (**B**) photographs of Glogau type IV photoaging with combination of ablative resurfacing, BTX-A and fillers

for perioral rejuvenation as they have been misinformed about the outcomes. Thorough consultation and setting realistic expectations are particularly critical here, with the emphasis on fillers and BTX-A as adjunctive procedures. The approach to perioral rejuvenation is almost identical to those patients with Glogau photoaging III, with the exception being that the minimally invasive procedures should be performed after definitive surgical and/or ablative procedures. The surgical approach is beyond the nature of this chapter and is discussed elsewhere. A subset of these patients benefits from ablative resurfacing prior to minimally invasive perioral rejuvenation.

Severe photodamage is best addressed with ablative resurfacing, of which pulsed erbium and pulsed carbon dioxide laser resurfacing are the most effective and precise modalities. Medium-depth and deep-chemical peels and dermabrasion are also effective by experienced physicians. The postoperative recovery of these procedures typically varies from 1–6 months and the final effects are evident after 1 year. Despite ablative resurfacing, the perioral region may still manifest significant areas that can be addressed with BTX-A and fillers. These include lip atrophy, persistent vertical lip rhytides, and lower melolabial folds and drooping (Fig. 5.14). The authors typically wait 6 weeks after ablative resurfacing to address perioral

rejuvenation with fillers and BTX-A injections. A more conservative approach is to wait 6 months to 1 year, as that is when the complete collagen remodeling is evident, particularly with lip rhytide results. The addition of BTX-A injections and fillers augment the effects of ablative laser resurfacing (Fig. 5.15).

The main pitfall in this patient group is appropriate treatment. While fillers and BTX-A injections may have some benefit, the extent of damage is too severe for these to be the sole modality of treatment. As with Glogau type III patients, adequate correction and use of fillers is critical. For optimal results, these patients are best treated after surgery and/or ablative procedures and the ideal time for biologic fillers is 6 months after the resurfacing.

CONCLUSIONS

Perioral rejuvenation is approached by multiple minimally invasive procedures. Guidelines using Glogau photoaging classifications can provide a reasonable algorithm for appropriate procedures. Glogau photoaging I patients are primarily treated with structural fillers for lip augmentation and superficial fillers for treatment of fine lines.

Glogau photoaging II patients are primarily treated for vertical lip rhytides, superficial melolabial rhytides, and early vermilion atrophy. BTX-A addresses isolated superficial vertical rhytides. Superficial direct placement of fillers and concurrent vermilion augmentation are indicated for vertical rhytides and lip atrophy. Superficial fillers address early melolabial folds and corner of mouth drooping. Nonablative lasers and pulsed light have a limited role as an isolated modality and produce better results when combined with BTX-A and fillers. Nonablative fractional resurfacing in the midinfra-red range produces more consistent and reproducible results and may be appropriate for monotherapy but definitely shows synergy when BTX-A and fillers are added. Glogau photoaging III patients are ideally suited for complete perioral rejuvenation and benefit from higher volumes of correction and approaching the perioral area as an entire cosmetic unit. Aggressive nonablative fractional resurfacing is appropriate as monotherapy in these patients and as in type II, has better results with BTX-A and fillers. Deeper placement of fillers and layering techniques with superficial fillers produce a complete result in these patients. Glogau photoaging IV patients should be first addressed surgically and/or with ablative procedures prior to minimally invasive treatments. Prototype fractional ablative devices may be more suitable in these patients also.

FURTHER READING

Baker TJ, Gordon HL 1979 Chemical peeling as a practical method for removing rhytides of the upper lip. Annals of Plastic Surgery 2:209–212

Bjerring P, Clement M, Heickendorff L, Egevist H, Kiernan M 2000 Selective non-ablative wrinkle reduction by laser. Journal of Cutaneous Laser Therapy 2:9–15

Elson ML 1988 Clinical assessment of Zyplast implant: a year of experience for soft tissue contour correction. Journal of the American Academy of Dermatology 18:707–713

Friedman PM, Mafong EA, Kauvar AN, Geronemus RG 2002 Safety data of injectable nonanimal stabilized hyaluronic acid gel for soft tissue augmentation. Dermatologic Surgery 28:491–494

Fulton JE Jr, Rahimi AD, Helton P, Watson T, Dahlberg K 2000 Lip rejuvenation. Dermatologic Surgery 26:470–474

Gonzalez UM 1992 The sensuous lip. Aesthetic Plastic Surgery 16:231–236

Holmkvist KA, Rogers GS 2000 Treatment of perioral rhytides: a comparison of dermabrasion and superpulsed carbon dioxide laser. Archives of Dermatology 136:725–731

Kesselring UK 1986 Rejuvenation of the lips. Annals of Plastic Surgery 16:480–486

Lemperle G, Gauthier-Hazan N, Lemperle M 1998 PMMA-microspheres (Artecoll) for long lasting correction of wrinkles: refinements and statistical results. Aesthetic Plastic Surgery 22:356–365

Lowe NJ, Maxwell CA, Lowe P, Duick MG, Shah K 2001 Hyaluronic acid skin fillers: adverse reactions and skin testing. Journal of the American Academy of Dermatology 4:930–933

Manstein D, Herron GS, Sink RK, Tanner H, Anderson RR 2004 Fractional photothermolysis: a new concept for cutaneous remodeling using microscopic patterns of thermal injury. Lasers Surg Med 34:426–438

Sadick NS 2003 Update on non-ablative light therapy for rejuvenation. A review. Lasers in Surgery and Medicine 32:46–49

Semchyshyn N, Sengelmann RD 2003 Botulinum toxin A treatment of perioral rhytides. Dermatologic Surgery 29:490–495

Wall SJ, Adamson PA 2002 Augmentation, enhancement, and implantation procedures for the lips. Otolaryngologic Clinics of North America 35:87–102

6 Augmentation with Autologous Fat

Lisa M. Donofrio

INTRODUCTION

Thorough evaluation and management of the aging face requires that the cosmetic dermasurgeon look past obvious superficial changes that have occurred with photoaging and begin with assessing the changes in morphologic structure that occur as a result of chronologic aging. The purpose of this chapter is to instruct the reader in the differences between surface aging changes such as wrinkles and deeper aging changes that occur in fat and bone that lead to misdraping of the skin envelope.

In the first decade of life the soft tissue structures of the face are round and cherubic. Owing to the abundance of fat in the cheek, there is an accentuation of the nasolabial and labiomental creases. Fat distribution is in 'pockets' and easily grabbed between thumb and forefinger. The maxillary height appears short when compared with the orbital height, leading to a visual diminution of the lower third of the face. This bony relationship as well as the abundance of fat seen in the medial cheeks is responsible for the presence of jowls seen in infants and young children (Fig. 6.1). In the young adult, however, there is an esthetic balance in the facial bones of the upper and lower cranial skeleton so the soft tissues drape harmoniously. The fat is abundant but unlike the infant face is smoothly and diffusely distributed. There is a continuum of the fat within and between cosmetic units of the face, so the distribution of fat appears balanced and homogeneous. In the youthful face there are many points of highlight and rare areas of shadow. Owing to the density of the fat compartments, the face projects away from the underlying bony framework forming light reflecting arcs. In profile two arcs distinguish a young face: the forehead arc, which lifts the skin away from the frontal bones diving into the superior lid crease, and the midface arc, traveling from the lower lid tarsus through to the mandible acting as a strut to 'tent' the skin of the cheek anteriorly (Fig. 6.2). Additionally the jawline is arced from mastoid to mastoid and curved in its superior to inferior dimensions forming a distinct yet rounded border with the neck (Figs 6.3 and 6.4). Animation in the young face shows the mimetic muscles to work independently of the skin. Contraction of the muscles of facial expression results in little if any surface convolutions due to the thickness of the subcutaneous tissue and the proportion of required muscular force (Fig. 6.5).

By contrast, an aging face displays loss of the anterior projection of the forehead, brow, and midface leading to relative skin excess with displacement in the dependent direction (Fig. 6.6). There is often a discrepancy in areas of the face that appear to have too much or too little fat. This topographically leads to 'hills and valleys,' the hills representing areas of fat excess, the valleys fat atrophy. These atrophic/hypertrophic fat patterns are markedly discernible in the aging face of overweight individuals. It seems that with an increase in body fat, the face also stores fat in distinctive areas of the lower midface, lateral malar area, submental area, and lower central cheek lateral to the nasolabial fold (NLF). All other areas of the face show atrophic patterns with involution and collapse of soft tissue. Very lean individuals may show panfacial atrophy without any hypertrophy (Fig. 6.7). The suborbital area however can show either an atrophic variant with hollowing and demarcation of the orbital ridge, or a hypertrophic variant with prominent suborbital fullness. It is important to realize that even the hypertrophic pattern of suborbital aging is due to loss in volume of the upper malar fat pad and interruption of the cheek/eye continuum rather than a true hypertrophic event. These suborbital patterns appear to occur independent of total body fat and may instead represent a genetic variant. The combined visual effect of areas of hollowing bordering areas of fullness is to give the aged face a shift in shape from the roundness and arcs of youth to a face replete in shadows and irregular contours. These overall morphologic patterns are so important in the practitioner's ability to determine the age of a person that they use them independent of surface characteristics such as wrinkles and photoaging. The interaction between the mimetic muscles and the skin is intimate in the aging face. Owing to the diminution in the thickness of the subcutaneous fat, the muscle lies in close juxtaposition with the skin surface. Since the required

Soft Tissue Augmentation

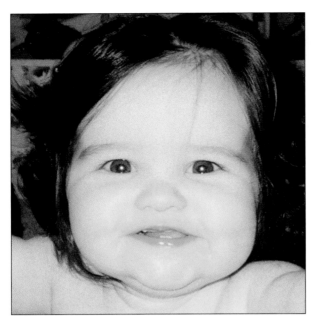

Fig. 6.1 Owing to the abundance of cheek fat, a child's face displays prominent nasolabial and labiomental folds

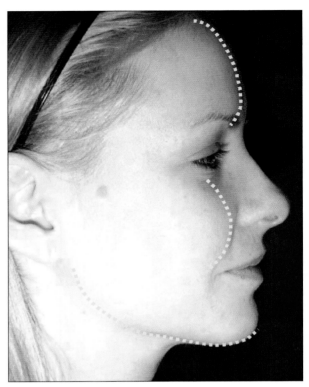

Fig. 6.2 The young face in profile

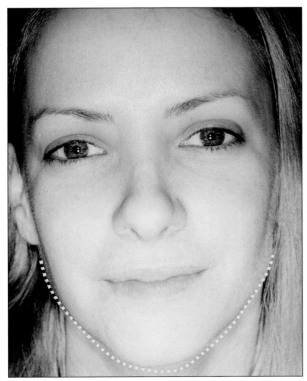

Fig. 6.3 The young face en face

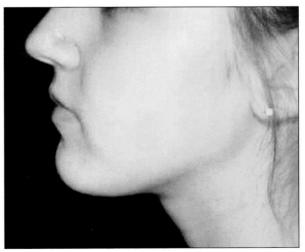

Fig. 6.4 A young neck displays 'rounded angularity' as it dives into the neck

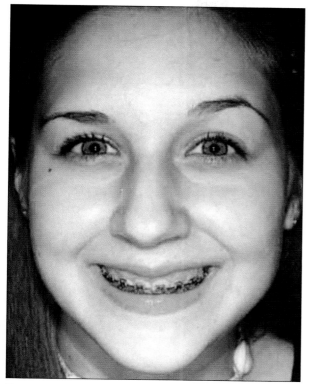

Fig. 6.5 Animation in the young face

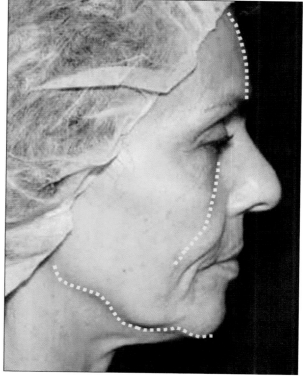

Fig. 6.6 The aging face in profile

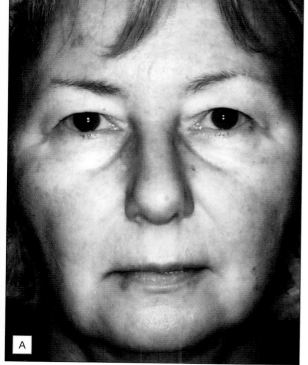

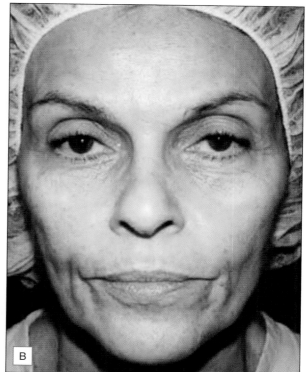

Fig. 6.7 (**A**) The heavy aging face. (**B**) The lean aging face

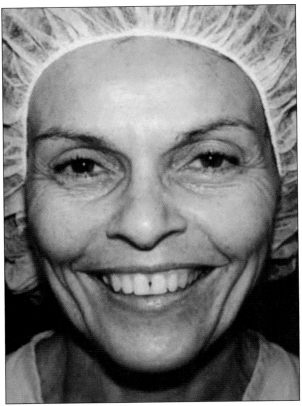

Fig. 6.8 Animation in the aged face

muscular force relative to the skin thickness is low, the skin tugs along with each contraction (Fig. 6.8). It is interesting to note that the cosmetic use of botulinum toxin decreases the muscular load on the skin, restoring a balanced proportion between the muscular force and the skin thickness reminiscent of that seen in youth.

The above mentioned volumetric changes in facial structure that occur with aging are due mostly to the changes that occur in the fatty compartments of the face. There is no change in the size of facial muscles with age so mimetic muscles as a structural element play little if any role in the aging process. Since the major morphologic shift in the aging face happens secondarily to changes within the fat, then redistributing fat back to patterns seen in youth is undoubtedly the most reasonable approach to rejuvenate the senescent face. The term 'fat rebalancing' will be used in this chapter to denote the end result of either solely adding fat to atrophic areas of the face or as a combination of microsuction of the hypertrophic areas in combination with transplantation to the atrophic areas. Patients who have a lean frame and therefore a lean face will require only fat transplantation, whereas those patients who are overweight may also require suctioning of the hypertrophic fat distribution areas in the face. Fat transplantation as described in this chapter will take place in the deep tissue planes of the face with the use of blunt

cannulas, preferably in a panfacial manner. When using fat in this way the face changes its three-dimensional contours, returning to a more youthful countenance (Fig. 6.9).

• Patient selection

Any patient desiring a more youthful appearance is a candidate for structural fat rebalancing. Because there is no skin excision, there are no telltale scars occurring around the hairline and so fat rebalancing is an excellent rejuvenating treatment for men as well as women (Fig. 6.10). To ensure the selection of patients with a favorable outcome it is important to truly understand how they want to look after a cosmetic procedure. Patients who desire to look like themselves 'only younger', or 'more refreshed', or 'less tired' have excellent expectations and most likely will be happy with fat rebalancing. However patients who apply posterior traction on their facial skin to demonstrate what is desired should be referred out for the more ascetic look of a traditional face lift. Results obtainable with fat rebalancing are much more dramatic if patients can return for between four and six 'touch up' procedures, completing the rejuvenation in a staged manner. Patients who can only schedule enough time to do a single procedure will most likely be disappointed unless that procedure is performed in an overly aggressive manner, increasing both the likelihood of misplacement of the fat and long-term edema. Since even a mild to moderately aggressive fat rebalancing session can leave the patient bruised and swollen for 1–2 weeks, patient selection should be also based upon their ability to take time off from work or social obligations. Structural fat rebalancing can be successful and dramatic in patients of all ages, however patients in the age range 35–50 are the most ideal candidates for fat rebalancing for the simple reason that they have less to correct. It also stands to reason that the response of the overlying skin envelope, either to contract if fat is removed or stretch if fat is added, may be much more predictable in a younger aged patient, especially one with minimal photoaging. Severe photoaging is a contraindication to any microsuction since skin with profound solar elastosis tends to show surface irregularities with even the most minimal fat removal. Other contraindications to fat rebalancing are lack of sufficient fat for extraction or poor skin tone in the 'donor' area, and serious chronic medical problems such as advanced organ disease, elevated PT/PTT (natural or iatrogenic), and acute infection. Patients with a past history of pulmonary embolus or deep vein thrombosis need to be evaluated on a case-by-case basis, taking into account the amount of fat being suctioned, their hormonal status, and their activity level postoperatively.

• Expected benefits

Following a series of six to eight structural fat rebalancing sessions, patients can generally expect to capture the shape of their face when they were 10–5 years younger

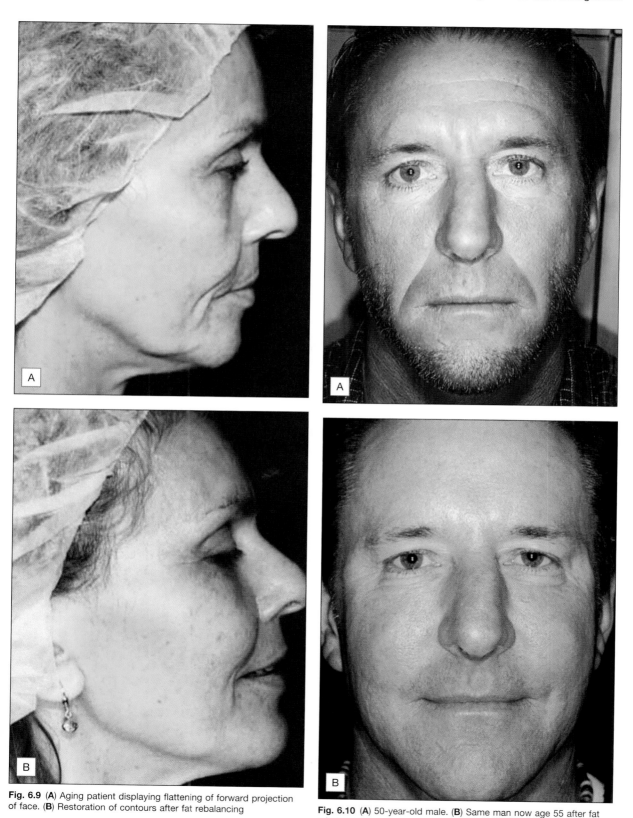

Fig. 6.9 (**A**) Aging patient displaying flattening of forward projection of face. (**B**) Restoration of contours after fat rebalancing

Fig. 6.10 (**A**) 50-year-old male. (**B**) Same man now age 55 after fat rebalancing

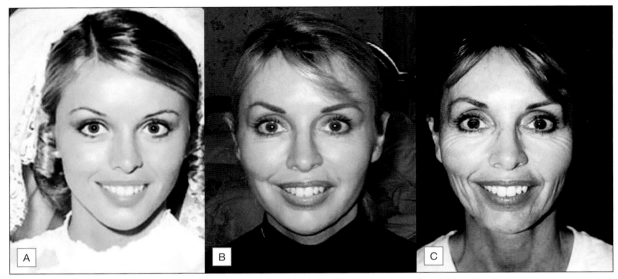

Fig. 6.11 All three photographs are of the same woman. **(A)** Age 20. **(B)** Age 50 after fat rebalancing. **(C)** Age 49

(Fig. 6.11). Segmental use of either microsuction on the face or limited area fat transfer should also be done in a staged, progressive manner and will take a minimum of four sessions to achieve balance. Since most patients can only view themselves in two dimensions it often takes critical analysis by looking at baseline photographs to appreciate the changes in profile after one or two sessions. When structural fat grafting is used to correct iatrogenic defects from face lifts or blepharoplasties, the results are dependent on the degree of fat deficit, the resultant tension on the skin, and the amount of subcutaneous scar tissue. Some deficits may be uncorrectable, for example the case when an overaggressive blepharoplasty has resulted in scleral show from too much skin removal. Fat can replace fat; fat cannot replace skin. Excellent long-term retention of fat grafts when placed for structural correction is well documented in the literature, however there are individual patients who do not retain the transplanted fat for unknown reasons. Retention rates vary and are most likely technique and operator dependent. Since there are no objective study designs other than the assessment of serial photographs, discussion of this nature may at this time be speculative.

Fat restructuring of the face occurs with the help of blunt-tipped 17–20 gauge cannulae as described later. Unlike fine placement of dermal fillers, fat infiltration incurs a blunt traumatic injury. Ecchymosis and edema usually lasting 5–10 days is common on the initial fat transplantation procedure or for the touch-ups when fat is placed in the periorbital area. Therefore patients need to be counseled on the expected down-time as well as delayed optimization of cosmetic appearance. Since the final results take between four and eight rebalancing sessions, the amount of total impact on the patient's lifestyle

will depend on whether fresh fat is harvested from the body on each transplant visit or whether previously extracted, banked and stored frozen fat is utilized.

Fat extraction takes place via local tumescent anesthesia. Supplemental oral benzodiazepines are helpful to quell preoperative anxiety. Owing to the profound safety profile and excellent anesthetic qualities of tumescent anesthesia alone, parenteral anesthetic agents are not recommended. This can be a daunting prospect for the prospective fat rebalancing patient and a certain level of anticipation of discomfort is required. The order of magnitude of discomfort is somewhat dependent on the chosen donor site. Abdomens are the most tender of harvest sites. Since nearly the entire face is addressed, panfacial local anesthesia by the use of nerve blocks or local infiltration will be required. Most patients, however, find the procedure quite tolerable as long as the local anesthesia is buffered, and describe it to be similar in discomfort to a trip to the dentist.

OVERVIEW OF TREATMENT STRATEGY

• Treatment approach

The goal of fat rebalancing is to reconstruct the arcs that project the face forward, re-establish the soft curve of the jawline, project the skin away from the midface and form an interface between the mimetic muscles and the skin. Other treatment approaches would be to enhance the cheekbones, reduce the appearance of dark shadows suborbitally caused by tear trough deformities, and redrape the skin of the eyelids via direct infiltration of fat. Fat rebalancing does not address photoaging changes such as skin texture, telangiectasias, or solar lentigos directly, but many fat transplant surgeons have noticed improvements in these surface characteristics presumably secondary to the pluripotent effects of stem cells and/or the effects of estrogen contained within the fat graft. Ancillary use of botulinum toxin is helpful in decreasing the mobility of underlying musculature in the periorbital, perioral and forehead areas. Although never studied scientifically, this could enhance 'take' of the fat grafts. Off-label use of botulinum toxin injections is also suggested when horizontal forehead furrows are present and the patient has neither the desire nor the surplus of fat to address this large surface area with autologous fat grafts.

• Major determinants

Patients desiring skin redraping achieved through fat rebalancing are generally looking for a natural-appearing rejuvenation procedure and are trying to avoid the 'pulled' or 'done' look of traditional lifts. They may also be quite aware of the loss in volume that has occurred with aging and are concerned that a face lift will hollow them out more. The fact that only local anesthesia is used in fat rebalancing is enormously attractive to many patients afraid of general sedation. Because of the lack of need of anesthesia personnel and operating room time, the cost of fat rebalancing when done in an office setting can be significantly lower than a traditional face lift. Other desirable attributes of the fat rebalancing are the lack of peripheral scars and the gradual nature of the changes achieved. Patients choosing face lifts or blepharoplasty are usually looking for a tighter, sculpted outcome. They may be overweight with a very full face and the thought of adding any fat to their face appears distasteful to them. The degree of volume enhancement and skin projection achieved with fat transfer is unique and difficult and costly to achieve with 'purchased' injectables such as collagen or hyaluronic acid. However, for simple lip augmentation or superficial correction of either the NLF or labiomental crease, both collagen and hyaluronic acid are viable choices. The hyaluronic acids may also be used when filling tear trough deformities and superior brow arches. Given the option, the majority of patients opt for filling with fat since it offers a hypoallergenic, natural, large volume, long-lasting alternative.

• Patient interviews

The patient interview is the most important part of the fat rebalancing procedure. Most patients seek fat rebalancing as a way to rejuvenate their aging face without looking too different or 'operated on'. In addition, many patients seek out fat rebalancing as a way to correct unwanted changes that have occurred to their face as a result of prior cosmetic surgery, especially as a corrective technique for hollowing secondary to blepharoplasty. The most important question to ask the patient is: 'what bothers you about your aging face?' and then come up with a cause–effect treatment strategy from there. For example, a patient who complains about jowling will often display superior and

lateral cheek atrophy as well as a corpulent body habitus. Since the hypertrophic fatty changes that occur in the lower third of the face are most times secondary to weight gain with aging, it is unrealistic for the patient to think that she can look as she used to without returning to a similar weight. So the second most important question often becomes: 'how has your weight changed in the last 10–15 years?' Patients who have gained a lot of weight can still benefit from filling atrophic areas of the face with or without microsuction of the hypertrophic areas, but may not obtain the striking results seen in patients whose weight has remained constant. Most patients will explain that they simply 'want to look like they used to look' but more often than not have no real objective idea of what they used to look like. Therefore it is helpful to ask the patient to bring a photograph from a time between 10 and 15 years ago when they liked how they looked. Again, remember to always compare the weight of the patient during the time of that photograph with the current weight. A patient who has had full cheeks her whole life and only through atrophic aging has gained the sculpted look in the buccal area she desires, may ultimately be a better candidate for a traditional face-lifting procedure than fat rebalancing. However if the patient and dermasurgeon agree that fat rebalancing is the optimal approach it is still possible to give her what she finds attractive by maintaining the relative relationship of the hollowed buccal area to the cheekbone with filling. That way the benefits of anterior projection of the midface can be achieved without making the face look too wide or full. The irony of fat transfer is that the patients who need it most are often the ones with too little to give. Unfortunately very lean patients or those without adequate donor sites due to multiple prior liposuctions must often be turned away from the procedure. However, even small amounts of fat can make a dramatic impact in the periorbital area in the correction of hollowing or in a flat, atrophic central cheek. These areas are often top priority for filling in very thin patients.

Nowhere are young photographs as helpful as when discussing rejuvenation of the periorbital area. Patients often seek skin removal through blepharoplasty as a way to regain the loss of lid show as a result of aging. However, skin redundancy in the upper lids is a result of fat loss with relative skin excess. The truth is that young faces have less lid show than their aging counterparts, and the patient interview becomes the perfect opportunity to point this out (Fig. 6.12). Most patients really do want to recapture what they had in youth with fat replacement of the upper lid, however some with very deep-set eyes find the added weight of fat in the brows unpleasant. Occasionally these patients need to seek traditional blepharoplasty but often are quite pleased with the brow elevation achieved with filling the forehead alone while avoiding the direct upper lid/brow filling. Evaluation of the suborbital areas requires the patient be classified into one of two aging patterns: atrophic suborbital aging, where the suborbital area is hollow often with apparent demarcation of

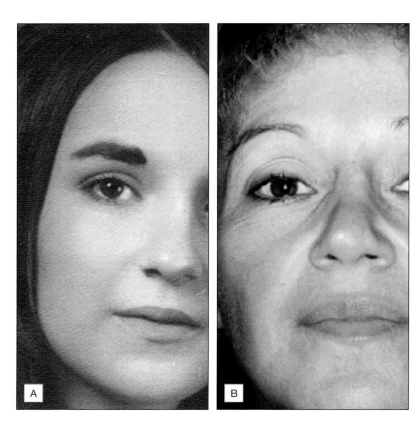

Fig. 6.12 Same woman. (**A**) Age 16. (**B**) Age 50. Note the increase in lid, shown with aging

the bony orbit, and hypertrophic suborbital aging, with protrusion of the suborbital fat anterior to the relationship with the inferior cheek mass. Atrophic suborbital aging is true atrophy of the suborbital fat, whereas hypertrophic suborbital aging is actually atrophy of the cheek without atrophy of the orbital fat and is most likely a false relative hypertrophy. Box 6.1 contains key questions to ask patients on the initial interview.

TREATMENT TECHNIQUES

• Equipment

The following equipment is recommended when performing fat rebalancing of the face:

❖ Coleman extractor (Byron, Tucson, AZ, USA)
❖ 10 mL Luer lock syringes, for manual collection and storage of fat
❖ A centrifuge that revolves at 3400 rev/min. Options include older model centrifuges that have removable domes or centrifuges made especially for spinning 10 mL syringes containing fat (Byron)
❖ Disposable plastic Coleman caps (Byron) or reusable stainless steel caps (Miller Medical, Mesa, AZ, USA) for centrifugation of 10 mL syringes

---

Box 6.1 Key questions to ask at patient interview

❖ Have you had cosmetic surgery before?
❖ Were you happy with the results?
❖ What bothers you about your face as it has aged?
❖ How has your weight changed over the past 20 years?
❖ Did you like the way you used to look?
❖ What didn't you like about your face when it was younger?

❖ 1 mL Luer lock syringes. These are used exclusively for controlled injection of fat into the face
❖ Female–female transfer device
❖ 17–20 g blunt infiltration cannulae. Coleman or Donofrio infiltration cannulae (Byron) for placing or removing fat in the face
❖ An alarm backed freezer at a temperature of −10 to −30°C (if fat is to be frozen for later use).

• Treatment algorithm

DRAWING ON THE FACE

Following the initial treatment plan determined in the patient interview/consultation the markings are trans-

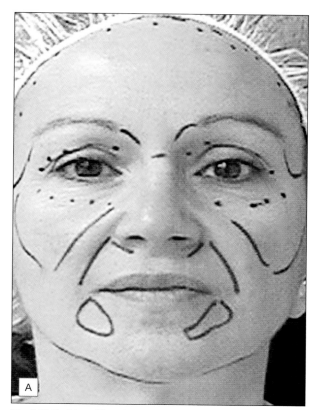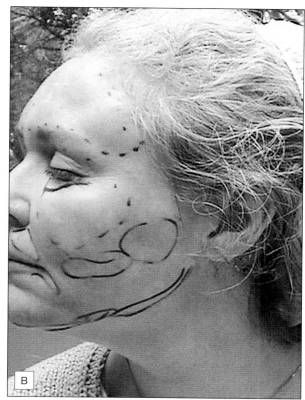

Fig. 6.13 Facial markings for fat rebalancing. (**A**) Front view. (**B**) Side view

ferred to the face with either a laundry marker or gentian violet pen. It is helpful to also mark out bony landmarks that may assist in local anesthesia infiltration or play a role in the placement of the fat as well as premarking any baseline asymmetry. Having the patient gaze up accentuates the inferior orbital ridge and tear trough if present, facilitating marking these areas. When drawing for upper eyelid filling, the dermasurgeon manually lifts the eyebrow until no lid redundancy remains, then draws a line where the 'new' supratarsal crease is demarcated by the shape of the globe. The mandibular markings are drawn by first palpating and marking the anterior border of the mandible and then drawing a line 1 cm below from mastoid to mastoid. The dermasurgeon may also wish to mark out any fullness in the jowl as a way to avoid this filling or remember to suction this area. To accentuate the atrophy occurring on the lateral cheek and jawline, have the patient lie supine and draw the line of demarcation for later filling posteriorly. After marking the face, the dermasurgeon may wish to estimate the amount of fat that will be required to fill each area by thinking in terms of elliptical measurements such as teaspoons (5 mL) or tablespoons (15 mL). Some dermasurgeons find it helpful to then transfer these thoughts to the blueprint or onto the face directly. Other markings should include areas of shadow

and highlight as they will affect the fat transfer (Fig. 6.13).

PATIENT PREPARATION

Patients are prophylaxed starting the day before surgery with either cephelexin 500 mg bid or erythromycin 500 mg bid. Ciprofloxacin 500 mg bid can also be used as an appropriate antibiotic. Antibiotics are continued including the day of the procedure and for a total of 7 days. Premedication on the day of the procedure includes 40 mg of prednisone PO and 5–10 mg of oral diazepam if needed. The donor site to be liposuctioned is prepared with a solution of Hibicleans and sterile water and the face is washed with antibacterial soap. Preoperative photographs are taken from multiple angles. It is also helpful to take photographs of the patient in animation and repose. Patients are placed onto a sterile, draped operating table covered with a sterile sheet.

FAT EXTRACTION

The patient and dermasurgeon must decide on an appropriate donor site. In females fat from the hips or lateral thighs is preferable to that of the abdomen due to the relative ease of extraction, the greater comfort of the

Soft Tissue Augmentation

Box 6.2 Tumescent fluid used for fat rebalancing

- ❖ 500 mg lidocaine (lignocaine)
- ❖ 1 L lactated Ringers solution
- ❖ 1 mg epinephrine (adrenaline)
- ❖ 12.5 meq sodium bicarbonate

patient, and the paucity of fibrous tissue encountered on extraction. Fat extracted from this area may also have the potential for greater lipogenic activity. The donor site is encircled with a marking pen in a way that would benefit the patient cosmetically. Designated skin markings are done with the patient standing. Autologous fat is harvested for the fat transfer procedure under local tumescent anesthesia. Every effort to make the procedure as sterile as possible is attempted by the use of sterile gloves, gown and mask by the dermasurgeon and a sterilely draped operating table. Lactated ringer's solution is augmented with lidocaine (lignocaine), epinephrine (adrenaline), and sodium bicarbonate in the concentrations specified in Box 6.2. This gives a solution with a final volume of lidocaine of 0.05%. The lidocaine is intentionally kept at a low concentration since it has been shown to be inhibitory to the function of adipocytes. With the patient in the recumbent position, entry sites on the skin of the donor area are made with a 1.5 mm punch tool. The tumescent solution is then infiltrated into the adipose tissue of the donor site via a mechanical infiltration pump or by hand infiltration with a 60 mL syringe. Infiltration can be accomplished with a blunt multiholed cannula or with an 18 gauge spinal needle. The endpoint for true tumescence is tissue turgidity. This also guarantees a bloodless adipose sample. It is necessary to wait for 20 minutes after infiltration for hemostasis to occur before attempting to harvest the fat. Fat collection is accomplished with an open-tipped cannula (Coleman extractor, Byron) on a 10 mL syringe (Fig. 6.14). Only manual negative pressure is applied by withdrawing the plunger on the syringe while the cannula is passed back and forth in the deep fat (Fig. 6.15). When the syringe is full, the cannula may be left in place changing only the syringe. Full syringes are left upside down in a sterile test tube tray or specimen cup. For most full-face fat rebalancing sessions a total of 50–100 mL of fat is needed. More is collected if surplus fat is to be frozen and stored for later use. It is preferable to briefly centrifuge the syringes of fat for 20 seconds to remove the extracellular tumescent fluid and separate out the supranatant triglyeride layer. Special screw-on caps that are disposable (Byron) or autoclavable (Miller Medical) are recommended during centrifugation for a tight seal. After spinning the fat, the infranate is squeezed off and the compacted adipocytes are transferred to 1 mL syringes via a female-to-female device, stopping short of the triglyceride layer.

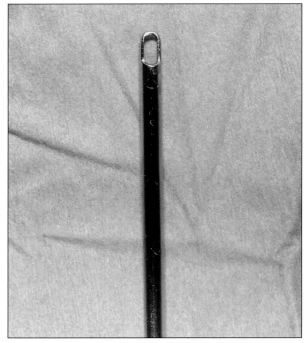

Fig. 6.14 Open-tipped extraction cannula (Byron, Tuczon, AZ, USA)

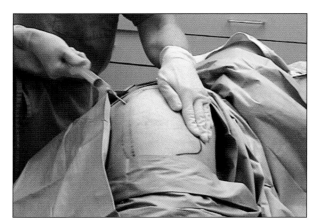

Fig. 6.15 Fat extraction

FACIAL ANESTHESIA

The patient's comfort is paramount to a successful procedure. Facial anesthesia should be carried out slowly while verbally soothing and distracting the patient. Patients are encouraged to bring headphones or a favorite CD to make the experience less unpleasant. In addition, vibratory devices can be utilized to floodgate neighboring pain signals. Facial blocks with 1% xylocaine are used when appropriate in the infraorbital, mental, supraorbital and supratrochlear areas. The majority of the anesthesia takes place via local infiltration of 0.5% lidocaine (lignocaine)

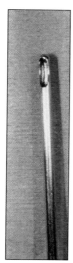

Fig. 6.16 Blunt infiltration cannula

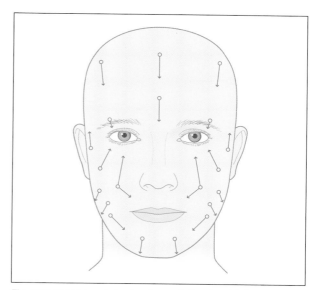

Fig. 6.17 Recommended entry sites and direction of infiltration

4:1 with sodium bicarbonate. To infiltrate broadly, 30 gauge 1 in needles are used. Injections are kept in the deep fat to minimize ecchymosis, especially in the lateral orbit and temple. In the perioral area an intraoral route of anesthesia is less uncomfortable than the percutaneous route. In this area it is only necessary to fill the superior and inferior labial vestibule superficially to achieve adequate lip anesthesia. The author prefers to use 4% prilocaine without epinephrine in this area administered via a dental injection syringe and cartridge.

GENERAL TECHNIQUE

All infiltration of fat is with blunt 17–20 gauge cannulae attached to 1 mL syringes of fat (Fig. 6.16). This not only offers superb control over the placement of minute droplets of fat, but also keeps the procedure safe by minimizing injection pressures and the risk of canalizing vessels. Blunt instrument infiltration allows the recipient tissues to 'spread' apart, thus anchoring the fat, rather than 'coring' out a tunnel as is the possibility with a sharp large bore needle. It also allows the dermasurgeon the freedom of placement in the periorbital area where sharp instruments run a high risk of perforation of the orbital septum or periocular vessels. Entry sites are made at various locations on the face to allow for easy access with an 18 gauge Nokor needle (Becton Dickinson, Franklin Lakes, NJ, USA) (Fig. 6.17). The dermasurgeon enters, bevel down on the cannula, weaving the cannula in a back and forth motion depositing approximately 0.05 mL of fat per stroke. Therefore, it should take 20 passes to empty a 1 mL syringe. All injection of fat takes place retrograde. Holding the 1 mL syringe with attached cannula in the dominant hand, the dermasurgeon uses the thenar eminance of this hand to push in the plunger in 'spurts' on the withdrawal phase of the movement through the tissue.

Unless otherwise specified below, infiltration of fat occurs in all levels of subcutaneous tissue, starting deeply adjacent to mucosa or bone and working up through muscle and subcutaneous fat taking advantage of multiple entry sites and weaving fat in a crosshatched three dimensional lattice.

FOREHEAD AUGMENTATION

The goals of forehead augmentation are to project the skin of the forehead anteriorly, thus achieving a lifting of the brow, and to form an interface subcutaneously to attenuate the pull of the frontalis muscle on the skin. All forehead infiltration is perpendicular to the brow, i.e. parallel to the fibers of the frontalis muscle. Incisions are best made at multiple places in the hairline. The temple and glabella as well as the brow/lid complex can all be addressed through these incisions. Fat is deposited subcutaneously in the supragaleal plane anterior to as well as in and under the frontalis muscle. Visible ridging is common, and requires smoothing out with firm pressure in all directions. For the temple a deep level of infiltration (subtemporalis muscle) can be most easily accomplished with a curved No. 7 Amar cannula (Miller Medical, AZ USA). Entering from the superior temporal hollow, the cannula is 'racheted' under the temporalis muscle (Fig. 6.18A). Typically the forehead can hold 6–12 mL of fat, and the temples 1–3 mL each (Fig. 6.18B).

BROW AUGMENTATION

As described earlier, brow filling can take place via an entry site at the hairline or from one just above the eyebrow. Fat is placed in 'droplets' depositing the base of the drop at the newly marked supratarsal crease and then

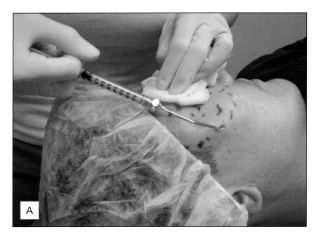

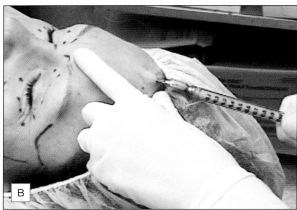

Fig. 6.18 (A) Curved Amar #7 cannula. (B) Forehead infiltration

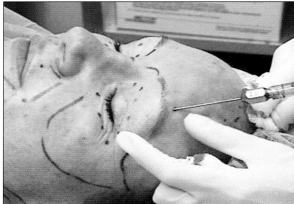

Fig. 6.19 Brow augmentation

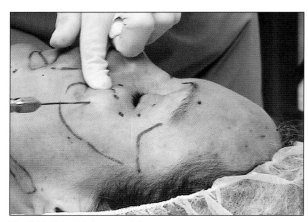

Fig. 6.20 Suborbital augmentation

pulling the 'tail' of the drop superiorly. Augmenting this area serves to advance the brow forward, filling up skin redundancy by applying an internal tenting force on the skin. The brow can take a total of 1–2 mL of fat and should be tapered to blend seamlessly with the neighboring temple and forehead (Fig. 6.19).

SUBORBITAL AUGMENTATION

The plan for augmentation of the suborbital area depends on whether the patient displays the atrophic or the hypertrophic variant of aging in this area or whether augmentation is being performed to correct an overaggressive blepharoplasty. In the case of atrophic aging an incision is made at a point midway between the midpupillary line and the lateral canthus 2 cm out from the orbital rim. Fat is placed in linear threads throughout the suborbital area maintaining a perpendicular alignment to the lid margin. Fat is placed under the orbicularis oculi muscle in smaller than 0.05 mL aliquots using only blunt cannulae (Fig. 6.20). Fingers of the nondominant hand protect the globe at all times. Often it is necessary to make a second incision

just lateral to the NLF with which to access the medial portion of the suborbital area, again in a plane under the orbicularis muscle (Fig. 6.21). This is the preferred incision site for bolstering the arcus marginalus with fat to support the lower lid and eliminate scleral show from blepharoplasty. For very fine detail work in the suborbital area a short, blunt 20 g cannula can be used. In this scenario, fat is threaded in minuscule amounts with multiple passes required to deposit even 0.1 mL. The author does not recommend placement of fat anterior to the orbicularis oculi muscle due to the substantial risk of irregularities possible in this plane. Hypertrophic suborbital aging requires filling of the cheek and will be discussed later.

CHEEK AUGMENTATION

Certainly the most dramatic changes achievable by fat transfer are simply by restoring the profile arc of the midface to an aging individual. Not only does this small change return a critical point of highlight to the 'apple' of the cheek, but also it serves to tent out the skin of the

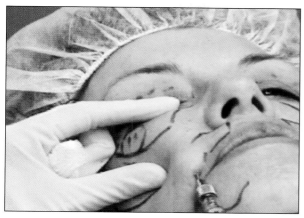

Fig. 6.21 Suborbital augmentation

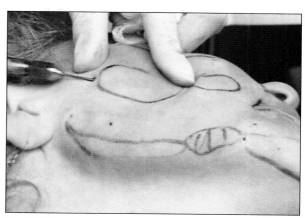

Fig. 6.23 Buccal augmentation

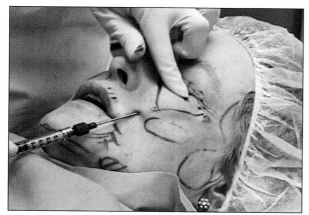

Fig. 6.22 Central malar augmentation

LATERAL FACIAL AUGMENTATION

To restore a harmonious balance to the augmented face and to prevent a 'chipmunk cheek' appearance often seen with central facial filling, the technique of 'backfilling' can be utilized. This involves filling the perimeter of the face including the temples, lateral cheek and jawline. From an incision anterior to the tragus the lateral cheek and jawline can be augmented with 5–8 mL of fat utilizing the anterior border of the parotid fascial insertion as a landmark. This technique is especially helpful in patients requiring multiple fat transfer procedures and insures a natural appearance.

PERIORAL AUGMENTATION

Involution in the perioral area with resultant collapse, shriveling and lengthening of the upper lip is a common manifestation of both fat atrophy and bony reabsorption secondary to chronologic aging. Fat replacement pushes the cutaneous portion of the lip forward, so that it appears shorter. It also interrupts the skin–muscle interaction that leads to a contracted pursed look. Fat replacement in the chin can soften or even alleviate the dimpling secondary to aging in patients with a past history of acne in this area. The cutaneous portion of the upper and lower lip is best reached by an incision in or lateral to the nasolabial and labiomental crease, or from an incision at the angle of the mouth. The direction of infiltration is parallel to the border of the lip, extending from the upper vermilion to the subnasal area and lower vermilion down to the chin (Fig. 6.24). Infiltration amounts of 1–2 mL of fat per side upper and lower for a total of 4–8 mL in the entire cutaneous perioral area is normally required. If desired the mucosal portion of the lip can be augmented with 2–4 mL either with a 20 gauge sharp needle into the vermilion border or bluntly with an 18 gauge cannula from an incision site lateral to the NLF (Fig. 6.25).

midface, in essence lifting skin inferior to it. In the case of hypertrophic suborbital aging, the goal is to advance the cheek to the level of the suborbital protuberance or beyond, so that the orbital area appears to recede. From an incision in the base of the NLF, or just lateral to it, fat is placed diffusely in the central cheek superiorly to the level of the tear trough, fanning out laterally (Fig. 6.22). Then from an incision inferior and lateral to the zygomatic arch, fat is deposited parallel to the arch and perpendicular to the previous placement. Fat is placed in multiple layers starting underneath the zygomaticus muscles, coming up through the muscles, then subcutaneously. Finally, the area of the buccal fat pad is restored to its youthful fullness by either one of the above incisions or one inferior to the buccal hollow (Fig. 6.23). Placement amounts vary, but it is very common to place 7–15 mL in these areas to re-establish anterior projection of the midface.

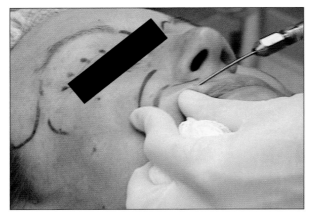

Fig. 6.24 Cutaneous upper lip augmentation

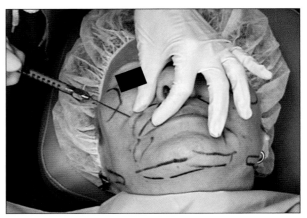

Fig. 6.26 Nasolabial fold augmentation

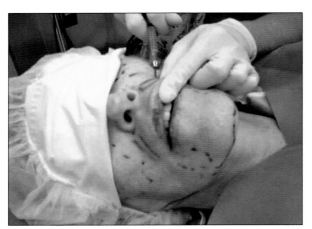

Fig. 6.25 Mucosal upper lip augmentation

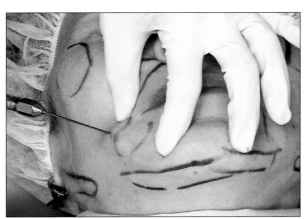

Fig. 6.27 Labiomental crease augmentation

NASOLABIAL AND LABIOMENTAL CREASE AUGMENTATION

Often amelioration of the NLF is achieved by the anterior projection achieved through filling of the central cheek area, and the advancement of the cutaneous portion of the lip that makes up the medial NLF. However if additional augmentation into this fold is desired, an incision site lateral to the fold through which 1–2 mL of fat is placed perpendicularly is preferable to fat placement parallel in the fold (Fig. 6.26). The same holds true for the labiomental crease, where filling of the lateral cheek and buccal area redistributes the skin redundancy that forms this fold. When additional filling is desired, as it often is in this area, 1–2 mL of fat can be placed through an incision lateral to the fold, being careful to pull the tail of the fat droplet across the fold so as not to accentuate the insertion of the retaining ligament in this area (Fig. 6.27).

JAWLINE AUGMENTATION

To restore the 'rounded angularity' characteristic of a young jawline, 8–20 mL of fat is placed in the submandibular area. Incision sites are perpendicular to the arc of the jawline so that the fat is placed in droplets wrapping around the inferior surface of the mandible (Fig. 6.28). The level of placement is superficial at the level of investment of the platysma muscle. Care must be taken to place the fat evenly. If it appears to be forming clumps then an approach through a parallel incision to smooth out the area may be necessary. Enhancement of the chin can also be accomplished through one of the anterior incisions, approaching this area laterally (Fig. 6.29). Placement of 1–2 mL of fat in this area is usually sufficient, but difficult due to the tough fibrous tissue present subcutaneously.

MICROLIPOSUCTION

As discussed earlier, in certain patients with adequate skin tone, it may be desirable to microliposuction the hyper-

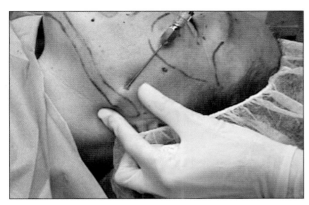

Fig. 6.28 Mandibular augmentation

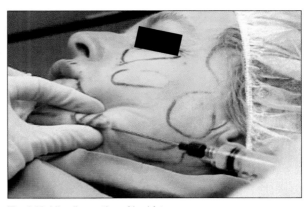

Fig. 6.30 Microliposuction of jowl fat

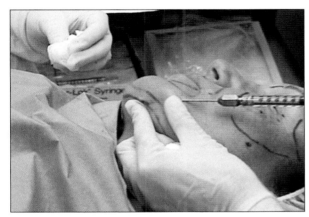

Fig. 6.29 Chin augmentation

Box 6.3 Common pitfalls of fat transplantation

❖ Underestimating the amount of fat it will take to cause volume change and tissue shifting
❖ Assuming that the change early on is due to fat and not edema
❖ Transplanting too much fat in one session
❖ Using sharp instruments
❖ Filling only the folds
❖ Filling only the central third of the face

---

trophic fat deposits of the lower face to achieve true fat rebalancing. This can be accomplished with a 17 gauge cannula attached to a 10 mL syringe. By pulling back on the plunger negative pressures can be created and suction accomplished. This technique can be used in the areas lateral to the NLF, lateral to the labiomental crease, and in the jowl (Fig. 6.30). It is prudent to undercorrect, staying in a deep plane. Typically 0.5–1 mL only of fat is removed from each area, and so repeat suction is required. In addition to erring on the side of caution, staging the suction procedures allows time for the skin to recontract to smaller insults. 18 g or 20 g cannulae that are used to place the fat are too small for efficient manual fat extraction.

• Pearls for successful fat rebalancing

The number one mistake made by fat transfer dermasurgeons is underestimation of the amount of fat it takes to affect a volume change and tissue shift. It is helpful therefore to think in elliptical terms like teaspoon and tablespoon measurements to visualize the volume of fat it

would take to cause projection in the desired plane. It is common for an atrophic cheek to require upwards of 15 mL (i.e. 1 tbsp) of fat placed in one or multiple sessions to recapture the anterior projection reminiscent of youth. Since the blunt trauma incurred by the fat transfer cannulae causes prolonged edema, it is also common to assume that the change in volume early on is due to the transplanted fat. This leads to a false assumption, and once the edema subsides, the supposition that the fat has been absorbed. The other common mistake made with fat transfers is to fill only the folds. A good test as to whether this would indeed correct the problem is to ask the patient to lie down, and examine the fold from this angle. If it is flattened, then only redraping of neighboring tissues and not direct filling will ameliorate this fold. Once the dermasurgeon starts thinking spatially in three dimensions this comes as second nature and panfacial fat rebalancing becomes the treatment of choice. Common pitfalls of fat transplantation are summarized in Box 6.3.

• Side effects, complications, and alternative approaches

The most common sequelae of panfacial fat rebalancing are edema and ecchymosis lasting 2–14 days. Patients seem to have more down-time from the first procedure than from subsequent touch up procedures. Small nodules or tracts of fat or edema can persist in the periorbital area

Soft Tissue Augmentation

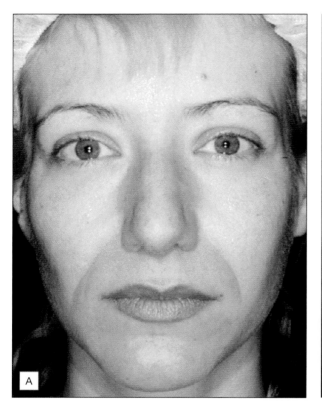

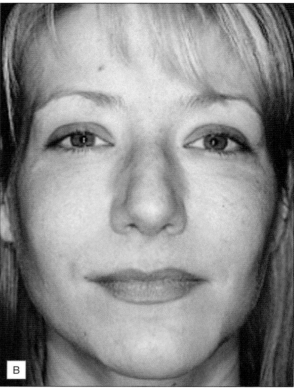

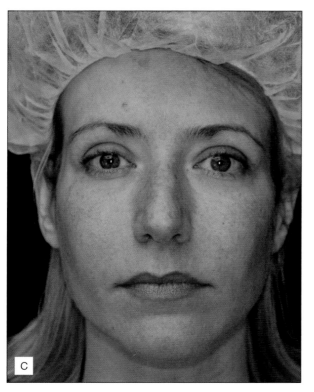

Fig. 6.31 (**A**) Age 32. (**B**) Age 37, at $2^1/_2$ year follow up after fat rebalancing series (**C**) Age 40, after backfilling to restore balance

and often require feathering via perpendicular cannula passes on a follow-up visit. Persistent uncorrectable irregularities are uncommon with judicious placement in experienced hands. Hard persistent nodules representative of sterile fat cysts require dilute steroid injections, or even incision to resolve. Postinflammatory pigmentation or hemosiderin pigmentation is occasionally encountered and can be treated with time or laser light sources. The author has encountered two patients who complained of prolonged pain in the temple and lateral zygomatic area following fat transfer in a deep structural plane, two patients with dimpling at the entry sites on animation and one patient with muscular fasciculations of the lip levator that resolved after 3 months. Also of note is one patient with apparent necrotic fat (on aspiration) that had migrated approximately 5 cm from the area of placement. Other rarely noted side effects are infection, eruption of herpetic lesions periorally, and submandibular lymph node enlargement. A review of the literature reveals such serious and disconcerting side effects as middle cerebral artery infarction, blindness, and abscess formation. The etiology of these events is unclear, but appears to be related to high-pressure injections of fat through a large syringe or sharp needle with retrograde flow into the internal carotid system. It is imperative therefore that fat be transferred with only blunt instruments in the presence of locally infiltrated epinephrine (in the anesthesia) using 1 mL syringes during the withdrawal stroke of the movement.

Retention rates are variable in the literature and appear to be site specific and operator dependent. Long-term retention of fat has been documented by many authors using a multilayer transplantation technique. Poorest retention is seen in the lips and perioral area probably due to the multiple dynamic and intrinsic muscular forces that contribute to folds in this area. The periorbital area and cheek have the best retention followed by the lateral jawline, forehead, and buccal area. Patients desiring further correction in low retention areas are often encouraged to augment with hyaluronic acid fillers, however these small volume fillers are not capable of the dramatic tissue shifts achievable with fat rebalancing in the structural plane (Figs 6.31–6.33).

• Postoperative course and follow up

Intramuscular or oral steroids are recommended immediately postoperatively to minimize postoperative edema. Ice packs should be applied to the face frequently, for the first and second postoperative day. The harvest sites are covered with absorbable dressings to wick off the tumescent drainage and then a compression elastic garment such as a girdle or Lycra biking shorts applied. When washing the face and body following the procedure, only sterile water should be used to minimize the risk of naturally occurring mycobacteria in the tap water supply. Structural fat rebalancing is most successful when done in repeated stages. Touch-up procedures can be scheduled at 1–3-

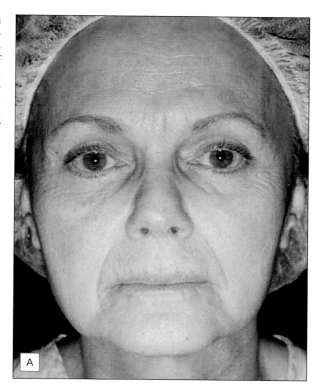

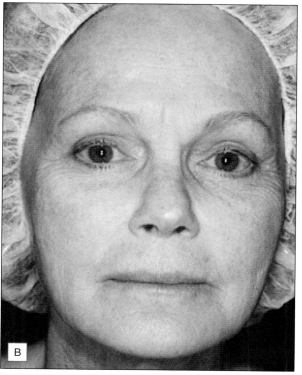

Fig. 6.32 **(A)** Age 53. **(B)** Age 56, at 1½ year follow up after fat rebalancing series

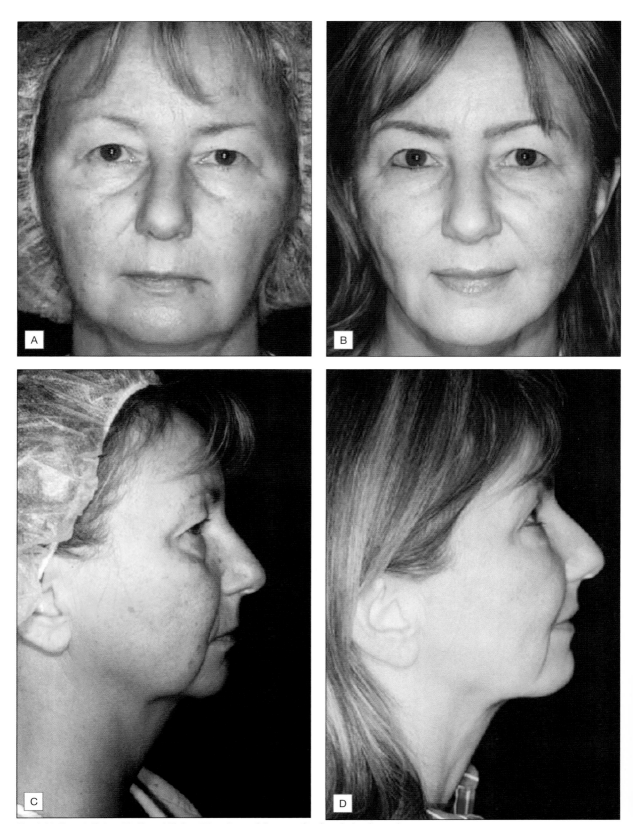

Fig. 6.33 (**A** and **C**) Age 50. (**B** and **D**) Age 55, at 2 year follow up after fat rebalancing series

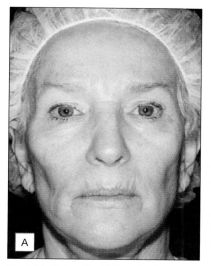 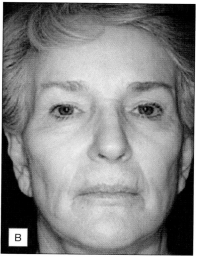 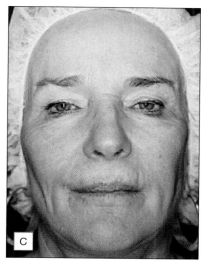

Fig. 6.34 (A) Age 50. (B) After first fat rebalancing session with fresh fat. (C) After two more sessions using only frozen fat, at 1 year follow up

month intervals until the desired correction is achieved. These touch-up sessions may be accomplished with either fresh fat harvested in the manner above, or previously frozen fat (Fig. 6.34). The use of frozen fat is highly controversial. It remains uncertain at this time whether frozen fat has the potential for long-term augmentation but many surgeons who routinely augment with previously frozen fat comment on its ability for long-term correction. If fat is to be frozen for future use, the fat should be frozen in 10 mL syringes after decanting infranate, but with triglycerides intact, meticulously labeled with patient's name, date of procedure, and social security number. Fat should be slowly frozen by placing it at −20°C, moved to temperature monitored and alarmed freezers for long term storage at −20 to −30°C, and then rapidly thawed when ready to use. Long-term sterility of frozen fat has been shown for up to 2 years.

FURTHER READING

Bertossi D, Kharouf S, d'Agostino A, et al 2000 Facial localized cosmetic filling by multiple injections of fat stored at −30°C. Techniques, clinical follow-up of 99 patients and histological examination of 10 patients. Annales de Chirurgie Plastique et Esthétique 45:548–555

Carraway JH, Mellow CG 1990 Syringe aspiration and fat concentration: a simple technique for autologous fat injection. Annals of Plastic Surgery 24:293–296

Carruthers A, Carruthers J 1998 Clinical indications and injection technique for the cosmetic use of botulinum A exotoxin. Dermatologic Surgery 24:1189–1194

Carruthers A, Carruthers J, Cohen J 2003 A prospective, double-blind, randomized, parallel-group, dose-ranging study of botulinum toxin type A in female subjects with horizontal forehead rhytides. Dermatologic Surgery 29:462–467

Coleman SR 1995 Long term results of fat transplants: controlled demonstrations. Aesthetic Plastic Surgery 19:421–425

Coleman SR 1997 Facial recontouring with liposculpture. Clinics in Plastic Surgery 24:347–367

Coleman SR 2001 Structural fat grafts: the ideal filler? Clinics in Plastic Surgery 28:111–119

Danesh-Meyer HV, Savino PJ, Sergott RC 2001 Case reports and a small case series; ocular and cerebral ischemia following facial injection of autologous fat. Archives of Ophthalmology 119:777–778

De Ugarte DA, Ashjian PH, Elbarbary A, Hendrick MH 2003 Future of fat as raw material for tissue regeneration. Annals of Plastic Surgery 50:215–219

Donofrio LM 2000 Structural lipoaugmentation: a pan-facial technique. Dermatologic Surgery 26:1129–1134

Donofrio LM 2003 The technique of periorbital lipoaugmentation. Dermatologic Surgery 29:92–98

Dreizen NG, Framm L 1989 Sudden unilateral visual loss after autologous fat injection into the glabellar area. American Journal of Ophthalmology 107:85–87

Egido JA, Arroyo R, Marcos A, Jimenez-Alfaro I 1993 Middle cerebral artery embolism and unilateral visual loss after autologous fat injection into the glabellar area. Stroke 24:615–616

Feinendegen DL, Baumgartner RW, Schroth G, Mattle HP, Tschopp H 1988 Middle cerebral artery occlusion and ocular fat embolism after autologous fat injection in the face. Journal of Neurology 245:53–54

Feinendegen DL, Baumgartner RW, Vaudens P, et al 1998 Autologus fat injections for soft tissue augmentation in the face; a safe procedure? Aesthetic Plastic Surgery 22:163–167

Flynn TC, Narins RS 1999 Preoperative evaluation of the liposuction patient. Dermatologic Clinics 17:729–734

Fulton J, Suarez M, Silverton K, Barnes T 1998 Small volume fat transfer. Journal of Dermatologic Surgery and Oncology 24:857–865

Goldman MP, Marchell N, Fitzpatrick RE 2002 Laser skin resurfacing of the face with a combined CO$_2$/Er : YAG laser. Dermatologic Surgery 26:102–104

Gosain A, Amarante MT, Hyde JS, Yousif NJ 1996 A dynamic analysis of changes in the nasolabial fold using magnetic resonance imaging : implications for facial rejuvenation and facial animation surgery. Plastic and Reconstructive Surgery 98:622–636

Gosain AK, Klein MH, Sudhakar PV, Prost RW 2005 A volumetric ananlysis of soft-tissue changes in the aging midface using high-resolution MRI: implications for facial rejuvination. Plastic and Reconstructive Surgery 115:1143–1152; discussion 1153–1155

Hanke CW 2001 The tumescent facial block: tumescent local anesthesia and nerve block anesthesia for full-face laser resurfacing. Dermatologic Surgery 27:1003–1005

Hudson DA, Lambert EV, Bloch CE 1990 Site selection for auto-transplantation: some observations. Aesthetic Plastic Surgery 14:195–197

Jackson RF 1997 Frozen fat – does it work? American Journal of Cosmetic Surgery 14:339–343

Klein JA 1990 The tumescent technique; anesthesia and modified liposuction technique. Dermatologic Clinics 8:425–437

Lawrence N 2000 New and emerging treatments for photoaging. Dermatologic Clinics 18:99–112

Lee DH, Yang HN, Kim JC, Shyn KH 1996 Sudden unilateral visual loss and brain infarction after autologous fat injection into the nasolabial groove. British Journal of Ophthalmology 80:1026–1027

Lilleth H, Boberg J 1978 The lipoprotein-lipase activity of adipose tissue from different sites in obese women and relationship to cell size. International Journal of Obesity 2:47–52

Markey AC, Glogau RG 2000 Autologous fat grafting: comparison of techniques. Dermatologic Surgery 26:1135–1139

Moore JH, Kolaczynski JW, Morales LM, et al 1995 Viability of fat obtained by syringe suction lipectomy: effects of local anesthesia with lidocaine. Aesthetic Plastic Surgery 19:335–339

Narins RS, Brandt F, Leyden J, Lorenc ZP, Rubin M, Smith S 2003 A randomized, double-blind, multicenter comparison of the efficacy and tolerability of Restylane versus Zyplast for the correction of nasolabial folds. Dermatologic Surgery 29:588–595

Nguyen A, Pasyk KA, Bouvier TN, Hassett CA, Argenta LC 1990 Comparative study of survival of autologous adipose tissue taken and transplanted by different techniques. Plastic and Reconstructive Surgery 85:378–386

Niechajev I, Sevcuk O 1994 Long term results of fat transplantation: clinical and histologic studies. Plastic and Reconstructive Surgery 94:496–506

Ostad A, Kageyama N, Moy RL 1996 Tumescent anesthesia with a lidocaine dose of 55 mg/kg is safe for liposuction. Dermatologic Surgery 22:921–927

Pessa JE, Zadoo VP, Mutimer KL, et al 1998 Relative maxillary retrusion as a natural consequence of aging combining skeletal and soft-tissue changes into an integrated model of midfacial aging. Plastic and Reconstructive Surgery 102:205–212

Pessa JE, Zadoo VP, Yuan C, et al 1999 Concertina effect and facial aging: nonlinear aspects of youthfulness and skeletal remodeling, and why, perhaps, infants have jowls. Plastic and Reconstructive Surgery 103:635–644

Schiffman MA, Mirrafati S 2001 Fat transfer techniques: the effect of harvest and transfer methods on adipocyte viability and review of the literature. Dermatologic Surgery 27:819–826

Shoshani O, Ullman Y, Shupak A, et al 2001 The role of frozen storage in preserving adipose tissue obtained by suction-assisted lipectomy for repeated fat injection procedures. Dermatologic Surgery 27:645–647

Sommer B, Sattler G 2000 Current concepts of fat graft survival: histology of aspirated adipose tissue and review of the literature. Dermatologic Surgery 26:1159–1166

Teimourian B 1988 Blindness following fat injections. Plastic and Reconstructive Surgery 82:361

7 Fillers Working by Fibroplasia

Jean Carruthers, Alastair Carruthers

INTRODUCTION

The original concept with the modern era of tissue augmentation was that by injecting collagen into the skin this would be incorporated into new collagen producing long-lasting correction. However, it rapidly became apparent that injectable collagen was principally a passive space occupier. This concept continued and was amplified in the current use of hyaluronic acid-derived fillers, which were originally proposed to be just passive. Recent research has shown that this is not entirely true and they do induce a degree of fibroplasia. Over the past decade however, the thinking has swung back toward intentionally inducing fibroplasia to make the filling more effective and also increase its longevity?

Dr Gottfried Lemperle, a plastic surgeon working initially in Germany, conceived the notion of using a well-tolerated substance used in bone cement and in hard contact lenses- polymethyl methacrylate (PMMA) suspended as microparticles in atelomeric bovine collagen. The initial product was called Arteplast and the particles were irregularly shaped. A second-generation product Artecoll followed with beads as round and polished as possible and of a more uniform size and the third generation (which is now approved by the FDA as ArteFill) has further refined the bead technology. The concept of injecting the permanent filling bead, which will gradually stimulate new collagen formation in a transitory collagen vehicle, has been very successful in giving increased longevity of response. The attentiveness to the shape, size and surface characteristics of the beads has allowed the product to be used safely.

Radiesse uses the same conceptual bimodal technology, but the beads are made of perfectly smooth spheres of calcium hydroxylapatite and the vehicle is biodegradeable carboxymethyl cellulose. With Radiesse, the concept has been altered somewhat in that the beads are long lasting, but unlike the PMMA beads in ArteFill, they are not permanent. Nevertheless, since fillers lasting 6 months and more have appeared, the filler market has approximately trebled. Radiesse treatments can last over a year and clinically Radiesse induces more fibroplasia than Artecoll.

Sculptra, or Poly-L-Lactic acid is injected in a dilute aqueous suspension and has been approved by the FDA for the amelioration of HIV related facial lipoatrophy but is approved for cosmetic indications in Canada and Europe. The same concept- of using a safe particulate product to stimulate neocollagenesis underlies its effectiveness. Several staged treatments are used and the effect is based on new collagen formation in both the dermis and the subcutaneous space. Thus subjects with dramatic thinning of facial skin as well as volume loss may receive a combined benefit.

Microdroplet medical grade 1000 centistoke viscosity silicone oil has lately undergone a "rehabilitation" in that it is now recognized that the autoimmune problems related to the use of silicone oil were no commoner in the silicone treated population than the non-silicone treated group. The Orentreich microdroplet technique makes it one of the safest of the neocollagenesis fillers although large volume "lake" injections are associated with a greater likelihood of migration and of granuloma formation. Much work has been done on the use of this exciting product to restore normal facial contours in individuals suffering from HIV related facial lipoatrophy; in Canada and the U.S. it is legal to use this product as an off-label indication except in Nevada.

We believe that use of these collagen-stimulating fillers will continue to increase as we understand them better.

A FILLERS WORKING BY FIBROPLASIA: ARTEFILL

Polymethylmethacrylate Microspheres in a Suspension of Atelomeric Bovine Collagen

Alastair Carruthers, Jean Carruthers

ArteFill (Artes Medical Inc., San Diego, CA) is the latest generation of the Artecoll used in Canada and Europe for over 8 and 12 years, respectively. It is a suspension of polymethylmethacrylate (PMMA) microspheres of 32–40 µm diameter in a 3.5% bovine collagen delivery vehicle, containing 0.3% lidocaine (Lemperle 2003). After implantation, the collagen solution slowly dissipates, leaving behind the nonbiodegradable PMMA microspheres that induce fibroplasia and become encapsulated by endogenous collagen. With its October 2006 FDA approval, ArteFill will be the only permanent filler approved for use in the United States for facial use.

ArteFill is injected into the immediate subdermis or at the deepest dermal level and thus targets deeper folds and rhytides. Applied by a skilled clinician, ArteFill is a powerful and effective filling agent that yields excellent results and does not require repeated touch-up treatments. However, its permanence demands that great care be taken in choosing the appropriate patients who are comfortable with the risks associated with the injection of permanent materials. Usually at least two to three injection sessions spaced several weeks to months apart are required. Since the product is permanent, it is important to select patients carefully and treat cautiously; partial correction, followed by re-injection after a few months, will produce a smoother, more natural appearance than initial overcorrection. Because of the collagen component, skin testing is required prior to injection.

CLINICAL EFFICACY

According to Lemperle et al, ArteFill has many advantages in the cosmetic field, including indications similar to those of collagen and hyaluronic acid, ease of injection, permanent stimulation of connective tissue and collagen deposition, and a long-lasting esthetic effect. Furthermore, since 1994, ArteFill has been used to fill horizontal forehead lines, glabellar rhytides, nasolabial folds (NLFs), perioral lip lines, and acne scars, and to sculpt the face in an estimated 200,000 patients with a high level of patient satisfaction (with optimal results achieved approximately 3 months post treatment). Although ArteFill has been used in Europe and Canada for lip augmentation, the FDA advisory panel recommended this region not be treated.

Despite the learning curve of injection technique associated with the injection of PMMA microspheres, some consider ArteFill superior to collagen for the treatment of a number of facial areas (Thaler 2005). In a randomized, multicenter FDA study of 251 patients who received ArteFill or collagen (Zyderm II or Zyplast; INAMED Aesthetics, Santa Barbara, CA) for the treatment of NLFs, glabellar rhytides, radial upper lip lines, and mouth corners, wrinkles treated with ArteFill improved significantly versus collagen at 3 and 6 months, as measured by the masked-observer Facial Fold Assessment Scale (FFAS) (Cohen and Holmes 2004). In addition, patient satisfaction ratings were higher in the ArteFill group ($P < 0.001$). At 3 months post-treatment, ArteFill was superior to collagen for NLFs ($P < 0.001$), mouth corners ($P = 0.001$), and overall cosmetic result ($P < 0.001$); at 6 months, results in the ArteFill group remained significantly better than collagen for NLFs ($P < 0.001$) and overall results ($P < 0.001$). In the ArteFill group, 12-month follow-up was obtained for 111 subjects (86.7%) and showed persistence of significant wrinkle correction in all treatment areas and for overall results. Cohen et al (2006) found in a subgroup of 69 patients who received ArteFill and was recalled 4–5 years later, investigator FFAS ratings at 4–5 years were improved from baseline by 1.67 points ($P < 0.001$).

COMPLICATIONS

The first clinical trials using PMMA microspheres (Arteplast) began in 1989; Lemperle et al reported that of 587 patients using Arteplast, 2.5% developed granulomas subsequently treated with intralesional corticosteroids or surgically excised. Early granulomatous reactions have been blamed on electrostatic charges; after improvements and purification of the microspheres in 1994, the rate of granulomas associated with the second generation

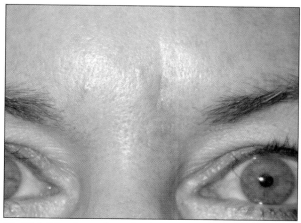

Fig. 7A.1 Artecoll granuloma showing erythema and induration in the glabella

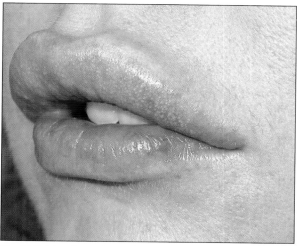

Fig. 7A.2 Artecoll granuloma of the upper lip presenting 4 years after 4 injection sessions of ArteFill

(Artecoll), was reported to be less than 0.01% in over 200,000 patients. According to Gelfer et al, additional refinement of ArteFill is expected to further decrease the incidence of granulomas.

Granulomas have been reported long after injection, though most respond, albeit slowly, to intralesional triamcinolone injections according to Alcalay et al, Saylan, and Conejo-Mir et al. Other treatment modalities given in Gelfer et al include the use of anti-mitotic agents, systemic allopurinol and corticosteroids, oral antibiotics, and nonsteroidal anti-inflammatories. The authors have documented ten cases of true granuloma formation over a period of 8 years treated with a variety of modalities reported by Carruthers and Carruthers, and Gelfer et al; the subsequent eventual resolution of many of their cases led to a hypothesis by Gelfer that some occurrences of granuloma may resolve spontaneously and do not require any treatment (Fig. 7A.1). However, subjects usually demand treatment; a conservative and supportive approach is recommended (Figs 7A.2 and 7A.3). Aggressive use of intralesional corticosteroids can cause significant atrophy and erythema and is not recommended.

Other complications as reported by Saylan include nodule formation, beading, and ridging causing disfigurement reversible only by surgical excision. Beading, palpability, and visibility of the implant has occurred with lip injections. In the FDA trial of 251 patients who received ArteFill or collagen, adverse events (redness, swelling, and injection site lumpiness) were more common among those treated with collagen (38 events compared to 27 in the ArteFill group), and no granulomas were reported in the group of patients who received ArteFill according to Cohen (2004). In the follow-up trial, also reported by Cohen (2006) of 69 patients 4–5 years later, five patients reported six late adverse events that occurred from 2–5 years after the initial injection. Four of the adverse events were mild cases of lumpiness and two were severe (a

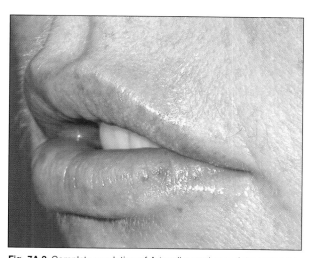

Fig. 7A.3 Complete resolution of Artecoll granuloma of the upper lip 1 year after conservative therapy with intralesional triamcinolone

nodular, minimally inflammatory to noninflammatory reaction in both NLFs).

Some clinicians feel that most adverse effects are due to poor technique or patient selection. Pollack emphasizes the steep learning curve and recommends a conservative approach, using small amounts of the filler and a long interval between injections. Lumpiness usually results from overenthusiastic use of the filler to produce immediate and complete correction, rather than the slow, careful approach. Patient selection is of utmost importance. The best candidates are those with well-defined wrinkles and furrows and little dermatochalasis and elastosis; patients with thick sebaceous skin and large pore size or extremely thin and loose skin may be poor candidates. Moreover, successful treatment with ArteFill requires careful technique, with injection into the upper levels of the subdermis. Intradermal placement can result in beading or ridging, while injection into the muscle can lead to nodule formation. In the experience of the authors, a minor degree of beading is common with lip injections, and this can be reduced by injection of botulinum toxin type A into the orbicularis oris prior to ArteFill treatment. Injections should be avoided in areas of thin skin, such as the lower eyelid and neck, or for crow's feet (except single crow's feet in patients with thick skin).

FURTHER READING

Alcalay J, Alkalay R, Gat A, Yorav S 2003 Late-onset granulomatous reaction to Artecoll. Dermatologic Surgery 29:859–862

Carruthers A, Carruthers JD 2005 Polymethylmethacrylate microspheres/collagen as a tissue augmenting agent: personal experience over 5 years. Dermatologic Surgery 31:1561–1564

Cohen SR, Holmes RE 2004 Artecoll: a long-lasting injectable wrinkle filler material: Report of a controlled, randomized, multicenter clinical trial of 251 subjects. Plastic and Reconstructive Surgery 15:964–976

Cohen SR, Berner CF, Busso M, et al 2006 ArteFill: A long-lasting injectable wrinkle filler material – summary of the US Food and Drug Administration trials and a progress report on 4- to 5-year outcomes. Plastic and Reconstructive Surgery 118(3 Suppl):64S–76S

Conejo-Mir JS, Sanz Guirado S, Angel Munoz M 2006 Adverse granulomatous reaction to Artecoll treated by intralesional 5-fluorouracil and triamcinolone injections. Dermatologic Surgery 32:1079–1081

Gelfer A, Carruthers A, Carruthers J, et al 2007 The natural history of polymethylmethacrylate microspheres granulomas. Dermatologic Surgery 33:614–620

Lemperle G, Romano JJ, Busso M 2003 Soft tissue augmentation with Artecoll: 10-year history, indications, techniques, and complications. Dermatologic Surgery 29:573–587

Pollack S 1999 Some new injectable dermal filler materials: Hylaform, Restylane, and Artecoll. Journal of Cutaneous Medicine and Surgery 3(Suppl 4):S27–S35

Saylan Z 2003 Facial fillers and their complications. Aesthetic Surgery Journal 23:221–224

Thaler MP, Ubogy ZI 2005 Artecoll: The Arizona experience and lessons learned. Dermatologic Surgery 31:1566–1574

B FILLERS WORKING BY FIBROPLASIA: RADIESSE

Calcium Hydroxyapatite Microspheres Suspended in Carboxy Methyl Cellulose Vehicle

Jean Carruthers, Alastair Carruthers

INTRODUCTION

Synthetic calcium hydroxylapatite (CaHA; Radiance FN, Radiesse; BioForm Inc., Franksville, WI) is a high-density, low-solubility bioceramic compound suspended in an aqueous gel carrier. After injection, the gel is absorbed and replaced with surrounding tissue structure, forming a long-lasting implant composed of CaHA and natural tissue. Previously used for facial reconstruction, radiologic procedures, stress urinary incontinence, and vocal cord problems, CaHA demonstrates an excellent safety profile and biocompatibility record according to Flaharty and White, and Sklar, and appears to provide long-lasting improvement with a high level of patient satisfaction. Unlike other fillers, CaHA does not require overcorrection, but since the matrix of material acquires characteristics of the cells that populate it after injection, precise placement of the filler is required in order for the permanent correction to occur. Skin testing is not necessary prior to use.

CLINICAL EFFICACY IN FACIAL REJUVENATION

Facial rejuvenation with CaHA appears to be well-tolerated and effective in softening facial folds, filling depressed scars, and adding soft-tissue volume according to Flaharty (Fig. 7B.1), particularly in patients with HIV-related facial lipoatrophy, report Comite and Liu, and Silvers et al (Fig. 7B.2). In a study of 64 patients treated with CaHA over a 6-month period in various facial areas, all patients showed clinical improvement with high patient satisfaction, minimal and mild side effects, such as bruising or swelling, and a low incidence of lip nodules and tear-trough overcorrection (Sklar and White 2004). Effects persisted in all patients at the 6-month follow-up visit. Tzikas et al studied 90 patients who received subdermal injections with CaHA in the lips, nasolabial folds (NLFs), glabellar rhytides, marionette lines, prejowl depressions, acne scars, and surgical soft-tissue defects; 88% of patients rated overall satisfaction as good or excel-

lent at 6 months. Common side effects included transient pain on injection, erythema, edema, and ecchymosis. Of seven patients who experienced persistent visible mucosal lip nodules, four required intervention. Likewise, Roy et al evaluated 82 patients injected with CaHA for soft-tissue augmentation of the face (primarily melolabial lines.) The average response to the look and feel of the implant was overwhelmingly positive (4.6 on a scale of 1–5) for both physicians and patients at 3 months, with similar responses at 6 months.

Although touted as a long-term filler, clinical experience has not been able to establish longevity of the implant as yet. CaHA shows clinical, histologic and electron microscopic evidence of persistence at 6 months as reported by Marmur et al, but evidence given by Goldberg et al, Jacovella et al, Jansen and Graivier, and Silvers et al suggests a possible duration of 12–24 months. A recent survey of 609 patients who received CaHA for NLFs, marionette lines, oral commissure, cheeks, chin, lips, and radial lip lines completed follow-up patient satisfaction surveys at 6 months and again between 12 and 24 months as reported by Jansen and Graivier. A total of 155 patients completed 6-month surveys, while 112 provided long-term 12- to 24-month data. Average satisfaction at 6 months was 3.94 on a five-point scale (1 = least satisfied; 5 = most satisfied) using subjective self-evaluation of preoperative photographs; 89% and 83% stated that they would use the product again at 6 and 12–24 months, respectively. Nodules were the only reported side effects, occurring in 12.4% of those treated for lip mucosa augmentation and 3.7% of patients treated for radial lip lines. The incidence of nodules decreased when the implant volume decreased. In another patient satisfaction survey, 87% of 40 patients treated with CaHA for glabellar lines, the lips, the nose, the face, and the infraorbital region rated their level of satisfaction as acceptable or better at 18 months. Minimal adverse effects were observed by Jacovella et al. In patients with HIV-related lipoatrophy, early reports suggested improvements of 75–90% and persistence for up to 9 months as stated by Comite et al; however, a more recent

Soft Tissue Augmentation

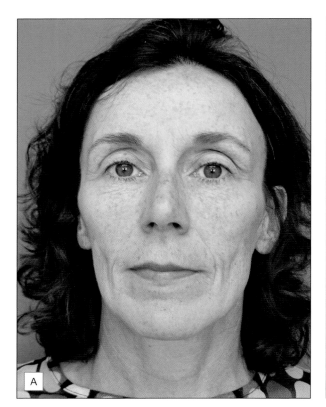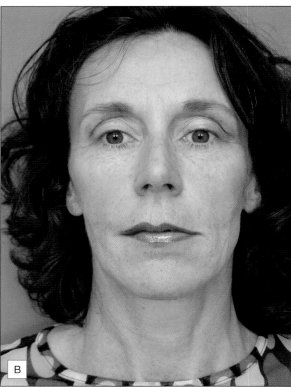

Fig. 7B.1 (**A**) Facial lipoatrophy in a healthy female marathon runner before treatment with 3 syringes of Radiesse. (**B**) Facial volume restoration immediately after treatment with subcutaneous Radiesse

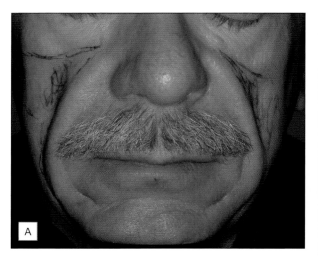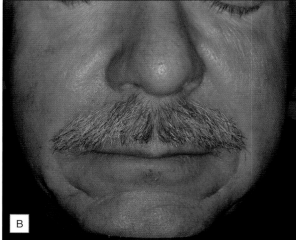

Fig. 7B.2 (**A**) Severe facial volume depletion due to HIV-related lipoatrophy before treatment. (**B**) Facial volume restoration in the same subject after 4 syringes in each cheek 8 × 1.3 cc = 10.4 cc volume total of Radiesse injected

long-term study reported in Silvers et al of 100 patients showed an impressive 91% of patients who were improved or better at 18 months following treatment.

COMPLICATIONS

Few data exist on potential complications or long-term safety of cosmetic CaHA. To date, there have been no reports of antibody formation or hypersensitivity. Erythema, edema, and ecchymosis are common but transient. Injection-related pain can be treated with acetaminophen. Injections should be placed deeply rather than superficially to avoid visible material. Nodule formation in the lips is the most commonly reported complication; some nodules will require treatment with either intralesional steroids or incision and drainage according to Gladstone and Morganroth, Sklar and White, and Tzikas. CaHA should not be used in its current formulation for lip augmentation; a newer formulation of this filler for this purpose is under current development.

REFERENCES

Comite SL, Liu JF, Balasubramanian S, Christian MA 2004 Treatment of HIV-associated facial lipoatrophy with Radiance FN (Radiesse). Dermatology Online Journal 10:2

Flaharty P 2004 Radiance. Facial Plastic Surgery 20:165–169

Gladstone HB, Morganroth GS 2003 Evaluating calcium hydroxylapatite for facial augmentation. Presented at the Annual American Society for Dermatologic Surgery Meeting. New Orleans, LA

Goldberg DJ, Amin S, Hussain M 2006 Acne scar correction using calcium hydroxylapatite in a carrier-based gel. Journal of Cosmetic Laser Therapy 8:134–136

Jacovella PF, Peiretti CB, Cunille D, et al 2006 Long-lasting results with hydroxylapatite (Radiesse) facial filler. Plastic and Reconstructive Surgery 118(3 Suppl):15S–21S

Jansen DH, Graivier MH 2006 Evaluation of a calcium hydroxylapatite-based implant (Radiesse) for facial soft-tissue augmentation. Plastic and Reconstructive Surgery 118(3 Suppl):22S–30S

Marmur ES, Phelps R, Goldberg DJ 2004 Clinical, histologic and electron microscopic findings after injection of a calcium hydroxylapatite filler. Journal of Cosmetic Laser Therapy 6:223–226

Roy D, Sadick N, Mangat D 2006 Clinical trial of a novel filler material for soft tissue augmentation of the face containing synthetic calcium hydroxylapatite microspheres. Dermatol Surg 32:1134–1139

Sklar JA, White SM 2004 Radiance FN: A new soft tissue filler. Dermatologic Surgery 30:764–768

Silvers SL, Eviatar JA, Echavez MI, Pappas AL 2006 Prospective, open-label, 18-month trial of calcium hydroxylapatite (Radiesse) for facial soft-tissue augmentation in patients with human immunodeficiency virus-associated lipoatrophy: one-year durability. Plastic and Reconstructive Surgery 118(3 Suppl):34S–45S

Tzikas TL 2004 Evaluation of the Radiance FN soft tissue filler for facial soft tissue augmentation. Archives of Facial Plastic Surgery 6:234–239

C FILLERS WORKING BY FIBROPLASIA: SILICONE

Chad L. Prather, Derek H. Jones

INTRODUCTION

Liquid injectable silicone (LIS) is a permanent soft tissue-augmenting agent that may be employed for an array of cutaneous and subcutaneous atrophies. When appropriately administered with the microdroplet serial puncture technique, LIS demonstrates superiority over temporary fillers in meeting several of the criteria that would define the 'ideal filler', including versatility, consistency of results, natural feel, and superb cost-to-benefit ratio. Patients may obtain enduring correction of scars, rhytids, and depressions, as well as lasting augmentation of lips and other facial contour atrophies and deformities with LIS.

Yet silicone is also one of the least forgiving fillers. Experience and precise technique are required in order to achieve favorable outcomes. For this reason, LIS should only be used by physicians with extensive training, and in patients with clear treatment goals and sufficient insight into the expected course of gradual augmentation over multiple treatment sessions. Those patients who are uncertain of treatment aims, desire immediate correction, or seek trial augmentation are best treated with temporary fillers rather than LIS.

BASIC SCIENCE

'Silicone' (SI) describes the family of synthetic polymers containing elemental silicon (Si). Individual polymers exist in solid, liquid, or gel states and display varied chemical, physical, mechanical, and thermal properties. Manufactured silicone products also differ in purity, sterility, and biocompatibility. Polydimethylsiloxane is the liquid injectable silicone used for soft tissue augmentation. It exists as an odorless, colorless, nonvolatile oil, with a molecular structure consisting of repeating dimethylsiloxane units bounded by terminal trimethylsiloxane units (Fig. 7C.1).

LIS viscosity is a function of dimethylsiloxane chain length and is measured in centistokes (cs), with 1 cs equal to the viscosity of water. Commercial LIS products intended for human injection are formulated to a known viscosity based upon the mean chain length, with longer chains comprising more viscous products. LIS viscosity remains stable after implantation and does not change at human body temperatures.

Silicone's mechanism of augmentation results from a combination of displacement of dermal and subcutaneous connective tissue (Fig. 7C.2) and stimulation of collagen formation around the implanted microdroplets. A local inflammatory reaction, consisting of an early neutrophilic infiltrate, and later macrophage phagocytosis eventuate in tissue fibroplasia (Fig. 7C.3). Ultimately, a thin-walled collagen capsule surrounds and contains the microdroplet of silicone. LIS is not altered in vivo but may enter the reticuloendothelial system through phagocytosis. Migration to other areas of the body may also occur when large volumes of liquid silicone are injected, but such 'drift' has never been reported using small volumes of pure liquid silicone, as with the microdroplet serial puncture technique.

HISTORY

Prior to FDA approval of bovine collagen in 1981, liquid silicones were the injectable filler of choice due to ease of use, natural texture, and long-lasting results. However, as anecdotal reports of granuloma formation and migration mounted, liquid silicone gradually decreased in popularity. It reached its nadir in the early 1990s, when the FDA banned all forms of silicone for the purpose of cosmetic implantation due to concerns over possible toxicity and systemic reactions in patients with silicone breast implants.

Yet legal use of injectable LIS was restored in 1997 after the FDA approved Silikon-1000 (Alcon, Fort Worth, TX) for intraocular treatment of retinal detachment in tandem with passage of the FDA Modernization Act, which granted physicians the right to employ authorized medical devices in an 'off-label' manner. The FDA has since further clarified that 'off-label' injection of FDA-

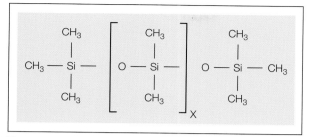

Fig. 7C.1 Linear molecular structure of polydimethylsiloxane. Repeating dimethylsiloxane units are flanked by terminal trimethylsiloxane units

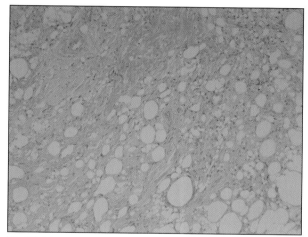

Fig. 7C.2 Histology of silicone at 3 months, showing the small droplets, which manifest as clear spaces after processing, interspersed between collagen bundles in the deep dermis. (Courtesy of Drs Sol Balkin and W. Dean Wallace)

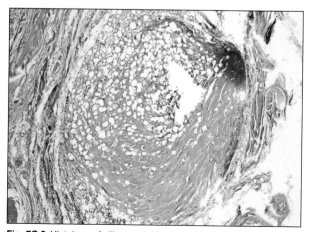

Fig. 7C.3 Histology of silicone at 19 years, showing round to oval spaces surrounded by dense fibrosis. (Courtesy of Drs Sol W. Balkin and W. Dean Wallace)

approved LIS products for soft tissue augmentation is legal if it is based on the unique needs of an individual patient and is not marketed or advertised for that purpose. In 2001 and 2003, the FDA approved clinical studies of SilSkin (Richard James Development Corp., Peabody, MA), an injectable, highly purified 1000 cs oil intended for soft tissue augmentation, for limited investigational study in the cosmetic improvement of nasolabial folds (NLFs), labiomental folds, mid-malar depressions, and HIV-associated lipoatrophy. These studies are currently ongoing.

CONTROVERSY AND LONG-TERM DISPOSITION

The last three decades have seen much debate in the literature regarding the safety and risks of LIS for soft tissue augmentation, with both critics and advocates largely citing anecdotal data rather than rigorous, controlled trials. However, for the past 5 years, multicenter investigational studies examining its efficacy and benefits have been underway. These studies, combined with several recently published series by authors with extensive use, are beginning to provide important, objective data and a clearer picture of the true risks of augmentation with LIS performed in a standardized and precautious manner.

Critics maintain that LIS is an intrinsically unpredictable implant, and cite several anecdotal reports of complications such as cellulitis, inflammatory nodules, granulomatous reactions, and product migration, though without substantiation of product purity or appropriate injection volume and technique in the published cases. On the other hand, proponents with extensive experience with LIS for soft tissue augmentation maintain that LIS is extremely safe, with minimal complications when used appropriately. Advocates stress the imperative need to adhere to the following three tenets when injecting LIS: (1) only pure, medical-grade LIS, approved by the FDA for injection into the human body should be utilized; (2) the microdroplet serial puncture technique must be rigorously adhered to; and (3) a timeline with limited per-session injection volumes and adequate spacing between treatment sessions must be observed. Deviation from these guidelines may significantly increase the risk of complications.

Several authors have recently reported of their excellent records of safety with prolonged use of LIS. Balkin reported his use of LIS as a soft tissue substitute for the loss of plantar fat in over 1500 patients, with 25,000 recorded silicone injections over 41 years. Long-term follow-up found that, even after long-term implantation, the host response to injections consisted of a 'banal and stable fibrous tissue formation'. Advocates such as Orentreich, Carruthers, and Jones have also published multiple reports of their extensive and successful experience with LIS, and reiterate that the three principles of product purity, appropriate technique, and proper protocol are imperative for success. Duffy, who has written extensively on the subject, gathers that LIS has been used for soft tissue augmentation worldwide for at least 40 years, and in at least 200,000 patients in the United States. He also pragmatically cautions that, while pure LIS may be a superior filler for the permanent correction of certain defects, physicians who use it must realize that its misuse, or the use of other materials masquerading as LIS, have created 'a pervasive climate of distrust and a veritable minefield of extraordinarily unpleasant medicolegal possibilities'. Such perceptions reiterate the importance of ongoing trials as they replace anecdotal reports with rigorously controlled data.

PATIENT SELECTION

Liquid injectable silicone is efficacious for tissue augmentation of NLFs, labiomental folds, mid-malar depressions, post-surgical defects and depressions, hemi-facial atrophy, lip atrophy, acne or other atrophic scarring, age-related atrophy of the hands, corns and calluses of the feet, healed diabetic neuropathic foot ulcers, and HIV or age-related facial lipoatrophy. LIS is contraindicated in those seeking augmentation of the breast, eyelids, or bound-down scars, and its safety has not been studied in pregnant women. The ideal patient is one with appropriate insight into the permanent and off-label nature of LIS, a realistic attitude regarding achievable results, in good physical health, and compliant with recommendations. Additionally, LIS is not meant to replace surgical re-draping, chemical or mechanical resurfacing, or 'relaxing' of dynamic rhytids with botulinum toxin.

BENEFITS

• Rhytids

LIS is considered an excellent tissue augmenting agent for the correction of several types of age-related rhytids, including NLFs, labiomental folds, and mid-malar depressions (Fig. 7C.4). An augmentative improvement of 30–90% may be expected with LIS, dependent upon the depth of original depression. However, in the authors' view, widespread use of LIS for this purpose should be reserved until long-term safety is demonstrated through clinical trials with the modern silicone products.

• Acne scarring

LIS is the only filler that achieves both immediate precision and permanence in improving broad-based, depressed acne scars. Barnett et al described LIS treatment of five patients with acne scarring who showed improvements at the initial treatment session that persisted over a 10-, 15-, and 30-year follow-up period (Figs 7C.5 and 7C.6). Additionally, he reported his 30-year experience in treating a few thousand patients for different types of acne scars, with no significant adverse reactions and fewer than

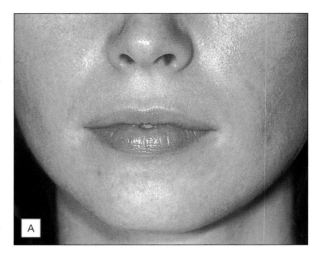

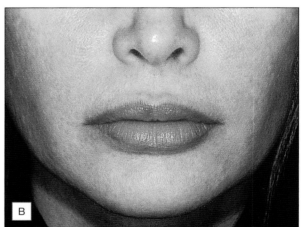

Fig. 7C.4 (**A**) Patient pre-treatment 1990. Patient was seen at 28 years of age with the earliest stages of NLFs. (**B**) Patient post-treatment (maintenance) 2004; 14 years later, NFL formation is absent at age 42. Improvement in both NLFs and lips has been maintained

10 having areas of overcorrection necessitating minor surgical correction (shave excision, light electrosurgery, or injections of low-concentration corticosteroid).

• HIV-associated lipoatrophy

The psychological effects of HIV-associated lipoatrophy may be devastating, with patients experiencing poor body image, low self-esteem, depression, social isolation, and career barriers. The permanence, natural feel, and low cost of LIS make it an ideal filler for correction of this potentially stigmatizing condition (Figs 7C.7 and 7C.8). Limited investigational study using SilSkin or Silikon-1000 for correction of HIV lipoatrophy is currently

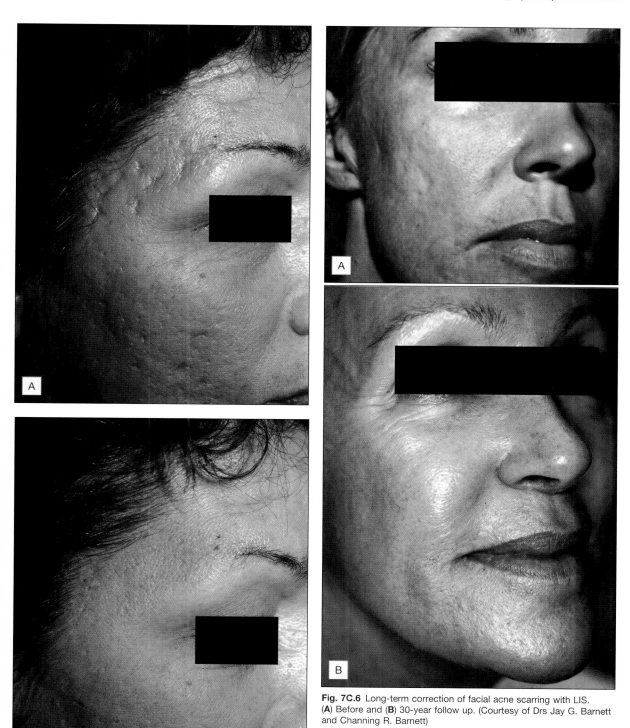

Fig. 7C.5 Immediate correction of facial acne scarring with LIS. (**A**) Before and (**B**) 10 minutes after treatment. (Courtesy of Drs Jay G. Barnett and Channing R. Barnett)

Fig. 7C.6 Long-term correction of facial acne scarring with LIS. (**A**) Before and (**B**) 30-year follow up. (Courtesy of Drs Jay G. Barnett and Channing R. Barnett)

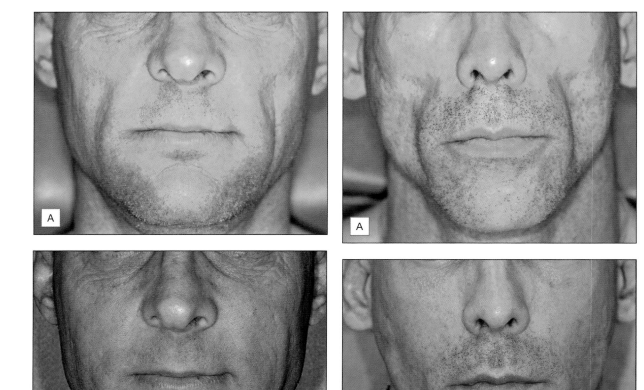

Fig. 7C.7 Improvement of Grade 1 HIV-associated lipoatrophy. **(A)** Before and **(B)** after two treatments (5.5 mL total)

Fig. 7C.8 Improvement of Grade 3 HIV-associated lipoatrophy. **(A)** Before and **(B)** after eight treatments (17 mL total)

underway, and over 1200 patients have been treated during the past 5 years. In one author's (DJ) experience treating over 600 patients, all have done well to date, without reports of adverse events beyond those transient and typically associated with any injection. In a recent report, data on 77 subjects with HIV lipoatrophy treated with LIS were analyzed to determine the number of treatments, the amount of silicone, and the time required to reach complete correction relative to initial severity. Each of these factors was found to be directly related to the initial severity of the lipoatrophy ($P < 0.0001$), as determined by the Carruthers' Facial Lipoatrophy Severity Scale (Fig. 7C.9). Supple, symmetrical facial contours were routinely restored, with all patients tolerating treatments well. No adverse events were noted.

INSTRUMENTATION

The preferred silicone for soft tissue augmentation in the United States is Silikon-1000, yet the more viscous Adatosil-5000 is also suitable. The silicone oil is drawn using sterile technique through a 16 gauge Nokor needle into a BD 1 cc Luer-Lok syringe to the 0.5 cc mark to allow for superior control of the plunger. Owing to the theoretical risk of contamination from the rubber stopper of the syringe after a long exposure period, LIS should be drawn into the injecting syringe immediately prior to treatment and never stored in the syringe. LIS is easily injected through a metal hub 27 gauge needle. The BD 3/10 cc insulin syringe may also be used for injection of LIS, but such syringes must be backloaded.

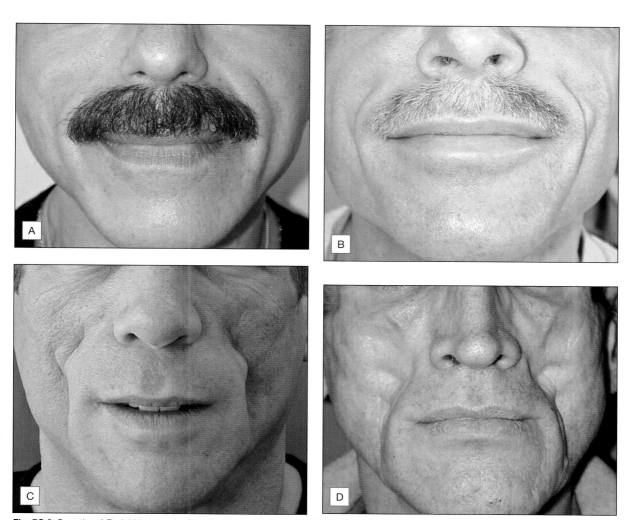

Fig. 7C.9 Carruthers' Facial Lipoatrophy Severity Scale. **(A)** Grade 1 is defined by mild, focal involvement, almost normal in appearance. **(B)** Grade 2, with deeper involvement, central cheek atrophy, and slight show of facial musculature. **(C)** Grade 3, even deeper and wider atrophy with prominent show of underlying facial musculature. **(D)** Grade 4, with extensive atrophy extending toward the orbit and facial contour over a wide area defined by the musculature. (Courtesy of Dr Carruthers)

PATIENT PREPARATION

Aspirin, nonsteroidal anti-inflammatory preparations, and anticoagulants should be avoided for 7–10 days prior to treatment. Written informed consent regarding risks, alternatives, LIS permanence, and the off-label nature of treatment must be obtained. Additionally, high-resolution pre-treatment photographs should be taken.

Make-up, if present, must be thoroughly removed to avoid implantation during injection. Next, the skin is thoroughly cleansed with an antibacterial cleanser and prepped with an iodine swab. With the patient seated under adequate procedural lighting, a marker is used to delineate areas to be treated. Precise marking is imperative in order to obtain appropriate correction, and this should be done

in both the smiling and resting facial positions (Fig. 7C.10). Marked areas are then anesthetized with topical lidocaine for 30 minutes under occlusion.

TECHNIQUE

In contrast to temporary fillers, where multiple injection techniques may be employed, LIS should only be injected by the microdroplet serial puncture technique, as described by Orentreich. Any other technique invites undesirable consequences, including pooling or beading of silicone in the injection tract, as well as the aforementioned problems of capsular escape and migration associated with macrodroplets of product.

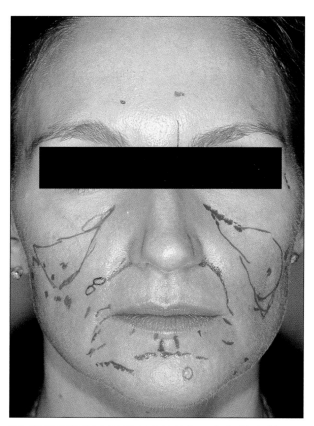

Fig. 7C.10 Typical pre-injection markings for patient with rhytides, depressions, and scarring

Table 7C.1 Microdroplet surface area curve

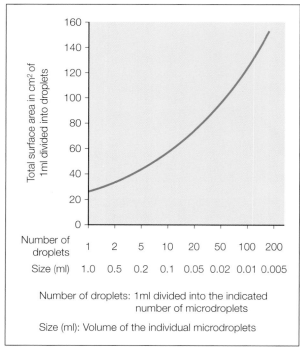

Number of droplets	1	2	5	10	20	50	100	200
Size (ml)	1.0	0.5	0.2	0.1	0.05	0.02	0.01	0.005

Number of droplets: 1ml divided into the indicated number of microdroplets

Size (ml): Volume of the individual microdroplets

The needle is inserted into the skin at intervals of 2–5 mm at the appropriate angle for optimal penetration and deposition into the subdermal plane. The angle of insertion varies with anatomic area: a more oblique (approaching perpendicular) angle should be used for areas of greater depth such as the lip or cheek, while a relatively acute (approaching parallel to the skin) angle is best for more superficial deposition over bony or vascular structures. Microdroplet injections of 0.005–0.01 mL should be placed into the immediate subdermal plane or deeper. The subdermal plane is usually about 5 mm beneath the skin surface, but varies according to skin thickness. To help prevent dermal tracking of LIS, the thumb should be removed from the plunger when inserting and withdrawing the needle. Except in the most experienced hands, intradermal injection should be avoided, as this may result in an undesirable 'beading' effect, particularly over bony structures such as on the forehead. Occasionally, however, controlled mid-dermal injection may produce the desired augmentative result, such as in certain acne scars and rhytids that lack dermal thickness.

The total volume and per session volume of LIS is dependent upon both the area to be treated and the desired level of correction. Per-session volumes should be limited to 0.5 cc for smaller areas such as the NLF, and no more than 2.0 cc for larger areas such as with facial lipoatrophy. Importantly, greater correction should be accomplished over a longer period of time rather than with a larger per-session volume. As a rule, double passes over the same treatment areas should be avoided. However, more experienced injectors may rarely treat with a second pass at a different subcutaneous level in order to build volume more quickly. As treatment endpoint approaches, the volume injected per visit will diminish, and the interval between treatments will lengthen until the final result is achieved.

Unlike with many temporary fillers, intentional overcorrection is to be avoided. Rather, under-correction with augmentation by serial treatment and gradual fibroplasia is the goal. Fibroplasia occurs on the surface of LIS microdroplets, and the amount of new collagen formed is directly proportional to the total surface area of the injected microdroplet implants (Table 7C.1). Since a given volume of LIS dispersed into many microdroplets provides a larger total surface area than would be provided by fewer, larger droplets, augmentation is greater with the microdroplet technique. More importantly, the microdroplet particles effectively eliminate product migration by stimulation of a collagen capsule capable of 'anchoring' the

---

Box 7C.1 Technique pearls for different esthetic regions

Premise: The mechanism of action of LIS as an augmenting agent is wholly different from that of most other fillers. Those accustomed to using temporary fillers may initially find the MDT counterintuitive and cumbersome. Comfort with the MDT will come with strict adherence to the technique and with time.

1. Exercise particular care in marking. NL folds are marked, usually wider at the nose, and injected in a random zigzag pattern to avoid repeating the same injection sites on future visits. Employ random placement of needle punctures while adhering to the 2–4 mm rule
2. Carefully blot topical anesthetic off skin to preserve original markings
3. Skin may be stretched to facilitate needle entry, or pinched to hold it away from underlying structures
4. Lips are usually injected at the 'wet line'. Finger pressure on the skin adjacent to the vermilion border will evert the wet line. Needle is perpendicular to lip surface
5. Be aware of bevel orientation, particularly when angle of injection is acute
6. Neck – stretch skin to facilitate needle entry. Bevel down, 45° angle (md ≤0.005 mL)
7. Periorbital lines (crow's feet) – very acute angle (~30°). Only the lightest touch on the plunger, i.e. ml ≤0.005 mL

---

microdroplet in place. With larger macrodroplets (>0.01 mL), the fibroplastic collagen to LIS ratio may not achieve adequate encapsulation to prevent the migration of silicone.

TREATMENT PROTOCOL

Treatment sessions are typically spaced 1 month apart in the early stages of treatment. Shorter intervals should only be used if different areas are being treated. While longer intervals pose no problem, augmentation will proceed at a slower rate. As final treatment goal approaches, longer intervals on the order of 2–6 months are appropriate to avoid overcorrection.

PEARLS (BOX 7C.1)

SIDE EFFECTS AND COMPLICATIONS

COMMON

Edema may result from the trauma of needle insertion, although it is typically milder than that seen with other injections and resolves within several hours to days. Edema itself can produce temporary correction of defects, and this confounding effect must be taken into account when judging cosmetic improvement. **Ecchymosis** may also occasionally occur due to needle puncture, vascularity of the underlying tissue, or the surface anticoagulant property of LIS. If anticoagulants were not discontinued prior to treatment, prolonged manual pressure is recommended in order to reduce the incidence and extent of ecchymosis.

Camouflaging make-up may be applied to areas of bruising immediately after treatment.

RARE

Moderate **erythema** of a few hours' duration may occur after injection, particularly in those with a history of urticaria. Rarely, persistent erythema may result from either impure materials or too superficial an injection. Topical or intradermal corticosteroids and pulsed-dye laser may help resolve persistent erythema. Brownish-yellow or bluish **discoloration** may also result from superficial injection or injection of impure material. Careful written and photographic documentation of pre-treatment dyschromia is recommended.

Overcorrection due to an excessive volume injected in one or several sessions violates a fundamental principle of the microdroplet technique. With intervals of 1 month or more between treatments, overcorrection of deeper tissues is rare. When present, overcorrection usually occurs as diffuse enlargement of the treated area.

'**Beading**' is the term used to describe small 1–5 mm firm papules that form at sites of injection due to fibroplastic collagen deposition around superficially implanted silicone. Such papules are not granulomas. Beading may rarely occur even after precautions are taken to avoid superficial injection. In some cases, beading is temporary and resolves without treatment over several months. Both beading and overcorrection may be treated with intralesional corticosteroid injection, microelectrodessication, punch excision, dermabrasion, or tangential shave excision. With corticosteroid therapy, improvement may be temporary, with overcorrection returning after waning therapeutic benefit.

Care must be taken to avoid injection of any augmenting agent, including LIS, into the intravascular space. The authors have not observed any tissue ischemia due to vascular injury from LIS.

Granulomatous inflammatory reactions to injected 'silicone' have been called 'siliconomas', a misnomer because neither silicone nor macrophages that phagocytose silicone multiply in a tumoral fashion (-oma). Critical scrutiny of reports of granulomatous reactions reveal that these cases fall into several causal categories: cases of overinjection, injection into contraindicated sites, injection of impure material, and injection of substances of unknown chemical composition. It is important to note that in such reports, the presence of unadulterated LIS was never conclusively established. Such cases have responded favorably to a variety of modalities, including imiquimod, high-potency corticosteroids, and antibiotics. The use of reflexion electron microscopy (REM) and electron dispersing X-ray (EDX) have recently been described as tools that may help establish the presence of silicone in injections of unknown composition. While useful, it should be noted that such tools are still unable to determine the presence or absence of adulterants in specimens that prove to contain silicone.

IDIOSYNCRATIC

Very rarely, instances of local, isolated, inflammatory reaction have occurred with LIS in the practices of experienced injectors. These are estimated to be on the order of 1 per 5000–10,000 treatment sessions, and appear as well-demarcated areas of moderate swelling and variable erythema. They have been noted to appear months to years after injection and to involve a small percentage of the area treated in an individual patient. Histopathology has revealed a nonspecific chronic inflammatory infiltrate, and intradermal testing with LIS was invariably negative.

Interestingly, such reactions have been frequently preceded by an infection at a local or distant site, such as sinusitis, furunculosis, otitis, or a dental abscess. This has led to the theory that the inert LIS may serve as a nidus for infection, with organisms encountering the silicone microdroplets either by local extension or via the circulation. Once colonized on the implant surface, bacteria may convert from a planktonic to a biofilm state, which entails encasement in a polysaccharide matrix. Duffy has thoroughly described the possible consequences of such biofilms on the surface of permanent implants, including resistance to clearance by antibiotics, frequent recurrence of inflammatory complications, and delayed host response up to several years after implant. As with other permanent implants, evident and occult infections, even when distant, should be considered contraindications to LIS implantation.

Such reactions have responded within weeks to intralesional corticosteroid injection and oral antibiotics such as minocycline, and treatment was repeated until resolution was complete. Response to etanercept has also been reported.

Drift, or migration, is defined as the movement of product to a site distant from original implantation. Drift is known to occur when large volumes are injected into a single site during a single treatment session. However, migration does not occur with the microdroplet technique, as the collagenous capsule of fibroplasia effectively anchors the microdroplet into place.

TROUBLESHOOTING

(See Table 7C.2)

CONCLUSION

LIS demonstrates a unique aptness for the correction of specific cutaneous and subcutaneous atrophies due to its versatility, permanence, excellent cost/benefit profile, and natural texture in vivo. Although it has been effectively employed for over 40 years, its use remains controversial due to a history of reported complications, most of which are confounded by unknown or impure product or improper technique. However, evidence continues to mount, demonstrating that modern silicone oils approved by the FDA for injection into the human body may be successfully used off-label, with a very low complication rate, when rigorously injected according to strict protocol, which includes using the microdroplet serial puncture technique with limited per-session quantities and adequately spaced treatment sessions. While the safety profile of newer LIS products should continue to be evaluated in long-term studies before the widespread, routine injection of LIS occurs, these are currently underway for the correction of HIV-associated lipoatrophy and for the improvement of NLFs, labiomental folds, and mid-malar depressions. As the armamentarium of subcutaneous and dermal fillers expands, LIS retains a unique position due to its permanence, and continued investigational study is warranted.

Table 7C.2 Troubleshooting	
Problem	**Possible causes**
Treatment progressing slowly	Injecting too deeply?
	Inadequate total volume/treatment?
Patient claims LIS is 'drifting'	Assuming use of MDT, point out facial redundancies prior to treatment to ensure that pre-existing redundancies are not erroneously attributed to LIS migration
Beading	Injection too superficially, or check if thumb is on plunger while inserting or withdrawing plunger. Treat with electrodesiccation
Dyschromia	Very superficial injection, usually into atrophic scars, which lack adnexal structures
Ecchymosis	Apply finger pressure to skin immediately after withdrawing syringe, discontinue use of anticoagulants prior to treatment when possible
Transient edema	Expected. Resolves over the course of several days

FURTHER READING

Alani RM, Busam K 2001 Acupuncture granulomas. Journal of the American Academy of Dermatology 45(6 Suppl):S225–S226

Ashley FL, Thompson DP, Henderson T 1973 Augmentation of surface contour by subcutaneous injections of silicone fluid: a current report. Plastic and Reconstructive Surgery 51:8–13

Assembly Bill 36, Ch. 82, Statutes of Nevada, 1975

Balkin SW 2005 Injectable silicone and the foot: a 41-year clinical and histologic history. Dermatologic Surgery 31:1555–1559

Barnett JG, Barnett CR 2005 Treatment of acne scars with liquid silicone injections: 30-year perspective. Dermatologic Surgery 31:1542–1549

Baselga E, Pujol R 1994 Indurated plaques and persistent ulcers in an HIV-1 seropositive man. Archives of Dermatology 130:785–786,788–789

Baumann LS, Halem ML 2003 Lip silicone granulomatous foreign body reaction treated with aldara (imiquimod 5%). Dermatologic Surgery 29:429–432

Benedetto AV, Lewis AT 2003 Injecting 1000 centistoke liquid silicone with ease and precision. Dermatologic Surgery 29:211–214

Blocksma R, Braley S 1973 Implantation materials. In: Grabb WC, Smith JW (eds) Plastic Surgery. 2nd edn. Little, Brown, & Co., Boston, pp 131

Bondurant S, Ernster V, Herdman R 1999 Institute of Health: National Academy of Medicine: Information for women about the safety of silicone breast implants. National Academy of Sciences, Institute of Medicine. Available at http://www.nap.edu/openbook/0309065321/html, accessed October 21, 2006

Brown LH, Frank PJ 2003 What's new in fillers? Journal of Drugs in Dermatology 2:250–253

Coleman S 2001 Injectable silicone returns to the United States. Aesthetic Surgery Journal 21:576–578

Collins E, Wagner C, Walmsley S 2000 Psychosocial impact of the lipodystrophy syndrome in HIV infection. AIDS Reader 10:546–551

Delage C, Shane JJ, Johnson FB 1973 Mammary silicone granuloma: Migration of silicone fluid to abdominal wall and inguinal region. Archives of Dermatology 108:105–107

Desai AM, Browning J, Rosen T 2006 Etanercept therapy for silicone granuloma. Journal of Drugs in Dermatology 5:894–896

Diamond B, Hulka B, Kerkvliet N, Tugwell P 1998 Summary of report of national science panel: silicone breast implants in relation to connective tissue diseases and immunologic dysfunction. Available at http://www.fjc.gov/BREIMLIT/SCIENCE/summary.htm, accessed September 2, 2006

Duffy DM 1998 Tissue injectable liquid silicone: new perspectives. In: Klein AW (ed.) Augmentation in clinical practice: procedures and techniques. Marcel Dekker, New York, pp 237–263

Duffy DM 2002 The silicone conundrum: a battle of anecdotes. Dermatologic Surgery 28:590

Duffy DM 2005 Liquid silicone for soft tissue augmentation. Dermatologic Surgery 31:1530–1541

Duffy DM 2006 Liquid silicone for soft tissue augmentation: histological, clinical, and molecular perspectives. In: Klein A (ed.) Tissue augmentation in clinical practice. 2nd edn. Taylor & Francis, New York, pp 141–237

Durst S, Johnson BS, Amplatz K 1974 The effect of silicone coatings on thrombogenicity. American Journal of Roentgenology, Radium Therapy, and Nuclear Medicine 120:904–906

Ellenbogen R, Rubin L 1975 Injectable fluid silicone therapy: human morbidity and mortality. Journal of the American Medical Association 234:308–309

Food and Drug Administration 1992 Physicians to stop injecting silicone for cosmetic treatment of wrinkles, Press Release P92–5. Available at http://www.fda.gov/bbs/topics/NEWS/NEW00267.html, accessed September 5, 2006

Fulton JE Jr, Porumb S, Caruso JC, Shitabata PK 2005 Lip augmentation with liquid silicone. Dermatologic Surgery 31:1577–1586

Jacinto SS 2005 Ten-year experience using injectable silicone oil for soft tissue augmentation in the Philippines. Dermatologic Surgery 31:1550–1554

James J, Carruthers A, Carruthers J 2002 HIV-associated facial lipoatrophy. Dermatologic Surgery 28:979–986

Jaques LB, Fidlar E, Feldsted ET et al 1946 Silcones and blood coagulation. Canadian Medical Association Journal 55:26

Jones DH 2002 Injectable silicone for facial lipoatrophy. Cosmetic Dermatology 15:13–15

Jones D 2002 Treatment of HIV facial lipoatrophy. Presented at the ASDS (American Society of Dermatologic Surgery)-ACMMSCO (American College of Mohs Micrographic Surgery and Cutaneous Oncology) Combined Annual Meeting; Oct 31–Nov 3; Chicago, IL

Jones D 2005 HIV facial lipoatrophy: causes and treatment options. Dermatologic Surgery 31:1519–1529

Jones DH, Carruthers A, Orentreich D, Brody HJ, Lai MY, Azen S, Van Dyke GS 2004 Highly purified 1000 centistoke oil for treatment of HIV-associated facial lipoatrophy. Dermatologic Surgery 30:1276–1286

Kagan HD 1963 Sakurai injectable silicone formula. Archives of Otolaryngology 78:663–668

Klein AW 2001 Skin filling: collagen and other injectables of the skin. Dermatologic Clinics 19:491–508

Kozeny GA, Barbato AL, Vertuno LL, et al 1984 Hypercalcemia associated with silicone-induced granulomas. New England Journal of Medicine 311:1103–1105

Lloret P, Espana A, Leache A, et al 2005 Successful treatment of granulomatous reactions secondary to injection of esthetic implants. Dermatologic Surgery 31:486–490

McDowell F 1978 Complications with silicones – what grade of silicone? How do we know it was silicone? [Editorial] Plastic and Reconstructive Surgery 61:892–895

Milojevic B 1982 Complications after silicone injection therapy in aesthetic plastic surgery. Aesthetic Plastic Surgery 6:203

Orentreich D, Leone AS 2004 A case of HIV-associated facial lipoatrophy treated with 1000-cs liquid injectable silicone. Dermatologic Surgery 30:548–551

Orentreich DS 2000 Liquid injectable silicone: techniques for soft tissue augmentation. Clinics in Plastic Surgery 27:595–612

Orentreich N, Durr NP 1985 The four R's of skin rehabilitation. In: Graham JAG, Kligman AM (eds) The Psychology of Cosmetic Treatments. Praeger, New York, pp 227

Parel JM 1989 Silicone oils: physiochemical properties. In: Glaser BM, Michels RG (eds) Retina. Vol. 3. Mosby, St Louis, pp 261–277

Pasternack FR, Fox LP, Engler DE 2005 Silicone granulomas treated with etanercept. Archives of Dermatology 141:13–15

Pearl RM, Laub DR, Kaplan EN 1978 Complications following silicone injections for augmentation of the contours of the face. Plastic and Reconstructive Surgery 61:888–891

Prather CL, Jones DH 2006 Liquid injectable silicone for soft tissue augmentation. Dermatologic Therapy 19:159–168

Price EA, Schueler H, Perper JA 2006 Massive systemic silicone embolism: a case report and review of literature. American Journal of Forensic Medicine and Pathology 27:97–102

Rapaport MJ, Vinnik C, Zarem H 1996 Injectable silicone: cause of facial nodules, cellulitis, ulceration, and migration. Aesthetic Plastic Surgery 20:267–276

Rapaport M 2002 Silicone injections revisited. Dermatologic Surgery 28:594–595

Selmanowitz VJ, Orentreich N 1977 Medical grade fluid silicone: a monographic review. Journal of Dermatologic and Surgical Oncology 3:597

Spanbauer JM 1997 Breast implants as beauty ritual: woman's sceptre and prison. Yale Journal of Law and Feminism 9:157–205

Spanoudis S, Koski G. Sci.polymers. Available at http://www.plasnet.com.au/plasnet5/11a_misc/poly-faq.html, accessed September 2, 2006

Wallace WD, Balkin SW, Kaplan L, Nelson SD 2004 The histological host response of liquid silicone injections for prevention of pressure-related ulcers of the foot: a 38-year study. Journal of the American Podiatric Medical Association 94:550–557

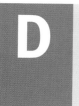

D FILLERS THAT WORK BY FIBROPLASIA: POLY-L-LACTIC ACID

Stephen H. Mandy

INTRODUCTION

Facial fat atrophy causes dramatic alteration in appearance and may result as a consequence of hereditary syndromes, disease or aging. In aging, it occurs as a part of a constellation that includes loss of elasticity, collagen degradation and bony reabsorption. This deflation due to volume loss results in further skin redundancy. Various classifications of lipoatrophy based upon anatomic considerations have been described by Ascher et al and Napdez and Park. Attempts at correction by tightening without addressing volume replacement results in a skeletonized appearance. Volume replacement has been accomplished by a wide variety of natural (fat, collagen, hyaluronic acid) and synthetic (acrylates, silicone and other polymers) fillers, both permanent and biodegradable. Poly-L-lactic acid (PLLA) represents a new family of fibroplastic fillers whose 'bulking effect' depends upon host response.

Injectable PLLA is a biocompatible, reabsorbable polymer that results in an intended foreign body inflammatory response, dermal fibroplasia and a slow metabolic degradation of the polymer microspheres as reported in Rotunda and Narins. Histological and clinical data given in Vleggaar and Vleggaar and Bauer suggests long-term effects, which may persist over 2 years (Figs. 7D.1 and 7D.2). Currently, PLLA is FDA-approved only for HIV-mediated lipoatrophy (as documented in Valantin et al), and all other applications are 'off-label', although double-blind clinical studies for cosmetic use are currently nearing completion. Numerous reports summarize the biological effects and treatment of lipoatrophy with PLLA (Rotunda and Narins).

PROCEDURE

Initially injectable PLLA was marketed in Europe as NewFill and was associated with a range of challenges that centered upon subcutaneous papules and nodules. According to Lowe, these most probably arose as the result of too concentrated a dilution, too large a volume of injec-tion, inappropriate areas for injection and injections that were too superficial. Originally the vial containing 150 mg of PLLA freeze-dried powder with excipients was diluted in 3 ml of sterile water. Current recommendations call for dilution with 5 ml or greater of dilutent. Many authors recommend 4 ml of sterile water or bacteriostatic saline and 1 ml of 2% lidocaine with epinephrine (which may reduce post-injection bruising). Some authors, including Vleggaar and Bauer, and Lam et al recommend greater dilutions (8–12 ml), in areas such as the hands and neck. The lyophilized powder should be reconstituted no less than 2 hours prior to injection, but most users now recommend 12–24 hours prior to use. Just before withdrawal from the vial PLLA needs to be vigorously shaken, and then again, in the syringe just prior to injection. Injection with a 1 cc luer-lok syringe and a 25 gauge 1 in needle affords excellent control. Smaller gauge needles are prone to blockage with the particulate material.

Topical anesthesia should be applied 20–30 minutes prior to treatment. Areas most frequently and successfully treated are the hollow of the cheek, nasolabial and prejowl folds, malar area, suborbital and temporal areas. The lips and nose are to be avoided. Unlike many 'immediate' fillers, PLLA is not injected directly into a fold to achieve correction, but rather in a matrix-like cross-hatching pattern (Fig. 7D.3). The pattern of injection is much like a scaffold or that of rebar in reinforced concrete, where an interlocking network is created as a foundation. PLLA is injected subcutaneously – not in the dermis – by means of a reverse threading technique, where the needle is passed at a 45-degree angle through the skin and then fully inserted in the subcutaneous plane parallel to the surface. The injection then places the PLLA upon withdrawal, usually in amounts of 0.1–0.2 cc per pass. In the temple and above the malar ridge it is injected in submuscular, small depot-like deposits of 0.05 ml. A fanning pattern of injection has been recommended by some, however, a single entry point for multiple passes increases the chance of too much material being deposited in a single area, leading to nodule formation. In the subocular hollow, a

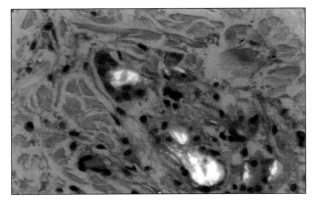

Fig. 7D.1 PLLA surrounded by histiocytes and macrophages

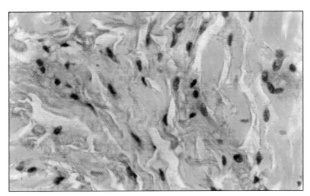

Fig. 7D.2 PLLA surrounded by new collagen

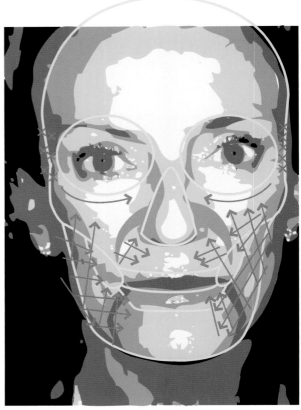

✕ = Depot technique   ↗ = Threading technique

Fig. 7D.3 Injection technique

successful technique for those comfortable injecting in the periorbital region is a reverse threading injection of small amounts (0.05–0.1 ml) beneath the orbicularis oculi and along the periosteum of the orbital rim (Fig. 7D.3).

Vigorous massage for 5 minutes to all injected areas immediately post-injection is important to assure proper dispersion in order to optimize results and avoid nodule formation. Patients should be instructed to massage daily for 1 week post treatment. The application of cold packs post injection is useful to limit bruising. Most patients require one vial per treatment session, and some, especially with significant lipoatrophy, require two vials. Injection sessions should be scheduled 4–6 weeks apart so that adequate time elapses to see volume enhancement. Three treatment sessions are often required to reach full correction.

RESULTS

Numerous reports, as published in Vleggaar, have indicated patient satisfaction in the range of 95%. Not only is volume replacement and duration excellent, but enhancement of skin texture and color are reported. Nonvisible subcutaneous papules are reported in approximately 3% of patients, and 30% of these resolved spontaneously in 3 months. As reported by Vleggaar, visible papules and nodules were seen in 1%, and rarely require intervention with subcision, intralesional saline or steroids (Figs 7D.4A–E). In rare instances, excision of a nodule may be prudent. Other adverse events, as with many injectables include edema and ecchymoses, and patients should be cautioned of this before injection. Avoidance of aspirin, NSAIDs and vitamin E prior to injection may be advisable.

A new off-label indication for the use of PLLA is as a pre-treatment of the deflated face prior to other modalities that might otherwise be unsuccessful because of the poor tissue quality or severe redundancy. This works especially well in conjunction with radiofrequency tightening, threadlifts and traditional face lifts when PLLA is injected in two or three sessions, at least several months previously (Fig. 7D.4C–E).

SUMMARY

Fibroplastic fillers represent a change in paradigm from previous direct fill agents used for volumetric restoration.

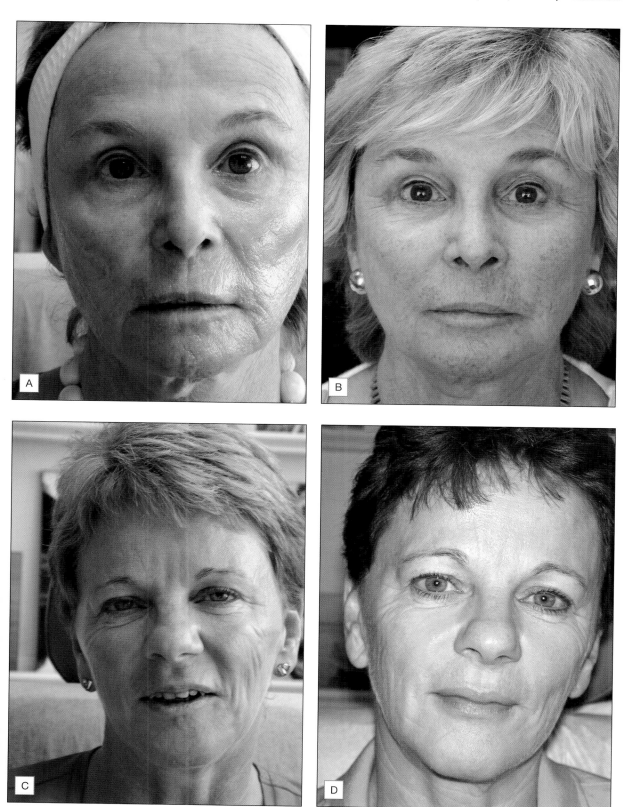

Fig. 7D.4 A and **C** Patients before receiving Sculptra, **B** and **D** patients after 3 vials of Sculptra

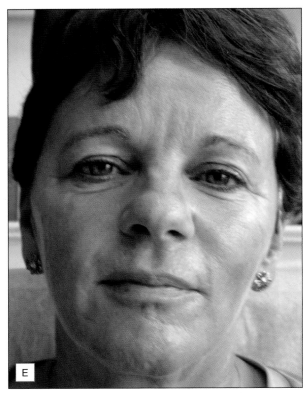

Fig. 7D.4 *Continued* E Patient after Sculptra and radiofrequency (thermage)

Although not offering instant gratification, often requiring 4–6 months to achieve correction, patient satisfaction remains high. The predictability and significant duration, up to 40 months, with injectable PLLA is also unique. Adequate dilution and placement, as well as proper technique followed by massage is essential to optimize outcomes and avoid nodules.

REFERENCES

Ascher B, et al. Full scope of effect of facial lipoatrophy: a framework of disease understanding. Dermatologic Surgery 32:1058–1069

Lam S, Azizzadeh B, Graivier M 2006 Injectable Poly-L-lactic acid (Sculptra): Technical considerations in soft-tissue contouring. Plastic and Reconstructive Surgery 118(3S Suppl):55S–63S

Lowe NJ 2006 Dispelling the myth: appropriate use of poly-L-lactic acid and clinical considerations. Journal of the European Academy of Dermatologic Venereology 20(Suppl 1):2–6

Napdez A, Park J 2006 A classification system for facial fat atrophy. American Journal of Cosmetic Surgery 23:122–126

Rotunda AM, Narins RS 2006 Poly-L-lactic acid: a new dimension in soft tissue augmentation. Dermatologic Therapy 19:151–158

Valantin M, et al 2003 Polylactic acid implants (New-Fill) to correct facial lipoatrophy in HIV-infected patients; results of the open-label study VEGA. AIDS 17:2471–2477

Vleggaar D 2005 Facial volumetric correction with injectable poly-L-lactic acid. Dermatologic Surgery 31:1511–1518

Vleggaar D 2006 Soft tissue augmentation and the role of poly-L-lactic acid. Plastic and Reconstructive Surgery 118(3S Suppl):55S–63S

Vleggaar D, Bauer U 2004 Facial enhancement and the European experience with Sculptra (poly-L-lactic acid). Journal of Drugs in Dermatology 3:542–547

8 Nasolabial Folds

Gary D. Monheit, Betty Davis

INTRODUCTION

The nasolabial fold (NLF) is the crease from the nose to the side of the oral commissure separating the cheek from the upper lip. Anatomically, the folds are the peripheral margin of the orbicularis oris muscle at the fusion of levator labii superioris medially and the zygomaticus major muscle laterally. The three branches of the levator labii superioris begin at the base of the nose, bottom edge of the orbit and zygomatic arch inserting into the skin of the upper lip. The zygomaticus major originates on the zygomatic arch inserting on the lateral mouth corner (Fig. 8.1). The repetitive action of these muscles over time contribute to the delineated NLF. As the zygomaticus major contracts and the lateral oral commissure rises to the cheekbone, a depression forms along the fold due to the bulging of the overlying cheek tissues. The NLF wrinkle gradually evolves from dynamic to static over time; as with any other rhytide, its axis always runs perpendicular to the direction of the muscular pull.

In addition to the dynamic factor of the lip elevators muscles, other factors contribute to the evolution of the nasolabial wrinkle fold. This includes soft tissue atrophy including loss of skeletal muscle and fat. Loss of suspension of the pad along with skin redundancy expands the fold to a deeper groove. In addition, the loss of dermal elasticity and collagen support increases the development of photoaging wrinkles along the nasolabial area. Because the skin loses elasticity with age, gravity's pull is most effective along the lower face from the nasolabial groove over marionette lines and including the jowls along the mandibular margin. These are the major factors of the aging process – loss of soft tissue volume, repetitive muscle contraction, cutaneous ptosis from loss of support and photoaging changes of elasticity (Fig. 8.2).

The prominence of the NLF is a major change revealing mid-face aging. The fold has a dynamic stage in earlier life and a static appearance with aging. This is shown with the newborn face, which has no fold, as well as the paretic face in which the fold disappears.

Treatment efforts are directed to correct these problems as follows: volume ptosis, repetitive muscle action and photoaging skin. Treatments are individualized in each patient relating to the degree of change within the fold and associated factors. This chapter will concentrate on volume correction with injectable fillers as this is the most common such treatment – correction. The other techniques will also be mentioned such as surgical corrections, resurfacing, and muscle relaxation with botulinum toxin (Botox), which can help as an adjunctive factor.

The gradual evolution of the NLF wrinkle from absence in the 20s, through mild and moderate grooves in the 30s and 40s to final severe grooves parallels the aging process. Quantitative scales of NLF prominence have been used to demonstrate the full evolution and guide the physician to proper therapy. The Genzyme six-point scale is an example of a measuring stick to determine groove level on a 0–5-severity level (Fig. 8.3). Early changes – 0 to 1 – are mainly dynamic as the fold is only exhibited with movement (Fig. 8.4). Moderate fold prominence exhibits malar fat pad depression at rest and is present because of early fat atrophy (Fig. 8.5). These individuals will get full correction with volume filling (Fig. 8.6). The more severe forms involve ptosis as well as volume loss and may not obtain the same degree of correction with injectable filling alone (Fig. 8.7). These subjects may require face-lifting procedures.

PATIENT SELECTION

When a patient seeks cosmetic treatment, it is important that they have realistic expectations. First of all, the physician needs to understand what the patient perceives as their chief esthetic concern. After this is accomplished, the physician should begin educating the patient as to the etiology and available treatment options. Changes in the skin due to inherent aging, actinic damage, and loss of subcutaneous tissue are variables different in each patient. This review is best done while a patient is looking into a mirror and subsequently reviewing the photographs.

Different treatment is required for each separate issue – rhytids caused by recurrent movement verses changes in the skin caused by increased laxity and gravity. When

Soft Tissue Augmentation

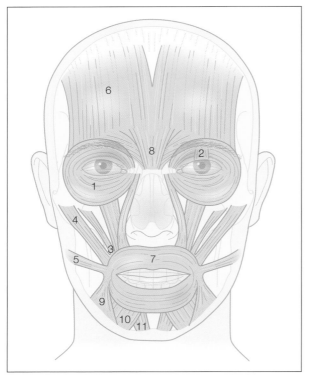

Fig. 8.1 Muscles of oral expression – sneering and smiling – contribute to the fold

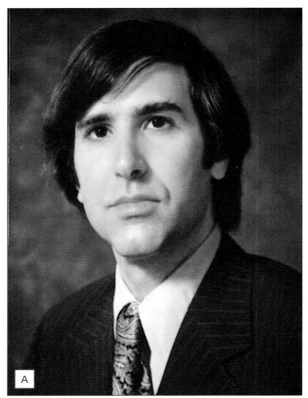

A

patients focus on prominent NLFs, it is best to begin with simple procedures that have little risk or down-time. Progression to more invasive procedures that require time for recovery is usual.

The ideal patient for soft tissue augmentation of the NLFs is a patient with moderate to moderately severe NLFs who wants smoothing of the contour of the mid-face, who understands the risks and benefits of the procedure, and who has realistic expectations. If a patient wants improvement more than soft tissue augmentation can offer or has a prominent cheek overhanging the NLF, a better option may be a face lift or a feather lift (Fig. 8.8). On the other hand, a patient who has signs of skin aging and wants augmentation may better be treated with a good skin care regimen and possibly a noninvasive laser or microdermabrasion procedure.

Procedures for correction of the nasolabial groove concentrate on the four major causes. The dynamic phase of wrinkles in many areas is corrected with Botox. The use of Botox in the perioral area in inexperienced hands may result in severe side effects by interfering with both

Fig. 8.2 (A and **B)** Changes in the NLF from dynamic expression to static ptosis: loss of soft tissue volume, repetitive muscle contraction, loss of support ptosis, photoaging skin changes, elastolysis

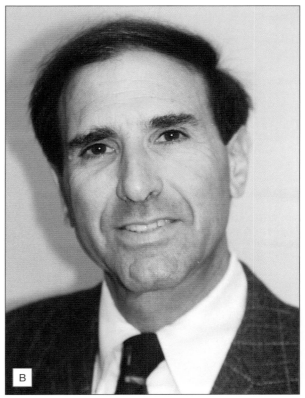

B

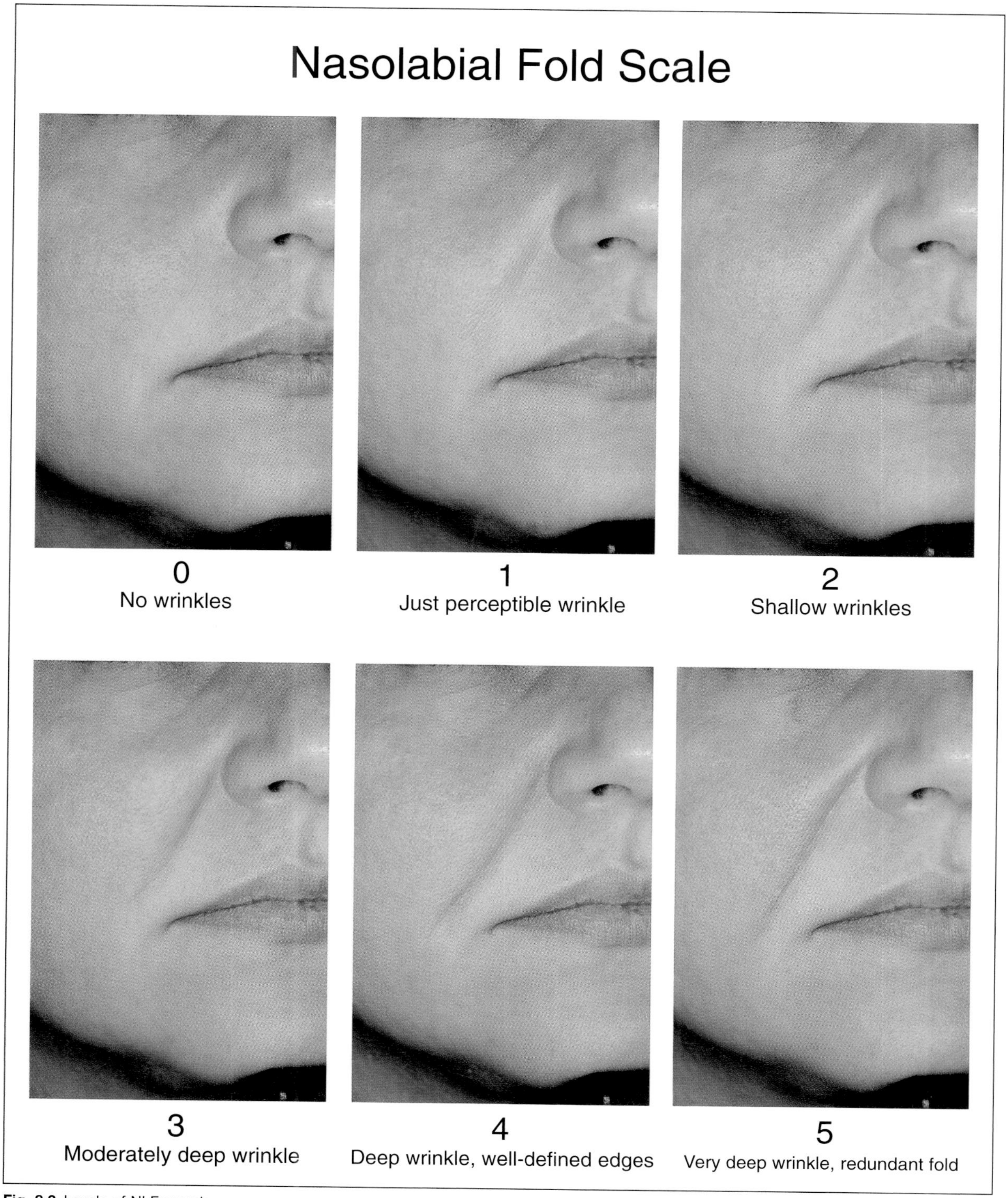

Nasolabial Fold Scale

0
No wrinkles

1
Just perceptible wrinkle

2
Shallow wrinkles

3
Moderately deep wrinkle

4
Deep wrinkle, well-defined edges

5
Very deep wrinkle, redundant fold

Fig. 8.3 Levels of NLF prominence

Soft Tissue Augmentation

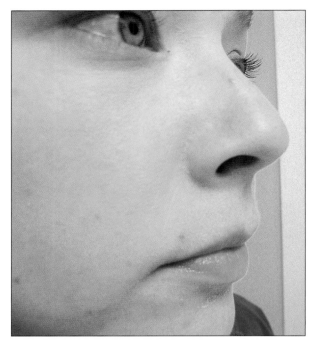

Fig. 8.4 Dynamic phase of NLF

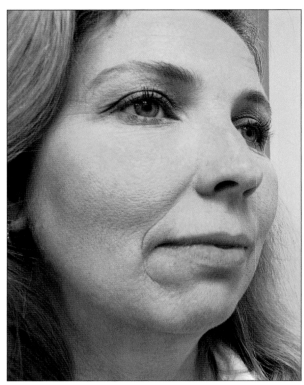

Fig. 8.6 Moderate to severe NLF with wrinkles from photoaging skin

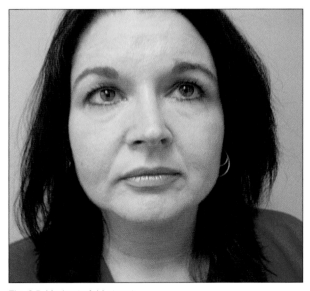

Fig. 8.5 Moderate fold at rest

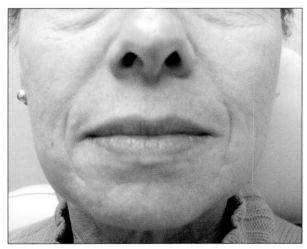

Fig. 8.7 Severe NLF with malar fat pad ptosis

function and expression. Inexperienced treatment may create an asymmetric paretic appearance and thus should be used with care around the zygomatous, levator labii or orbicularis oris muscles. Botulinim toxin A (BTX-A) can be used in the depressor anguli oris to elevate the lateral commissure as an adjunct to the insertion of filling material in the lower NLF and marionette lines. Two to five units of Botox (Botox Cosmetic, Allergan) are injected into the section of the depressor muscle just above the mandible. This procedure will give moderate enhancement of the filler esthetic (Fig. 8.9). Volume depletion may be corrected with injectable and surgically implanted filling materials. These may be temporary or permanent injectables including autologous fat, and solid implants.

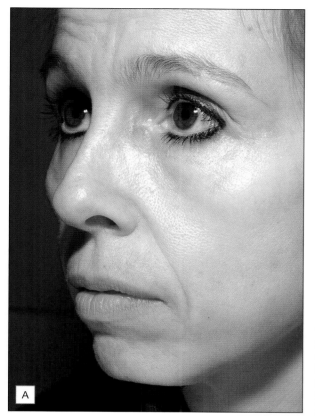
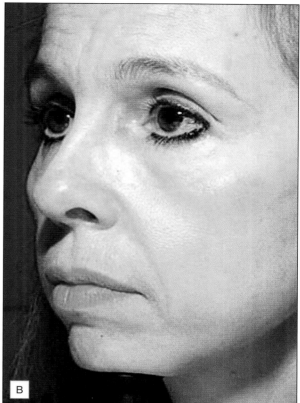

Fig. 8.8 Severe NLF with malar fat pad ptosis treated with Restylane filler and featherlift cheek suspension. **(A)** Before. **(B)** After

These procedures will be reviewed in detail for use in the NLF as volume replacement is the primary method of NLF correction.

Ptosis of the medial cheek is the most difficult factor to correct and may require a surgical approach. These include midface-lifting procedures such as subperiosteal midface lifts, endoscopic malar fat pad elevation, cable-suture fat pad elevations and short incision or traditional incision face lift. The technique of Sulamanidze – Aptos Threads – offers a novel nonsurgical approach to malar fat pad lifting to further correct severe NLFs. It is most commonly used in combination with injectable fillers (Fig. 8.10). The Aptos threads are not FDA-approved for use in the United States. Contour threads are a new and improved thread suspension lift which is FDA-approved and available in the United States. It is different from the floating Aptos threads in that it is anchored superiorly to the fascia in the temporal and frontal scalp. Used in concert with fillers, it will give excellent results to the severe and extreme NLFs (Figs 8.11 and 8.12).

Lasers can be used to correct photoaging skin along the NLF. CO_2 or erbium laser resurfacing are adjunctive techniques which can be used in combination with volume filling. Resurfacing techniques include nonablative lasers and most recently radiofrequency devices. All of these procedures can be used to correct skin defects around the fold and may be used in combination with volume filling.

The improvement achievable with soft tissue augmentation of the NLFs depends on the amount of the implant used, the type of implant, the frequency of implantation, and the intrinsic qualities of the NLF including the texture and quality of the fabric of the skin. The benefits of filler substances include softening NLFs by elevating the areas with the deficit of soft tissue. A lightening of the shadows created due to the aging face is seen in Table 8.1. A single implant or multiple implants can be used to attain the desired effect. If a patient presents with fine lines radiating from the NLFs, the best treatment would be to utilize an injectable filler specific for fine lines plus filling the NLFs with a heavier volume filler for deeper furrows.

Injectable soft tissue fillers are the primary choice for treatment of the NLF from minimal to severe. This chapter will briefly review the agents most commonly used and emphasize the techniques that work best in the NLF. Soft tissue augmentation is technique sensitive so

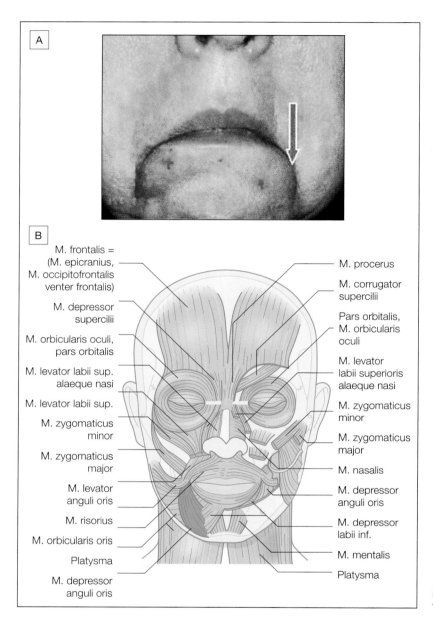

Fig. 8.9 Botox as an adjunctive procedure for NLF and lateral lip groove

Table 8.1 NLF prominence			
None to mild	**Mild to moderate**	**Moderate**	**Severe**
Muscular phase	Volume loss and photoaging skin	Moderate volume loss	Volume loss and ptosis

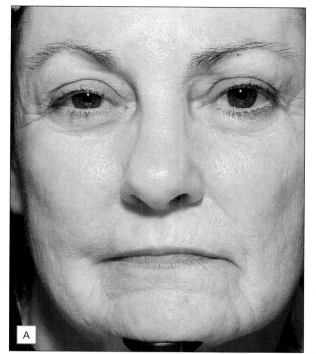

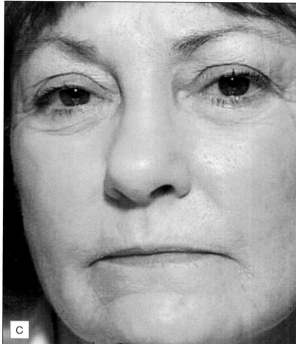

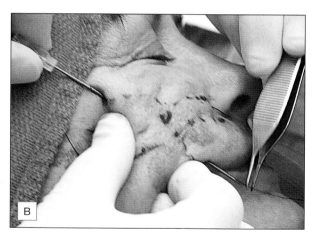

Fig. 8.10 Aptos Threads to elevate the NLF. (**A**) Before. (**B**) Threads in. (**C**) After

the individual procedure for each implant must be mastered (Table 8.2).

Injectable implants can be as effective as the product packaging claims as long as the implant is injected as directed on the package insert. Variables in efficacy can be noted if the material is injected into the subcutaneous tissue, causing much less augmentation compared to when it is injected correctly into the dermis. If the injectable implants are injected too superficially, beading or nodulation can occur. The beading will eventually decrease with time, decreasing fastest in areas with the most movement.

When injecting into the dermis and inserting the needle in a forward fashion, the injectable material can be extruded into an area of the dermis that is not the ideal site. Firm massage of the injected sites can help to smooth the contour of the injectable filler and guide the filler to a more optimal location.

Injecting material into the NLFs can cause considerable discomfort in some patients, with maximal discomfort occurring at the superior aspect of the NLFs. Some injectables contain an anesthetic, which helps with discomfort of the injection (Box 8.1). Countermeasures to avoid pain

Soft Tissue Augmentation

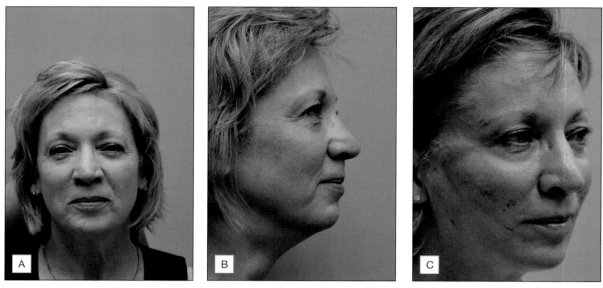

Fig. 8.11 Contour threads. (**A**) Before. (**B**) Before. (**C**) Immediately after injections of Radiesse and 12 contour threads

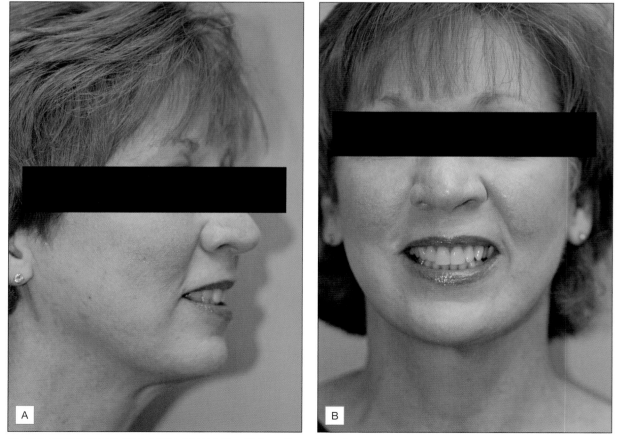

Fig. 8.12 Contour threads. (**A**) 3 months post insertion. (**B**) 3 months post insertion

Table 8.2 Fillers for the NLF

Biodegradable	Nonbiodegradable
Zyderm/Zyplast	Silicone
Cosmoderm/Cosmoplast	Artecoll
Isolagen	Profill
Fascian	Gortex
Hylaform	SoftForm
Restylane	
Juvéderm	
Newfill/Sculptra	
Dermal/fascial grafts	
Fat	

Box 8.2 Commonly used topical anesthetic agents

❖ Betacaine enhanced gel, BetaCaine Plus
❖ L.M. ×4 and L.M. ×5
❖ EMLA (lidocaine pritocaine) cream
❖ Ice or other cryoesthetic agents
❖ Vibratory counterstimulation

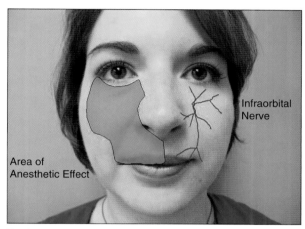

Fig. 8.13 Anesthetic distribution of the infraorbital nerve block

Box 8.1 Anesthesia guidelines for injecting fillers

Implants with lidocaine

❖ Zyderm/Zyplast
❖ Cosmoderm/Cosmoplast

Topical anesthesia
❖ Elamax
❖ Betacaine

Nerve blocks
❖ Infraorbital
❖ Mental

Counter nerve stimulation
❖ Vibrator

include topical anesthetics, ice, infraorbital nerve block, or simultaneous stimulation with a massaging apparatus. While it may be tempting to inject an anesthetic into the area to be treated, this can distort normal contours and should be avoided. Topical anesthetics help to decrease the pain of the needle puncture, but help minimally with the injection itself or the forward motion of the needle through the dermis. Infraorbital nerve blocks or counter nerve stimulation have mixed results, but do help to lessen the pain (Box 8.2, Fig. 8.13).

PATIENT INTERVIEW

A thorough medical history, family history, and physical exam should be done with each patient. Any history of collagen vascular diseases (CVDs) should be noted, as well as hypersensitivity to ingredients of the filler substance. Skin tests should be performed when indicated. Bleeding disorders or anticoagulation medications should be noted. Bruising occurs more frequently when an anticoagulant is used and the patient should be aware of this possibility. The patient should be asked to smile and sneer to evaluate dynamics and symmetry. Any asymmetries in the patient's appearance should be noted and brought to the attention of the patient and documented with pre-treatment photographs in the chart.

The cosmetic patient is questioned as to what bothers them most about their appearance. They are asked to make a 'wish list' including up to five aspects of their appearance they would like to have improved with the most important feature to be first on the list. The list is reviewed with the patient, having them demonstrate for us in the mirror exactly what is meant by each topic on their list. Treatment options are then reviewed with the patient, beginning with simple procedures and combined simple procedures with little down-time and ending with more long-lasting procedures requiring significant down-time. If the patient has not had augmentation procedures before, the current authors typically recommend beginning with a product that lasts the least amount of time so that the patient can decide if augmentation is right for them. Although permanent fillers have the advantage of fewer injection sessions to maintain a desired affect, there is less of a margin of error when injected and the products can shift over time and with muscular movement. As the face ages, the site first injected may not be the ideal site for injection 5 or 10 years later in life. Subjects should be aware of the possibility that the aging process may result in a later unnatural appearance from the permanent implant to the area. The cost of each procedure is reviewed with the patient and written information is given to the patient, who can either proceed with treatment or can schedule a future appointment after considering their treatment options.

TREATMENT TECHNIQUE

Every patient who is to be treated cosmetically reviews the treatment plan, and reviews the risks, benefits, and alternatives to the procedure as discussed. The patient must express understanding and sign an informed consent. Any last-minute questions are answered at this time. The patient's make-up is removed and the areas to be injected are cleansed with isopropanol and allowed to air dry. Photographs both distant and close-up are taken at this time including a frontal view, a 45-degree angle view from the right and left, and a side view. It is important when comparing photographs that each picture is taken in a similar fashion under similar lighting. Make-up should be removed in all pictures and a similar background should be used.

BIODEGRADABLE COLLAGEN

• Zyderm/Zyplast

Bovine collagen is the first dermal filler approved for usage in the United States. It has a 20-year record of safety as a dermal filler and is most commonly used on the NLF. Three types of bovine collagen are presently available: (1) Zyderm I (ZI) is a 3.5% by weight bovine collagen (35 mg/mL), (2) Zyderm II (ZII, which is 6.5% mg/mL), and (3) Zyplast. Zyplast 1.5 cross-linked bovine collagen, which constitutes an injectable latticework of bovine collagen, is more resistant to degradation with less immunogenicity. All of these products require skin tests to rule out allergy. Two intradermal injection tests should be performed at day 0, 2 weeks, and both evaluated in 6 weeks. The collagen is suspended in saline with 1% lidocaine. The products have different indications.

Zyderm I is primarily indicated for superficial defects while Zyderm II and Zyplast are used for deeper depressions and grooves. Zyderm I is placed in the papillary and upper reticular dermis. A quantity of 150–200% is required and the endpoint of injection is a 'peau d'orange' or blanching of the skin. Zyderm I is best used in combination with Zyplast or another heavier filler to correct the remaining fine wrinkles after the nasolabial groove is volume corrected (Fig. 8.14). This is a layering technique which will give a full correction to the dermal defect (Fig. 8.15).

Zyplast is a denser substance with greater longevity. It must be injected into the mid reticular to deep dermis and is especially useful for treatment of the NLF. Zyplast is placed at a mid- to deep-dermal level with a 30 gauge

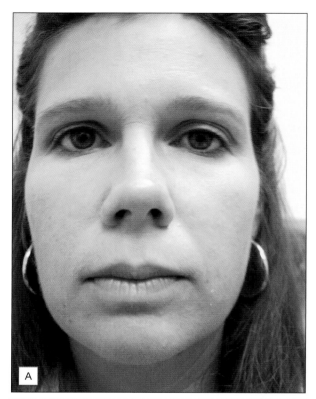

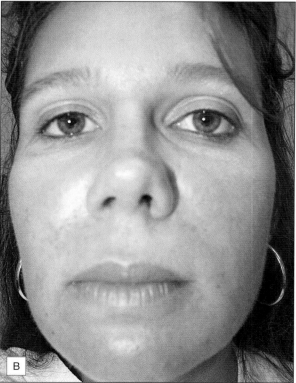

Fig. 8.14 Zyderm I + Zyplast layered in NLF – before and after

needle at a 10–20-degree angle to the skin surface. The material is deposited using a serial puncture technique.

There are variable techniques developed for NLF injections which are also applicable to other injectable fillers.

The three injection techniques most commonly used in the NLF are: serial puncture, threading and fanning (Fig. 8.16). The current authors find all three are useful for most injections. Serial puncture indicates the use of multiple injections into the mid-dermis going up to the NLF,

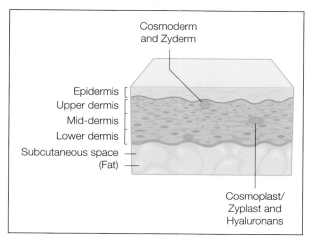

Epidermis

Upper dermis

Mid-dermis

Lower dermis

Subcutaneous space
(Fat)

Cosmoderm
and Zyderm

Cosmoplast/
Zyplast and
Hyaluronans

Fig. 8.15 Tissue compartment and choice of fillers

injected medial to the line/fold at a 30-degree angle. The injected implants are then massaged for even distribution. Threading technique uses a 1 in 30 gauge needle, which is advanced at a 30-degree angle below the depth of the NLF. The filler is then injected as the needle is slowly withdrawn. This fills the depth of the fold through the trough evenly. The fanning technique is used for diffuse volume filling and useful for the triangle at the superior aspect of the NLF as it approaches the alar rim. Multiple 30-degree mid-dermal pathways are formed out and from the groove to elevate the superior angle evenly. It is also useful for volume filling at the lateral lip commissure to elevate the corner of the NLF and marionette line. Zyplast injections should never be overcorrected and always within a mid- to deep- dermal level, avoiding the peau d'orange appearance seen with superficial dermal injections.

Two or more implant sessions at intervals no less than 2 weeks apart may be needed for maximal correction. Enhancement implants are performed at 4–12-month intervals to maintain full correction (Fig. 8.17).

Best results are obtained by combining Zyplast with Zyderm I for correction of all levels of dermis within the fold. The two materials are layered with Zyplast injected first to 100% correction of the deeper groove. *The author's choice* of techniques is to use the threading method first for volume filling and the deeper aspects of the groove. The serial puncture technique is then applied to areas of depression after full threading of the fold. Further volume filling is performed at the superior sulcus. It usually takes 1–2 cc of Zyplast to correct most NLF volume

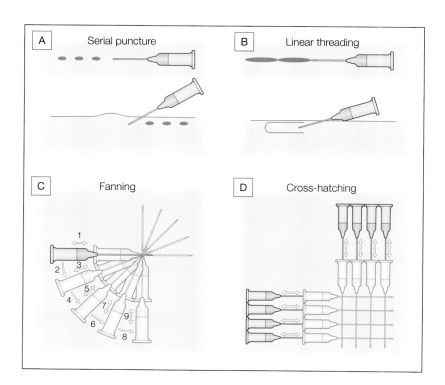

Fig. 8.16 Serial puncture, threading and fanning are all useful techniques for injecting collagen within the NLF

A Serial puncture

B Linear threading

C Fanning

D Cross-hatching

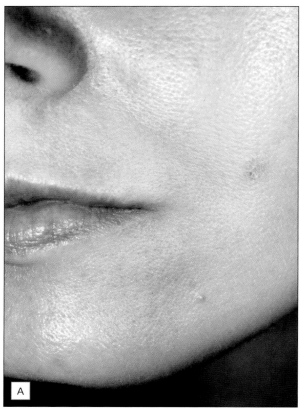
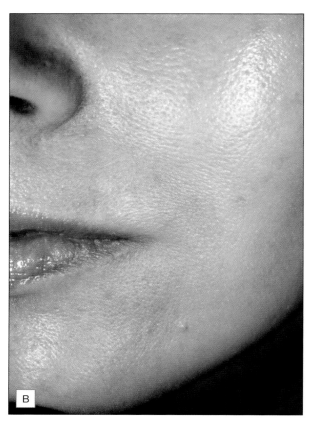

Fig. 8.17 Nasolabial lines and furrows

deficiencies. Then, Zyderm I is placed above the Zyplast for the remaining wrinkle within the fold and any accessory wrinkles. Massage is necessary after each injection to avoid nodulation and assure a smooth, natural implant.

Variation in longevity of augmentation is due to dynamic motion and mechanical stress along the NLF.

Though Zyderm/Zyplast is historically a reliable, forgiving product, disadvantages include the potential for allergy and need for skin tests prior to injection, the relative short duration and potential adverse events including nodulation, allergic potential, vascular infarction with deepest injection and the rare event of cystic formation.

CosmoDerm/CosmoPlast (Allergan) is a second-generation collagen filling agent produced as a human bio-engineered collagen. It is derived from dermal fibroblast cells seeded and incubated in a bioreactor to produce a human collagen product. The type I collagen is isolated from the dermal tissue, purified and mixed with lidocaine and phosphate-buffered saline. CosmoDerm I, II and CosmoPlast are used as injectable fillers in the NLFs similar to the methods of Zyderm I, II and Zyplast. No skin test

is required though and some clinicians believe the product may last slightly longer than Zyderm/Zyplast products. It also can be used in combination with other products including hyaluronic acid fillers. It has an excellent record of safety. It produces little swelling or bruising with the least amount of down-time of any filler presently available (Fig. 8.18). The most recently developed collagen product is Evolence or Dermical P-30. It is a formulation of porcine collagen in suspension at 35 mg/mL. Evolence represents an injectable matrix of highly cross-linked, homogenous type I telopeptides porcine collagen produced by Glymatix technology with ribose used as the cross-linked glyacation agent. Evolence has been formed to last up to 2 years in animal models and over 1 year in the initial European studies.

Evolence is especially effective for the NLF because of its stiff characteristics, which can fill even deep folds and give adequate support. It is injected with a 27 gauge needle using a perioral nerve block for comfort. There is mild to moderate inflammation but it gives a very natural correction early on (Fig. 8.19).

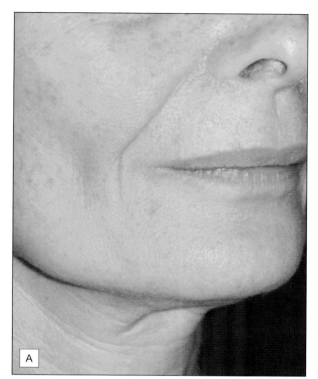

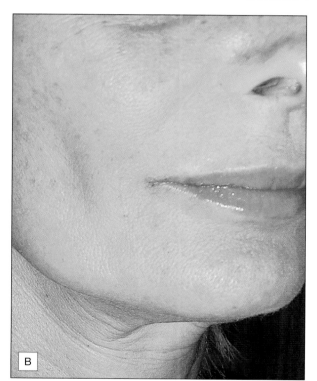

Fig. 8.18 CosmoPlast/CosmoDerm. (Courtesy of Dr Leslie Baumann) (**A**) Before. (**B**) 30 minutes after

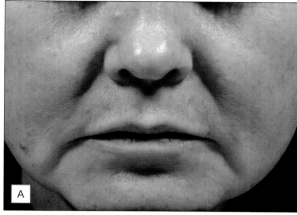

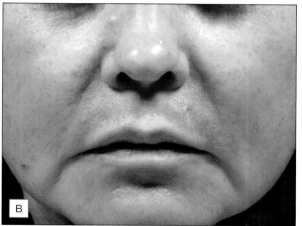

Fig. 8.19 Nasolabial lines treated with Evolence – 30. (**A**) Before. (**B**) After

HYALURONIC ACID: RESTYLANE (MEDICIS ESTHETICS), HYLAFORM (ALLERGAN/GENZYME), JUVÉDERM (ALLERGAN)

The hyaluronic acid products are the most recently approved family of injectable fillers for contour defects. These are especially applicable for the NLF, in which the unique viscoelastic properties and high water retention capacity fill the groove in a very natural manner. Hyaluronic acid is chemically, physically and biologically identical in the tissues of all species. It is biocompatible with little or no allergenicity. The body rapidly clears the hyaluronic acid molecule in 24–48 hours so that the product needs stabilization to be effective as a dermal implant. Restylane is a bacterial-based product while Hylaform is derived from chicken combs. Both products are purified and stabilized by cross-linking, producing a hydroscope gel that is gradually eliminated. Both Restylane and Hylaform

Soft Tissue Augmentation

have been approved by the FDA for intradermal injection to correct the NLFs. This is especially applicable since the NLF was the area chosen for the paired double-blind studies used for efficacy and safety of the products. Both studies used Zyplast as a control. The Restylane study compared products on either side of the face in a double-blind paired comparison. It was to demonstrate efficacy and longevity. The Hylaform study was a 'noninferiority' study with outcomes for efficacy at 4 months. Both products were successful with the following outcomes:

1. Both products achieved correction equal to or better than Zyplast at 4 months
2. Both products were declared safe with no need for skin testing
3. Both were declared safe and effective treatments for correction of NLFs.

Neither product has lidocaine; thus pretreatment topical anesthesia and/or local blocks are needed for patient comfort. The current authors prefer using topical betacaine or lidocaine infraorbital nerve block.

The products are packaged as a gel within a syringe with 0.7 mL product and a 30 gauge 0.5 in needle. They should be injected into the mid-dermis with only 100% correction (no overcorrection).

Restylane and Hylaform can be injected into the NLF by all three defined techniques: serial puncture, threading and fanning. The viscoelastic properties of the gel make it malleable for massage in the fold resulting in a very natural correction (Fig. 8.20). Juvéderm was approved as a family of hyaluronic acid fillers developed by Corneal Industries in Europe and FDA-approved in June 2006. It is processed differently from other HA fillers in that there are no distinctive particles but rather a homogenous gel that has a high degree of cross-linking. It makes Juvéderm a highly desirable filler for the NLF. Juvéderm Ultra (24 HV) can be injected through a 30 gauge needle in the mid-dermis with early natural results that last 6 months plus. Juvéderm Ultra Plus (30 HV) is a more highly cross-linked product which also gives a sustained correction but is designed as a deeper injection in the mid to deep dermis. The FDA clinical study compared Zyplast to Juvéderm in a split face randomized study that gave the following results:

1. Juvéderm gave longer lasting results than Zyplast, correction for at least 24 weeks
2. It has an excellent safety profile
3. It is preferred by patients for use on NLFs (Fig. 8.21).

The implant should not be placed superficially as it results in nodularity with a visibly bluish discoloration to the skin.

The hyaluronic acids are relatively free of side effects with a very small risk of allergic or inflammatory reactions. Rare granulomas have been reported from both products. This filler, like all the biodegradable products, is forgiving

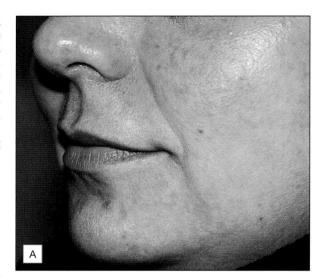

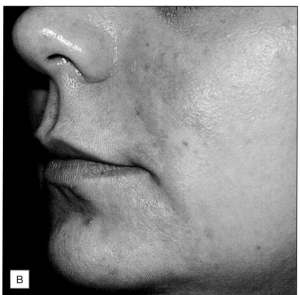

Fig. 8.20 Mid-dermal injection of Hylaform to correct NLF. (**A**) Before. (**B**) After

because it will be resorbed and side effects disappear with time (Fig. 8.22).

CALCIUM HYDROXYLAPATITE (RADIESSE: BIOFORM)

Calcium hydroxylapatite (CaHA) is an inorganic substance that mimics the structure of bone. In the United States, it is marketed as Radiesse. Radiesse is currently FDA-approved for use in oral maxillofacial defects and for soft tissue vocal fold augmentation and as a radiographic

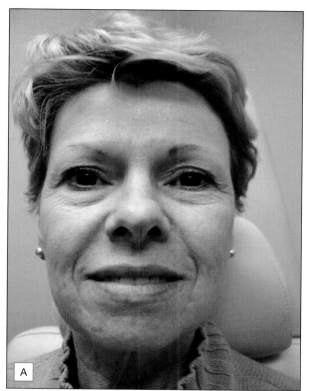

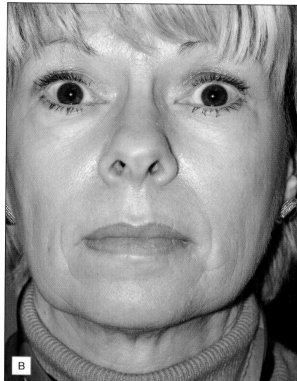

Fig. 8.21 Juvéderm Ultra Plus. (**A**) Pre-injection. (**B**) 7 months post injection

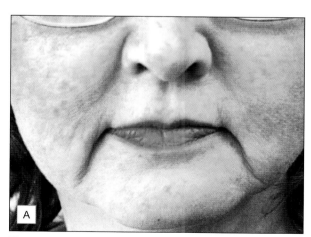

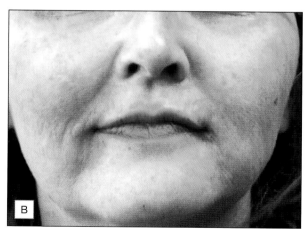

Fig. 8.22 Deep marionette lines treated with Restylane 0.7 cc within each fold. (**A**) Before. (**B**) After

tissue marker. CaHA is currently widely used in Europe as a soft tissue filler. Radiesse is not approved in the United States by the FDA for cosmetic applications and use for soft tissue augmentation is classed as off-label use.

In its soft tissue injectable form, CaHA microspheres are suspended in a sodium carboxymethyl cellulose absorbable gel, and it is injected into the dermis or subcutaneous tissue. As the gel is absorbed, collagen deposition into and around the microspheres causes collagen formation and enhances augmentation. It is expected to last between 2–5 years with breakdown products of calcium and phosphorous.

Radiesse has been used effectively for correction of NLF defects by deep dermal injection. A local nerve block is needed for its comfortable usage. The gel is injected through a 25 or 27 gauge needle and the correction is usually 1 : 1. It is advisable to undercorrect the fold as lumpiness and medial overcorrection can produce a deformity. Conservative correction with follow-up correction in 2–4 weeks is advisable. The pliability of the substances allows postinjection massage, minimizing irregularities or lumpiness which can occur. It is expected to last over 2 years (Fig. 8.23).

POLY-L-LACTIC ACID: SCULPTRA (NEW-FILL): DERMIK

Poly-L-lactic acid (PLLA) received conditional approval from an FDA advisory panel for treatment of HIV-related lipoatrophy under the trade name Sculptra in March 2004. However, the FDA has not yet approved Sculptra for general cosmetic use in the USA. Studies of this product are currently underway to gain FDA approval. PLLA has been marketed as New-Fill in Europe since November 1999.

PLLA is a synthetic polymer which is resorbable, biocompatible, and biodegradable. It has been used for several years in multiple medical devices and is a component of vicryl sutures. PLLA can be injected into the deep dermal tissue or subcutaneous tissue. The area to be filled should be undercorrected. After injection, gradual degradation takes place by hydrolysis while gradual deposition of collagen occurs.

The initial correction, due to implantation of the PLLA decreases over the next few days as the diluent is resorbed. The area treated with PLLA will then slowly refill as the tissue reacts to the implant. A gradual increase in the volume will continue to occur over the next few months.

The side effects of this material are similar to those of other injectables and include erythema, edema, and bruising at the injection site. Palpable but nonvisible subcutaneous nodules have been noted in some patients, which can resolve spontaneously. These nodules on the lip may be due to overcorrection. Massaging the treated area after injection may reduce the incidence of this side effect.

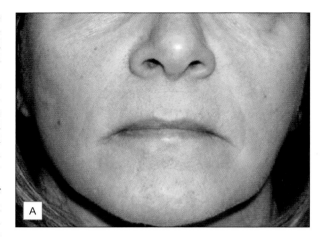

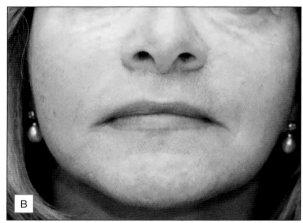

Fig. 8.23 Deep NLFs treated with Radiesse. (**A**) Before. (**B**) After

Rare cases of sterile abscess, late granuloma formation and hypersensitivity reactions have been reported.

Sculptra is injected with a different technique than the other wrinkle fillers. It is layered as a deep dermal and subcutaneous soft tissue filler that is used mainly to correct volume deficits rather than wrinkle correction alone. The technique of Vleggar demonstrates injection with a criss-cross pattern to lay down a uniform matrix for new collagen to be deposited in the deep dermis (Fig. 8.24). To correct NLFs, the entire lower facial area should be blended to augment tissue and provide a volume-enhancing effect. That not only corrects the furrow but also redefines the lost volume in surrounding skin and soft tissues (Fig. 8.25). A 27 gauge needle is used to implant the gel into deep dermis and subcutaneous tissue in a criss-cross pattern. No more than 1–2 ml is injected with undercorrection. The area is then massaged and iced to decrease inflammation. Two or three repeat procedures are performed for full correction. The product has been found to last 2–4 years.

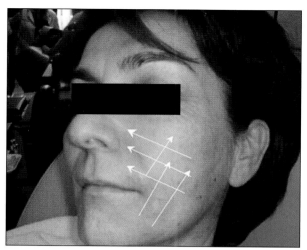

Fig. 8.24 Sculptra is a deep volume filler injected in a criss-cross pattern

Table 8.3 Nonbiodegradable synthetic fillers	
Injectables	**Solids**
Silicone	Gortex
Artecoll	SoftForm
Bioplastique	

NONBIODEGRADABLE FILLERS

Nonbiodegradable fillers include both injectables and solid products (Table 8.3). Over a period of time, the authors' patients do request longer lasting fillers and discuss permanence. There are both advantages and disadvantages of these products. Most importantly, the physician must understand that errors and complications are not forgiving and in some cases, not correctable.

• Silicone

Silicone is the oldest filling material in the United States, first used in 1930 and used for NLF augmentation since 1965 by Orentreich and Associates. The Dow Corning material had a viscosity of 360 cs, ideal for microdroplet deep dermal injection. The fine droplets are deposited as an undercorrection with only minimal change in the NLF. Collagen is laid down around the droplets and the process is repeated at 6-month intervals until the desired correction is obtained. Optimal correction has been followed for over 30 years by Orentreich and Barnett with good cosmetic correction. The patient though must be alerted to the fact that aging changes facial contour and the silicone may 'bead up' or change position as wrinkles and features fall. The most common complications seen are implant migration and nodulation. These are usually technique related (Fig. 8.26).

Dow Corning silicone is not approved by the FDA. Other forms of silicone, though, are presently approved for ophthalmic usage. These are: Adato-Sil (5000 cs) and Silikon (1000 cs). They are presently being used as dermal fillers in off-label usage.

ARTEFILL

ArteFill is a permanent injectable filler used to correct the NLF since 1994. Polymethyl-methacrylate (PMMA) microspheres are suspended in bovine collagen for intradermal injection. The product is manufactured by Rofil Medical International but presently is not FDA-approved. The product has had clinical trials in the United States under the name of ArteFill (Fig. 8.27). It has recently been approved in the United States by the FDA panel for use in front wrinkles, the NLF.

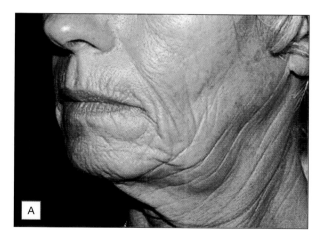

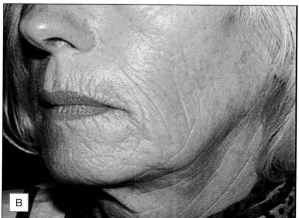

Fig. 8.25 Volume filling redefines facial features as well as fills wrinkle folds. (**A**) Before. (**B**) 10 months after treatment

Soft Tissue Augmentation

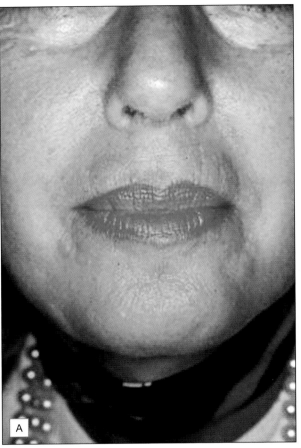
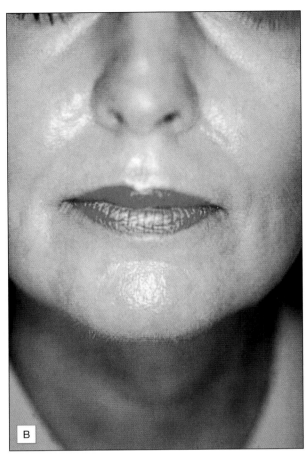

Fig. 8.26 Long-term nodulation – silicone (**A** and **B**)

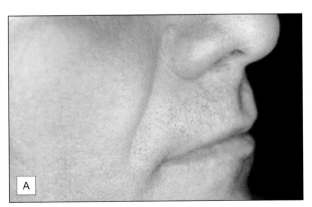
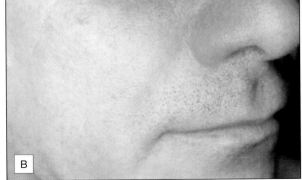

Fig. 8.27 ArteFill injection within the NLFs. (**A**) Before. (**B**) 3 years after

The suspension of bovine collagen and PMMA microspheres is injected into the deep dermis with 100% correction of the fold, yet not overcorrection. With 3–4 months, the collagen is degraded as new collagen is formed around the microspheres. The product is well indicated for deep NLFs for long-term correction.

ArteFill is designed for implantation into the deep reticular dermis. Implanting ArteFill is more technique sensitive than injecting collagen due to its viscosity and permanence. The viscosity of ArteFill is three times higher than that of Zyplast and therefore a greater and a constant pressure should be applied to the plunger of the syringe throughout the injection procedure. Also due to the increased viscosity, more pain occurs during injection compared to collagen. Before injecting, the injector should exert a firm and steady push on the plunger of the syringe to ensure that there is no blockage of the needle and that the material is moved to the tip of the needle and is ready for injection. The needle should be inserted into the deep reticular dermis tunneled just beneath the area to be filled while maintaining constant pressure on the plunger of the syringe.

The material should only be injected while withdrawing the needle since if infection on entering the tissue is as if you are injecting into a wall of tissue; material injected can move in any direction away from the needle tip, taking the path of least resistance. When injecting into the reticular dermis, a firm resistance is felt and a lifting of the skin is noticed. If the needle is in the subcutaneous tissue, the resistance will be much less and a much greater amount of product will be needed to achieve a lifting of the skin. If while injecting ArteFill a blanching occurs, the needle is placed too superficially. If this occurs, it is important to stop the injection immediately and massage the area with firm pressure, helping to deepen the injected material. At the end of implantation, massage all areas gently. If lumpiness is noted, massage more firmly. Patients should limit movement of the injected site for the next 3 days as ArteFill can be pushed deeper into the skin with pronounced movement during this time. The implant site can be taped for approximately 3 days, serving more as a reminder to try to keep the area still than as a dressing. The patients should be instructed that they may develop edema and erythema over the next few days.

The area should be allowed to settle for several weeks and the patient should then be re-evaluated to see if any further augmentation is needed. If further augmentation is needed, ArteFill should be injected in a layered fashion with care taken not to inject the material too superficially.

When correcting the NLFs with ArteFill, two to three strands are implanted in a parallel fashion 1–2 mm medial to the NLF. This is because NLFs are involved in many facial expressions. For the first 3 days after injection, ArteFill is more easily dislodged and due to muscular movement of this area can be moved laterally with facial expression during this time.

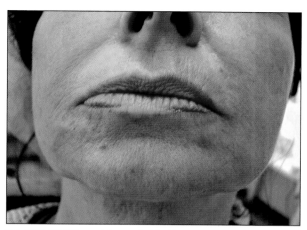

Fig. 8.28 ArteFill – nodules on lip injection

• Side effects/complications

The tolerability and acceptability of side effects due to Artefill is low due to the longevity of the implant and therefore the potential for nonresolving side effects. Although the PMMA microspheres are nonallergenic, allergic reaction can occur with Artefill as it can with any injectable collagen preparation. Even with a test-site, allergic reaction can occur.

True granuloma formation is a rare occurrence, occurring in less than 0.01% of patients and occurring 6–24 months after Artefill treatment. This side effect may not be reversible. In summary, Artefill is a permanent product with permanent results and permanent complications. Care must be taken to avoid the latter (Fig. 8.28).

AUTOLOGOUS FAT

As opposed to these injectable products, long-term correction can also be attained with fat injections. This is a more complicated surgical procedure involving fat harvesting, centrifuging and then injecting. There is downtime with significant swelling, inflammation and bruising, thus it is not a procedure to be taken lightly. In fact, the current authors like to try a simpler temporary filler first prior to fat injection procedures. This will show the patient the type of correction that can be obtained before this longer lasting procedure is performed. The following concepts have made fat injection a reliable and long-lasting procedure:

1. Fat is harvested atraumatically and handled in vitro carefully to preserve the live fat cells
2. Small aliquots of fat are injected into tissue using a layering technique – microlipoinjection
3. Fat is injected deeply into muscle and deep subcutaneous tissue for best survival.

Soft Tissue Augmentation

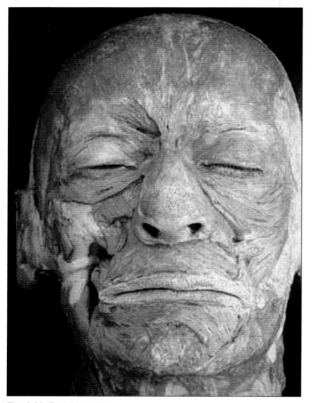

Fig. 8.29 Facial muscles

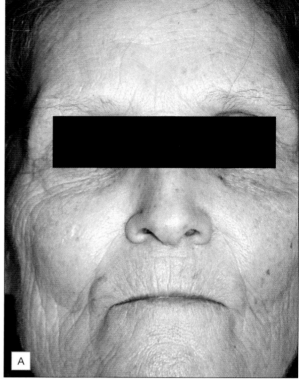

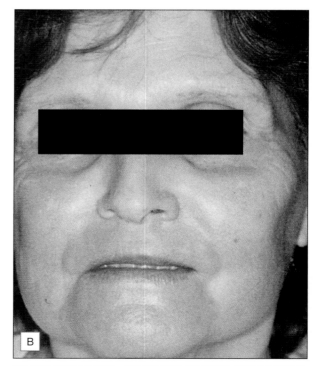

Fig. 8.30 FAMI injection – lips and folds. (**A**) Before. (**B**) 2-year result

The fat autograft muscle injection (FAMI) technique developed by Roger Amar is a reliable method of deep fat injection to correct the lower face and NLF. It involves a careful analysis of muscle and fat loss around the NLF with correction of fat into those areas of loss. For example, deep NLFs are corrected by microlipoinjection into the following muscles: levator labii, zygomaticus major, orbicularis oris. This is performed through the use of a specially designed cannula through which the fat is injected longitudinally through the muscle mass and fat above (Fig. 8.29).

The thin patient with severe folds and skeletonized lower face responds well to this operative procedure. The fat is injected through definitive incision sites for volume replacement of the lower face. Volume replacement will give long-lasting (1–5 years) correction of folds and a new contouring of the lower face (Fig. 8.30).

CONCLUSION

This chapter has explored the available techniques to correct the NLFs with emphasis on individualizing correction to meet each patient's needs.

FURTHER READING

Alam M, Hsu TS, Dover JS, Wrone DA, Arndt KA 2003 Nonablative laser and light treatments: histology and tissue effects – a review. Lasers in Surgery and Medicine 33:30–39 [Review]

Allevato MA, Pastorale E, Zamboni M, Kerdel F, Woscoss A 1996 Complications following industrial liquid silicone injection. International Journal of Dermatology 20:267–276

Anderson RD, Lo MW 1998 Endoscopic malar/midface suspension procedure. Plastic and Reconstructive Surgery 102:2196–2208

Atamoros FP 2003 Botulinum toxin in the lower one third of the face. Clinical Dermatology 21:505–512

Barr RJ, Stegman SJ 1984 Delayed skin test reaction to injectable collagen implant (Zyderm). The histopathologic comparative study. Journal of the American Academy of Dermatology 10:652–658

Barton FE Jr, Kenkel JM 1997 Direct fixation of the malar pad. Clinical Plastic Surgery 24:329–335

Baumann L, Frankel S, Welsh E, Halem M 2003 Cryoanalgesia with dichlorotetrafluoroethane lessens the pain of botulinum toxin injections for the treatment of palmar hyperhidrosis. Dermatologic Surgery 29:1057–1059

Berry J 2002 New-Fill for an old face. Posit Aware 13:34–35

Bisson MA, Grover R, Grobbelaar AO 2002 Long-term results of facial rejuvenation by carbon dioxide laser resurfacing using a quantitative method of assessment. British Journal of Plastic Surgery 55:652–656

Blitzer A, Binder WJ, Aviv JE, Keen MS, Brin MF 1997 The management of hyperfunctional facial lines with botulinum toxin. A collaborative study of 210 injection sites in 162 patients. Arch Otolaryngol Head Neck Surg 123:389–392

Bolognia JL, Jorizzo JL, Rapini RP 2003 Dermatology 1st edn. Mosby

Butterwick KJ, Lack EA 2003 Facial volume restoration with the fat autograft muscle injection technique. Dermatologic Surgery 29:1019–1026

Carruthers A 2003 History of the clinical use of botulinum toxin A and B. Clinical Dermatology 21:469–472

de Maio M 2003 Challenges in the mid and the lower face. Journal of Cosmetic Laser Therapy 5:213–215

Carruthers J, Carruthers A 2003 Aesthetic botulinum A toxin in the mid and lower face and neck. Dermatologic Surgery 29:468–476

Charriere G, Bejot M, Schnitzler L, Ville G, Hartmann DJ 1989 Reactions to a bovine collagen implant. Clinical and immunologic study in 705 patients. Journal of the American Academy of Dermatology 21:1203–1208

Chen JZ, Alexiades-Armenakas MR, Bernstein LJ, Jacobson LG, Friedman PM, Geronemus RG 2003 Two randomized, double-blind, placebo-controlled studies evaluating the S-Caine Peel for induction of local anesthesia before long-pulsed Nd : YAG laser therapy for leg veins. Dermatologic Surgery 29:1012–1018

Cheonis N 2002 New-Fill to treat facial wasting. BETA. 15:10–15

Clark DP, Hanke CW, Swanson NA 1989 Dermal implants: safety of products injected for soft tissue augmentation. Journal of the American Academy of Dermatology 21:992–998 [Review]

Day JN, Raabe A, Shiner AM, Wilkins EL 2002 Intradermal polylactic acid (Newfill) for treatment of severe HIV-associated facial lipoatrophy. HIV Medicien. 3:162

Donofrio L 2000 Fat distribution: a morphologic study of the aging face. Dermatologic Surgery 26:1107–1112

Donofrio L 2000 Structural autologous lipoaugmentation: a pan-facial technique. Dermatologic Surgery 26:1129–1134

Duffy D 1990 Silicone: a critical review. Advances in Dermatology 5:93–107

Duffy DM 1998 Injectable liquid silicone: new perspectives. In: Klein AW (ed.) Tissue Augmentation in Clinical Pratice: Procedures and Techniques. Marcel Dekker, New York, pp 237–267

Duranti F, Salti G, Bovani B, Calandra M, Rosati ML 1998 Injectable hyaluronic acid gel for soft tissue augmentation: A clinical and histological study. 24:1317–1325

Ellenbogen R, Rubin L 1975 Injectable fluid silicone therapy: human morbidity and mortality. JAMA 234:308–309

Eremia S, Newman N 2000 Long-term follow-up after autologous fat grafting. Dermatologic Surgery 26:1150–1158

Faigin G 1990 The Artist's Complete Guide to Facial Expression, Watson-Guptill Publications, New York, NY

Fernandez-Acenero MJ, Zamora E, Borbujo J 2003 Granulomatous foreign body reaction against hyaluronic acid: report of a case after lip augmentation. Dermatologic Surgery 29:1225–1226

Frank P, Gendler E 2001 Hyaluronic acid for soft-tissue augmentation. Clinics in Plastic Surgery 28:121–126 [Review]

Fournier P 2000 Fat grafting: my technique. Dermatologic Surgery 26:1117–1128

Friedman PM, Mafong EA, Friedman ES, Geronemus RG 2001 Topical anesthetics update: EMLA and beyond. Dermatologic Surgery 27:1019–1026

Friedman PM, Mafong EA, Kauvar AN, Geroneumus RG 2002 Safety data of injectable nonanimal stabilized hyaluronic acid gel for soft tissue augmentation. Dermatologic Surgery 28:491–494

Gogolewski S et al 1993 Tissue response and in vivo degradation of selected polyhydroxyacids: polylactides, poly(3-hydroxybutyrate), and poly(3-hydroxybutyrate-co-3-hydroxyvalerate). Journal of Biomedical Materials Research 27:1135–1148

Goodman G 1998 Botulinum toxin for the correction of hyperkinetic facial lines. Australasian Journal of Dermatology 39:158–163

Hanke CW 1998 Adverse reactions to bovine collagen. In: Klein AW (ed.) Tissue Augmentation in Clinical Practice. Procedures and Techniques. Marcel Dekker, New York, pp 145–154

Hanke CW, Higley HR, Jolivette DM, Swanson NA, Stegman SJ 1991 Abscess formation and local necrosis after treatment with Zyderm or Zyplast collagen implant. Journal of the American Academy of Dermatology 25:319–326 [Review]

Hertzog B 1997 L'Artefill: historique, composition et aspects histologiques: technique d'injection, comparasion avec les autres produits. Journal of Medicine Esthetics Chir Dermatology 24:253–237

Hirsch RJ, Dayan SH 2004 Nonablative resurfacing. Facial Plastic Surgery 20:57–61

Homicz MR, Watson D 2004 Review of injectable materials for soft tissue augmentation. Facial Plastic Surgery 20:21–29

Jacobson LG, Alexiades-Armenakas M, Bernstein L, Geronemus RG 2003 Treatment of nasolabial folds and jowls with a noninvasive radiofrequency device. Archives in Dermatology 139:1371–1372

Jacquet A, Depont F. Evaluation of the acceptability, innocuity and performance of a gel made of microspheres of polylactic acid, New-Fill, for the injection of vertical facial wrinkles in women. Internal Report, March Biotech Industry S A, Luxembourg

Jasin ME 2002 Achieving superior resurfacing results with the erbium : YAG laser. Archives of Facial Plastic Surgery 4:262–266

Klein AW, Elson ML 2000 The history of substances for soft tissue augmentation. Dermatologic Surgery 26:1096–1105 [Review]

Klein AW 2001 Skin filling. Collagen and other injectables of the skin. Dermatology Clinics 19:491–508, ix [Review]

Labow TA, Silvers DN 1985 Late reactions at Zyderm skin test sites. Cutis 35:154–6, 158

Larrabee Jr W, Makielski K, Henderson J 2004 Surgical Anatomy of the Face. 2nd edn. Lippincott Williams and Wilkins

Lemperle G, Morhenn V, Charrier U 2003 Human histology and persistence of various injectable filler substances for soft tissue augmentation. Aesthetic Plastic Surgery 27:354–366; discussion 367. Epub 2003 Dec 04

Lemperle G, Ott H, Charrier U, Hecker J, Lemperle M 1991 PMMA microspheres for intradermal implantation. I. Animal research. Annals of Plastic Surgery 26:57–63

Lemperle G, Romano J, Busso M 2003 Soft tissue augmentation with Artefill: 10-year history, indications, techniques, and complications. Dermatologic Surgery 29:573–578

Lemperle G, Holmes R. Larson FG 200 Granuloma formation and electrical surface charges after Bioplastique and Arteplast implantation. Aesthetic Plastic Surgery 24:74–75

Le Van P 1978 The causes and prevention of poor cosmetic results from injection of fluid silicone. Journal of Dermatologic Surgery and Oncology 4:328–332

Lombardi T, Samson J, Plantier F, Husson C, Kuffer R 2004 Orofacial granulomas after injection of cosmetic fillers. Histopathologic and clinical study of 11 cases. Journal of Oral Pathology and Medicine 33:115–120

Lowe NJ 2003 Arterial embolization caused by injection of hyaluronic acid (Restylane). British Journal of Dermatology 148:379; author reply 379–380

Lycka B, Bazan C, Poletti E, Treen B 2004. The emerging technique of the antiptosis subdermal suspension thread. Dermatologic Surgery 30:41–4; discussion 44

Mastruserio M, Pesqueira MJ, Cobb MW 1996 Severe granulomatous reaction and facial ulceration occurring after subcutaneous silicone injection. Journal of the American Academy of Dermatology 34:849–852

Many WL, Sawatzki K 1998 Fremdkerorperreaktion nach Implantation von PMMA (polymethylmethacrylat) zur Weichteilaugmentation. Z Hautkrhu, H + G 73:42

Markey A, Glogau R 2000 Autologous fat grafting: Comparison of techniques. Dermatologic Surgery 26:1135–1139

Moyle GJ, Lysakova L, Brown S, et al 2004 A randomized open-label study of immediate versus delayed polylactic acid injections for the cosmetic management of facial lipoatrophy in persons with HIV infection. HIV Medicine 5:82–87

Narins RS, Brandt F, Leyden J, Lorenc ZP, Rubin M, Smith S 2003 A randomized, double-blind, multicenter comparison of the efficacy and tolerability of Restylane versus Zyplast for the correction of nasolabial folds. Dermatologic Surgery 29:588–595

Nayak PL 1999 Biodegradable polymers: opportunities and challenges. J.M.S. Rev Macromol Chemistry and Physics C39:481–505

Owsley JQ 1995 Elevation of the malar fat pad superficial to the orbicularis oculi muscle for correction of prominent nasolabial folds. Clinical Plastic Surgery 22:279–293

Papadavid E, Katsambas A 2003 Lasers for facial rejuvenation: a review. International Journal of Dermatology 42:480–487. Review

Park MY, Ahn KY, Jung DS 2003 Botulinum toxin type A treatment for contouring of the lower face. Dermatologic Surgery 29:477–483

Orentreich NO 1983 Soft tissue augmentation with medical grade fluid silicone. In: Rubin LR (ed.) Biomaterials in Reconstructive Surgery. CV Mosby, St Louis 859–881

Rapaport MJ, Vinnik CH, Zarem H 1996 Injectable silicone: cause of facial nodules, cellulites, ulceration, and migration. Aesthetics in Plastic Surgery 20:267–276

Rudkin F, Miller TA 1999 Aging nasolabial fold and treatment by direct excision. Plastic and Reconstructive Surgery 104:1502–1505

Sattler G, Sommer B 2000 Liporecycling: a technique for facial rejuvenation and body contouring. Dermatologic Surgery 26:1140–1144

Schanz S, Schippert W, Ulmer A, Rassner G, Fierlbeck G 2002 Arterial embolization caused by injection of hyaluronic acid (Restylane). British Journal of Dermatology 146:928–929

Selmanowitz VJ, Orentreich N 1977 Medical grade fluid silicone: a monographic review. Journal of Dermatologic Surgery and Oncology 3:597–611

Sklar JA, White SM 2004 Radiesse FN: A New Soft Tissue Filler. Dermatologic Surgery 30:764–768

Sommer B, Sattler G 2000 Current concepts in fat graft survival: histology of aspirated adipose tissue and review of the literature. Dermatologic Surgery 26:1159–1166

Tanzi EL, Alster TS 2003 Single-pass carbon dioxide versus multiple-pass Er : YAG laser skin resurfacing: a comparison of postoperative wound healing and side-effect rates. Dermatologic Surgery 29:80–84

Valantin MA, Aubron-Oliver C, et al 2003 Polylactic acid implants (New-Fill) to correct facial lipoatrophy in HIV-infected patients: results of the open-label study VEGA. AIDS 21:2471–2477

Webster R, Hamdan U, Fuleihan N, et al 1986 Injectable silicone: its history and its current status. American Journal of Cosmetic Surgery 3:31

Weiss RA, McDaniel DH, Genonemus RG 2003 Review of nonablative photorejuvenation: reversal of the aging effects of the sun and environmental damage using laser and light sources. Seminars in Cutaneous Medical Surgery 22:93–106 [Review]

Wulf HC, Sandby-Miller J, Kobayasi T, Gniadecki R 2004 Skin aging and natural photoprotection. Micron 35:185–191

Yousif NJ, Matloub MD, Matloub H, Summers AN 2002 The midface sling: a new technique to rejuvenate the midface. Plastic and Reconstructive Surgery 110:1541–1553; discussion 1554–1557

Zelickson BD, Kist D, Bernstein E, et al 2004 Histological and ultrastructural evaluation of the effects of a radiofrequency-based nonablative dermal remodeling device: a pilot study. Archives in Dermatology 140:204–209

9 Pain Control in Cosmetic Facial Surgery

Joseph Niamtu, Kevin Smith, Jean Carruthers

INTRODUCTION

In cosmetic facial surgery practices, the majority of patients require regional anesthesia, topical or injected. The esthetic physician and surgeon can do a better job on a patient who is comfortable, relaxed and confident. The reputation for excellence in amelioration of pain and discomfort serves as an extraordinary internal marketing enhancer. Conversely, even the most talented cosmetic surgeon can produce negative marketing effects if they have the reputation of causing unnecessary physical or emotional discomfort.

This chapter is designed to teach basic methods of pain control for cosmetic facial surgical procedures. It is impossible within the scope of this text to provide full details on each technique, but after reading this chapter the doctor should be able to understand the most basic techniques of local anesthesia as well as the neuroanatomy involved in anesthetizing specific dermatomes related to the injection of fillers in the face. In some cases the focal application of ice for 30–60 seconds prior to administration of filler substances or Botox for hyperhidrosis of the palms produces good anesthesia and is preferred by patients to the use of injectable local anesthetics.

In addition to the mechanics of anesthesia, it is important to understand and use 'talkesthesia' – which helps us to earn and maintain the confidence of our patients. A well-informed patient who is confident of your skill and your care usually needs less anesthesia and analgesia. 'Talkesthesia' starts with the patient's first phone call to your office or visit to your website, and continues through to your final contact with the patient. 'Talkesthesia' includes all verbal and nonverbal communication by yourself, your staff, and your operating environment with the patient, and includes such things as music and art throughout your office and in your treatment rooms.

Pre-emptive analgesia can also reduce patient discomfort. The use of nonsedating analgesics and anxiolytics can greatly enhance patient comfort, and not interfere with their ability to drive home. For example, a combination of 800 mg of ibuprofen (e.g. two 400 mg Liquid Advil GelCaps) and 2 g of acetaminophen (2 oz pediatric liquid Tylenol) can produce additive analgesia, because ibuprofen blocks cyclooxygenase types 1 and 2, while acetaminophen blocks cyclooxygenase type 3. The liquid formulation allows for a good blood level to be reached within half an hour.

Propranolol (Inderal 40–80 mg po 1–2 hours before a procedure) is an excellent nonsedating anxiolytic. Propranolol is a very lipid-soluble beta blocker, so it crosses the blood–brain barrier efficiently, and reduces anxiety by blocking the beta receptors in the brain, in particular at the amygdala.

Pre-treatment with propranolol has also been shown to reduce the emotional content of memories of painful experiences, so that the memory is less vivid and is mainly intellectual. The principal contraindication to propranolol is that it should not be given to patients who suffer from asthma, because members of this class of medication can exacerbate asthma.

PATIENT SELECTION

Patient selection for any esthetic procedure includes an assessment of esthetic needs and expectations within the traditional medical framework of an assessment of general health, allergy, and previous response to analgesic medications. It is often helpful to inquire about previous dental work and the response to injected anesthetic.

EXPECTED BENEFITS

The expected benefits for local anesthetic techniques are primarily focused on the subjective comfort of the patient. The physician will be able to more completely address the esthetic concerns in a subject who is relaxed and comfortable. The safety profile and benefits of these techniques are high and the complication rate and risks are low.

Complications of anesthesia are related to individual patient susceptibility and to physician technique. The former can include allergic reaction, vasoconstrictor overdose, ineffective block, and extended anesthesia.

Soft Tissue Augmentation

Technique-related complications are largely avoidable and include hematoma, nerve damage, bruising, and intravascular injection.

• Sensory Dermatomes of the Head and Neck

The main sensory innervation of the face is derived from cranial nerve V (trigeminal nerve) and the upper cervical nerves (Fig. 9.1).

• Trigeminal nerve

The trigeminal nerve is the fifth of the 12 cranial nerves. Its branches originate at the semilunar ganglion (gasserian ganglion) located in the temporal bone. Three large nerves, the ophthalmic, maxillary, and mandibular, proceed from the ganglion to supply sensory innervation to the face (Fig. 9.2).

Often referred to as 'the great sensory nerve of the head and neck', the trigeminal nerve is named for its three major sensory branches. The ophthalmic nerve (V1), maxillary nerve (V2), and mandibular nerve (V3) are literally 'three twins' (trigeminal) carrying sensory information of light touch, temperature, pain, and proprioception from the face and scalp to the brainstem. The main branches of the trigeminal nerve supply sensation to the well-defined and consistent facial areas (Fig. 9.2). The inset in

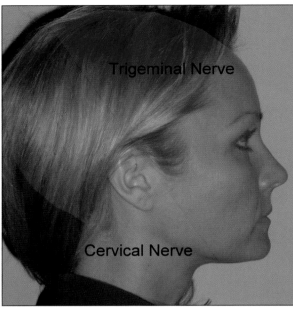

Fig. 9.1 The entire head and neck is supplied by the trigeminal and cervical nerves

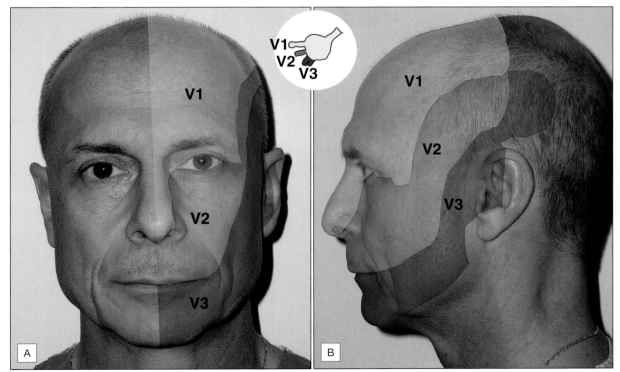

Fig. 9.2 (**A** and **B**) The main branches of the trigeminal nerve supplying sensation to the respective facial areas, The inset shows the trigeminal ganglion with the three main nerve branches

Figure 9.2 shows the trigeminal ganglion with the three main nerve branches.

• Ophthalmic nerve (V1)

The ophthalmic nerve, or first division of the trigeminal, is a sensory nerve only. It supplies branches to the cornea, ciliary body, and iris; to the lacrimal gland and conjunctiva; to part of the mucous membrane of the nasal cavity; and to the skin of the eyelids, eyebrow, forehead, and upper lateral nose (see V1 on Fig. 9.2). It divides into three branches: the frontal, nasociliary, and lacrimal. The frontal nerve divides into the supraorbital and supratrochlear nerves providing sensation to the forehead and anterior scalp.

Anesthetizing branches of V1 has clinical significance for procedures in the forehead, brow regions, and glabella.

• Maxillary nerve (V2)

The maxillary nerve or second division of the trigeminal is a sensory nerve that appears upon the face at the infraorbital foramen as the infraorbital nerve. At its termination, the nerve divides into branches which spread out upon the side of the nose, the lower eyelid, and the upper lip (see V2 on Fig. 9.2). Additional branches include the zygomaticotemporal, which supplies sensation to the skin on the side of the forehead and zygomaticofacial nerve, which supplies sensation to the skin on the prominence of the cheek (see V2 on Fig. 9.2). Anesthetizing branches of V2 has clinical significance for procedures in the temporal area, midface, nasolabial folds, and the upper lip.

• Mandibular nerve (V3)

The mandibular nerve supplies the teeth and gums of the mandible, the skin of the temporal region, part of the auricle, the lower lip, and the lower part of the face (see V3 on Fig. 9.2). Sensory branches of the mandibular nerve include the auriculotemporal nerve, which supplies sensation to the skin covering the front of the helix, and tragus (Fig. 9.2). The inferior alveolar nerve is the largest branch of the mandibular nerve. It exits the ramus of the mandible at the mandibular foramen. It then passes forward in the mandibular canal, beneath the teeth, as far as the mental foramen, where it divides into two terminal branches, the incisive and mental nerves. The mental nerve emerges at the mental foramen, and divides into three branches of which one descends to the skin of the chin, and two ascend to the skin and mucous membrane of the lower lip. The buccal nerve is a branch of V3 which supplies sensation to the skin over the buccinator muscle. Anesthetizing branches of V3 have clinical significance for procedures in the lower lip and perioral areas of the lower face.

TOPICAL ANESTHESIA

Despite the effectiveness of injectable anesthetics, the injection itself is often as painful as the procedure for which the anesthetic is used. This is especially true for minor procedures such as botulinum exotoxin injection and nonablative lasers. In these cases, topical anesthetics are useful to alleviate mild to moderate discomfort.

There are several commonly used topical anesthetics. Eutectic Mixture of Local Anesthetics (EMLA) is a 5% eutectic mixture of lidocaine (lignocaine) and prilocaine. One of the most widely used topical agents, it was briefly removed from the market recently due to a faulty child-resistant cap, but is now available once again with a redesigned child-resistant closure. EMLA provides suboptimal analgesia when applied for 30 minutes or less, but gives adequate dermal analgesia when applied under occlusive dressing for 60 minutes. Dermal analgesia continues for 15–30 minutes after its removal.

ELA-Max, which recently has been renamed LMX-5, is a 5% lidocaine (lignocaine) cream which uses a liposomal encapsulation system. Liposomes enhance the penetration into the skin, provide sustained release, and protect the drug from metabolic degradation. It appears superior to EMLA in providing analgesia when applied for 30 minutes.

Betacaine is also a combination of lidocaine (lignocaine) and prilocaine with an added vasoconstrictor, although the manufacturer has not revealed the exact proportion. The vasoconstrictive agent and the proprietary microemulsion delivery system speed the onset of the analgesia, and the petrolatum base makes the gel self-occlusive. The manufacturer recommends an application time of 30–45 minutes without occlusive dressing. This product is not approved by the FDA and must be purchased from the manufacturer.

Tetracaine gel, previously known as amethocaine in the UK, is a compounded, proprietary ester anesthetic with a recommended application time of 30–45 minutes under occlusion. Its advantage is the long duration of analgesia, up to 4–6 hours. A comparison study shows that tetracaine is more efficacious than lidocaine–prilocaine mixture when both anesthetics are applied for the same amount of time. However, unlike the amide anesthetics, allergic contact reactions to ester anesthetics are quite common.

The average time of application of topical anesthetics ranges from 30–60 minutes, which can be a frustrating rate-limiting step in clinical practice. S-Caine peel is a new development that may have a quicker onset. S-Caine peel is a eutectic lidocaine (lignocaine) and tetracaine (amethocaine) cream mixture that dries to a flexible film that easily peels off. This property precludes the need for extra time-consuming steps such as application of occlusive dressing and removal of the creams. Furthermore, adequate anesthesia is achieved in as little as 20 minutes of application. A recent double-blinded study concluded that S-Caine peel is superior to EMLA cream under occlusion for 30 minutes.

CRYOANESTHESIA

Cyroanesthesia refers to localized application of cold as a means of producing regional anesthesia. There are many sources of cold, but as a practical matter ice has turned out to be the most useful and safe source of cold when working on the skin. Because ice makes a transition to water at 0°C, the temperature of the tissue will not drop below 0°C, reducing the risk of excess cooling. The focal application of ice before and sometimes after painful procedures has been practiced for thousands of years – ice was one of the first forms of local anesthesia and analgesia.

Mechanisms of action of cryoanesthesia include:

1. Reduction in the sensitivity of pain receptors in the skin
2. Reduction in the rate of sensory nerve depolarization
3. Inhibition of both the release and the activity of:
   a. Inflammatory mediators, and
   b. Pain-mediating neurotransmitters such as substance P
4. Activation of the gate control of pain mechanism at the level of the spinal cord.

One author (KCS) found the focal application of ice to be of particular value prior to the administration of filler substances. In areas other than the lips (e.g. the NLFs), ice is applied to an area which includes the intended needle insertion point, the path the needle will follow under the surface of the skin, and (very importantly) to a 1 cm margin of skin around those areas. The optimum size for the surface of an ice cube which is in contact with the patient is about 3 × 5 cm.

To improve the grip on the ice cube, it is helpful to remove the ice cubes from the ice cube tray, apply a folded 2 × 4 inch piece of gauze (made from a 4 × 4 inch piece of 4 ply gauze) to the rounded surface of the ice cube, then put the ice cube back in the tray and freeze it for several hours so that the ice will bond to the gauze. These ice cubes can then be put into individual paper cups and stored in the freezer until they are needed (Figs 9.3 and 9.4).

Ice is applied for at least 30 seconds (sometimes 45 seconds) – and adequate duration of icing is ensured by watching a clock in the treatment room. If there is a fine line to be treated, it can be marked by pressing the needle into the line (as shown) while ice is applied. After the area to be treated has been iced for an appropriate duration, the ice is moved to skin several cm away from the area to be treated (or sometimes is applied to the next area to be treated, on the contralateral side of the patient's face). Application of ice nearby, during the injection, further reduces the patient's discomfort, probably by maximizing activation of the neural systems responsible for gate control of pain at the level of the spinal cord, in a manner similar to that observed when vibration is used. A detailed discussion of the neurophysiology of the gate control

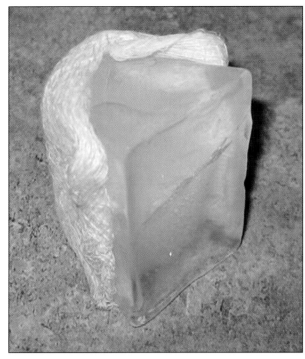

Fig. 9.3 Gauze applied to the rounded surface of ice

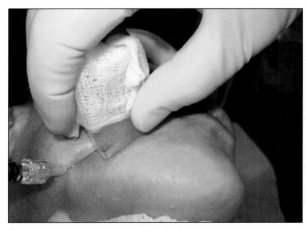

Fig. 9.4 Applying ice between 30 and 45 seconds

of pain can be found at http://dermatology.cdlib.org/102/therapy/anesthesia/comite.html (accessed 15 July 2006).

The duration of high-quality cryoanesthesia is about 10–15 seconds after ice is removed from the area to be treated. It is helpful to rub ice on the treated area for about 5 seconds immediately after the injection is completed, to attenuate any residual discomfort.

When treating the lips with filler substances, ice should be applied for 60 seconds before needle insertion. The lips are usually treated in a series of six applications of ice: starting with each lateral third of the lower lip, then the middle third of the lower lip, then the lateral thirds of the upper lip and finally the middle third of the upper lip.

Patients who have previously been treated with local anesthetics before administration of fillers prefer cryoanesthesia with ice because:

❖ 'Ice is more natural'
❖ No 'pins and needles' as the anesthetic wears off
❖ No 'hyper' feeling from adrenaline
❖ Total experience (anesthesia + treatment) hurts less
❖ Lower risk of bruising (as there are no injections of local anesthetic).

Both patients and the physician appreciate the fact that cryoanesthesia does not cause the distortion of facial features (either from volume of local anesthetic or from muscle relaxation secondary to regional anesthesia), which is seen so frequently with injectable anesthetics.

COMPARISON OF LENGTH OF NEEDLES COMMONLY USED FOR ADMINISTRATION OF FILLERS

The author (KCS) has found that the use of long needles further reduces patient discomfort and anxiety (Fig. 9.5). Patients report that needle *insertion* is the most stressful moment during the treatment process, regardless of the form of anesthesia. Advantages of long needles include:

❖ Long needles allow for a considerable reduction in the number of needle insertions, which also shortens the duration of the procedure.
❖ Because there are fewer needle insertions, there are fewer occasions when the needle passes through the vascular plexus in the papillary dermis, contributing to a reduction in the incidence and severity of bruising.
❖ The reduced number of needle insertions also helps to keep the needle tip sharp, reducing tissue trauma and associated discomfort.
❖ Long needles allow the physician to lay down a continuous bead of filler material, and to more precisely modulate the quantity of filler material delivered as the treated area is filled.

Figure 9.6 shows a comparison between the area which can be treated with a single insertion of a 27 gauge 1.25 in needle.

Typical l-o-n-g needles (B-D PrecisionGlide) routinely used for various products include:

❖ Restylane: 30 gauge 1 in or a 27 gauge 1.25 in
❖ Perlane, Juvéderm 24 HV, (Juvéderm Ultra) and Juvéderm 30 HV (Juvéderm Ultra Plus) Evolence, Radiesse: 27 gauge 1.25 in
❖ Artecoll: 25 gauge, 7/8 in to 1.5 in

The routine application of firm, steady pressure for 5 minutes (as measured on the clock in the treatment room), starting as soon as possible after the needle is withdrawn from the skin, has greatly reduced the incidence and severity of bruising in the author's practice (Fig. 9.7). Patients are pleased to participate in their care by holding pressure on the treated area.

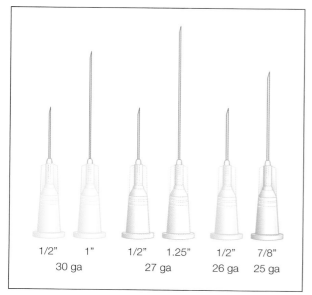

Fig. 9.5 Comparison of length of needles commonly used for administration of fillers

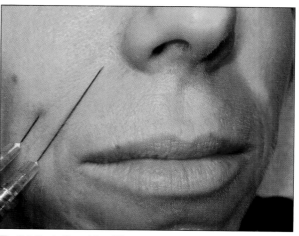

Fig. 9.6 Illustration of the different areas treated with a long needle compared with a short needle

Soft Tissue Augmentation

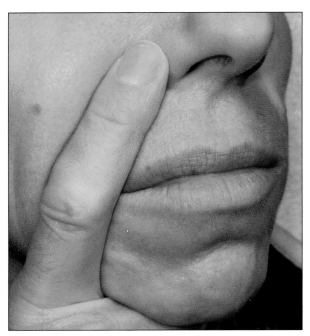

Fig. 9.7 Application of pressure on the treated area

VIBRATORY ANESTHESIA

Vibration has been used for many years to reduce pain in disciplines such as dentistry and physiotherapy, and is now becoming recognized as a simple, safe, and effective form of anesthesia in dermatology. Vibration anesthesia can be explained by the 'gate theory of pain control' popularized by Melzack and Wall in the 1960s. Noxious nerve impulses evoked by injuries are influenced in the spinal cord by other nerve cells that act like gates, either preventing the impulses from getting through, or facilitating their passage. Without vibratory modulation, noxious impulses are carried through small C fibers uninhibited through a 'gate' in the spinal cord that ultimately sends the signal to the brain. When applied simultaneously, vibratory stimulation excites large A fibers, which activates inhibitory interneurons at the gate and mitigates the perception of pain in the brain.

A variety of vibratory massagers can be used to produce effective vibratory anesthesia. A study has shown that pain sensitivity gradually declines as vibration amplitude increases, but no specific frequency is more effective in interference with nociception. The vibratory massager should be applied within 1–2 cm of the site to be treated for approximately 2–3 seconds prior to the injection or laser application and continued throughout the injection or laser application. A detailed discussion of vibratory anesthesia, with video clips illustrating various procedures, can be found at http://dermatology.cdlib.org/102/therapy/anesthesia/comite.html (accessed 15 July 2006).

INFILTRATIVE PERIPHERAL ANESTHESIA VERSUS REGIONAL NERVE BLOCK ANESTHESIA

Local anesthesia can be effectively obtained both by infiltrations and nerve blocks. Infiltrative local anesthesia applies to the injection of the local anesthesia solution in the area of the peripheral innervation distant from the site of the main nerve. An advantage of infiltrative anesthesia is that no specific skill is necessary, only the selected area of innervation is involved and vasoconstrictors can improve local hemostasis. A drawback of infiltrative local anesthesia is the distortion of the tissue at or around the site of injection, which may obscure the tissue detail required in cosmetic procedures such as filler injection.

• Nerve blocks

A nerve block involves placing the local anesthetic solution in a specific location at or around the main nerve trunk that will effectively depolarize that nerve and obtund sensation in the area of sensory distribution of that particular nerve. Advantages of nerve blocks include the fact that a single accurately placed injection can obtund large areas of sensation without tissue distortion at the operative site. Disadvantages of peripheral nerve block include the sensation of numbness in areas other than the operative site and the lack of hemostasis at the operative site from the vasoconstrictor component of the local anesthetic injection.

Individual anatomic variation is responsible for the sometimes unpredictable effect of peripheral nerve block. Nerves that innervate areas close to the midline may receive innervation from the contralateral side and require bilateral blocks. Some nerve blocks may also require infiltrative local anesthesia to obtain adequate pain control.

Since many nerves are accompanied by corresponding veins and arteries, preinjection aspiration should always be performed to prevent intravascular injection. Using local anesthetics with vasoconstrictors will prolong anesthesia, which may be undesirable for most patients who want to return to normal activities after filler injection. Prolonged anesthesia makes speaking and normal lip posture difficult, so most doctors only prefer to use shorter acting anesthetics so that the anesthetic effect persists through the injection sequence.

ANATOMIC ARRANGEMENT OF THE FACIAL FORAMINA

Successful nerve block anesthesia is largely dependent upon knowing the positions of the nerve foramina. The surgeon can take advantage of the alignment of the major facial foramina as they relate to a vertical line through the midpupillary line with the eye in the primary position of natural forward gaze (Fig. 9.8).

BLOCKING THE SCALP AND FOREHEAD

The use of fillers has recently expanded beyond the lips. Multiple areas of all sensory dermatomes may be sites for

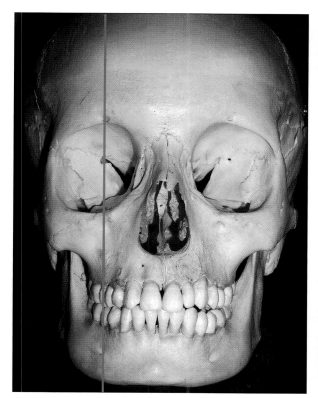

Fig. 9.8 The supraorbital, infraorbital and mental foramina are all in line with an imaginary vertical passing through the mid pupil

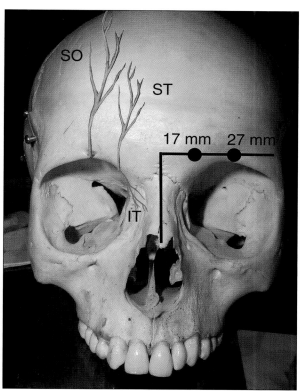

Fig. 9.9 The supraorbital nerve (SO) exits about 27 mm from the glabellar midline and the supratrochlear nerve (ST) is located approximately 17 mm from the glabellar midline. The infratrochlear nerve (IT) exits below the trochlea

the use of dermal fillers. Using filler agents in the glabellar area and frontalis lines may require local anesthesia of the frontal nerve to anesthetize the forehead.

Supraorbital nerve

The supraorbital nerve exits through a notch (in some cases a foramen) on the superior orbital rim approximately 27 mm lateral to the glabellar midline (Fig. 9.9). This supraorbital notch is readily palpable in most patients. After exiting the notch or foramen, the nerve traverses the corrugator supercilii muscles and branches into a medial and lateral portion. The lateral branches supply the lateral forehead and the medial branches supply the scalp.

Supratrochlear nerve

The supratrochlear nerve exits a foramen approximately 17 mm from the glabellar midline (Fig. 9.9) and supplies sensation to the middle portion of the forehead. The infratrochlear nerve exits a foramen below the trochlea and provides sensation to the medial upper eyelid, canthus, medial nasal skin, conjunctiva, and lacrimal apparatus (Fig. 9.9).

When injecting this area it is prudent to always use the nondominant hand to palpate the orbital rim to ensure that the needle tip is exterior to the bony orbital margin. To anesthetize this area, the supratrochlear nerve is mea-

sured 17 mm from the glabellar midline and 1–2 mL of local anesthetic are injected (Fig. 9.10A). The supraorbital nerve is blocked by palpating the notch (and/or measuring 27 mm from the glabellar midline) and injecting 1–2 mL of local anesthetic solution (Fig. 9.10B). The infratrochlear nerve is blocked by injecting 1–2 mL of local anesthetic solution at the junction of the orbit and the nasal bones (Fig. 9.10C; Fig. 9.11 shows the regions anesthetized from the above blocks).

INFRAORBITAL NERVE BLOCK

This block is one of the most commonly utilized facial blocks in order to anesthetize the upper lip and upper NLF for injection of fillers. Obviously, a bilateral block must be performed to achieve anesthesia on both sides of the lip.

The infaorbital nerve exits the infraorbital foramen 4–7 mm below the orbital rim in an imaginary line dropped from the midpupillary midline. The anterior superior alveolar nerve branches from the infraorbital nerve before it exits the foramen, and thus some patients will manifest anesthesia of the anterior teeth and gingiva if the branching is close to the foramen. Areas anesthetized include the lateral nose, anterior cheek, lower eyelid, and upper lip

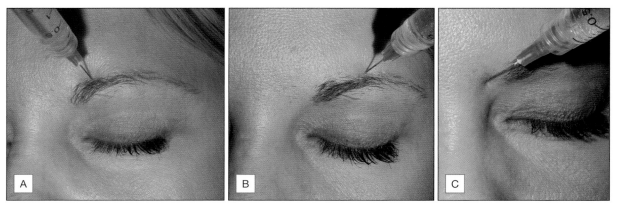

Fig. 9.10 (A–C) The forehead and scalp is blocked by a series of injections from the central to the medial brow

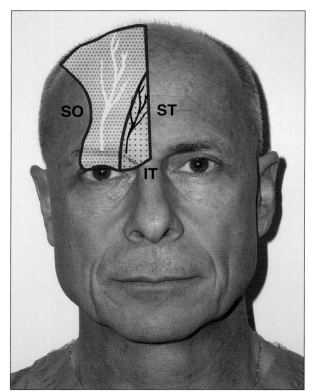

Fig. 9.11 The shaded areas indicate the anesthetized areas from supraorbital nerve (SO) and supratrochlear nerve (ST) and infratrochlear nerve (IT) blocks

on the injected side. This nerve can be blocked by intraoral or extraoral routes. To perform an infraorbital nerve block from an intraoral approach, topical anesthesia is placed on the oral mucosa at the vestibular sulcus just under the canine fossa (between the canine and first premolar tooth) and left for several minutes. The lip is then elevated and a $^1/_2$ in 30 gauge needle is inserted in the sulcus and directed superiorly toward the infraorbital foramen (Fig.

9.12). Bending the needle at a 45-degree angle upward can facilitate the needle insertion (Fig. 9.13). The needle needs only to approach the vast branching around the foramen to be effective. It is important to use the other hand to palpate the inferior orbital rim to avoid injecting superiorly the orbit. For the infraorbital block, 2–4 mL of 2% lidocaine (lignocaine) are injected in this area and the palpating finger can feel the local anesthetic bolus below the infraorbital rim, confirming the correct area of placement.

The authors find it important to ask the patient to open their eyes and look straight ahead when performing the infraorbital block. This way, the injector can see the pupil and better appreciate the position of the infraorbital foramen, which is 4–7 mm below the infraorbital rim in the midpupillary line.

The infraorbital nerve can also be very easily blocked by the transcutaneous facial approach and may be the preferred route in dental phobic patients. A 32 gauge $^1/_2$ in needle is used and is placed through the skin and aimed at the foramen in a perpendicular direction. Between 2 and 4 mL of local anesthetic solution is injected at or close to the foramen (Fig. 9.14). Again, the other hand must constantly palpate the inferior orbital rim to prevent inadvertent injection into the orbit. Care must be used in this approach to avoid superficial vessels that may cause noticeable bruising.

A successful infraorbital nerve block will anesthetize the infraorbital cheek, the lower palpebral area, the lateral nasal area, and superior labial regions as shown in Figure 9.15.

Anesthesia for esthetic lip augmentation

Although in theory a bilateral infraorbital block should anesthetize the entire upper lip, some patients may still perceive pain for various anatomic (or sometimes psychological) reasons detailed earlier in this article. The author recommends the injection of 1.0 mL of local anesthetic solution in the maxillary labial frenum (Fig. 9.16). Whether for psychological or physiological reasons, this seems to provide additional anesthesia. This can also be performed

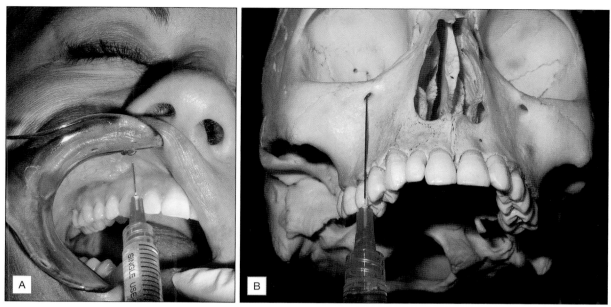

Fig. 9.12 (**A** and **B**) The intraoral approach for local anesthetic block of the infraorbital nerve

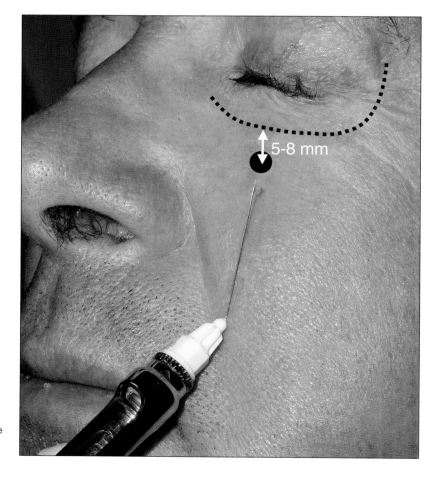

Fig. 9.13 Bending the 1½ inch 28 gauge needles at a 45-degree angle can facilitate the injection technique of the infraorbital nerve. Note the needle is shown outside the mouth for illustrative purposes only. The actual injection is intraoral

Soft Tissue Augmentation

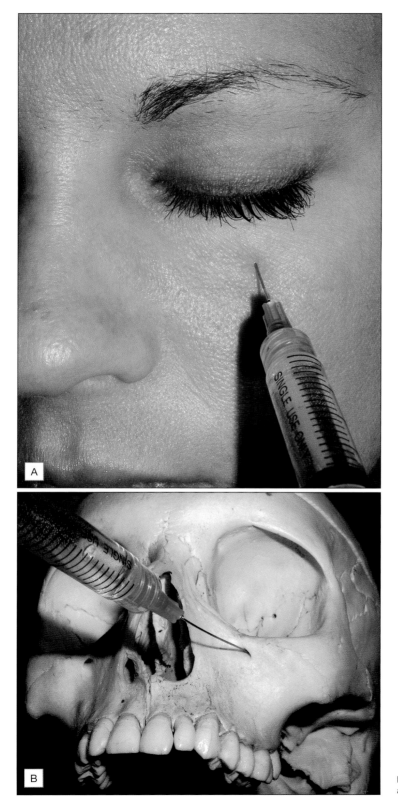

Fig. 9.14 (**A** and **B**) The facial approach for local anesthetic block of the infraorbital nerve

in the lower lip labial frenum area to augment bilateral mental blocks, as will be discussed later in this chapter. The combination of bilateral infraorbital and mental blocks and the just described infiltrative augmentation (when necessary) is an ideal technique for anesthetizing the lips for filler injection or lip implant placement.

Zygomaticofacial nerve

Two often overlooked nerves in facial local anesthetic blocks are the zygomaticotemporal and zygomaticofacial nerves. This may assist the injection of fillers in facial rhytides on the lateral temporal and lateral canthal areas or in the malar areas. These nerves represent terminal

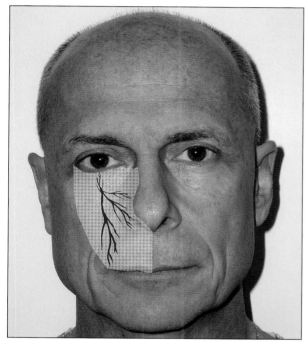

Fig. 9.15 Area of anesthesia from unilateral infraorbital nerve block

branches of the zygomatic nerve. The zygomaticotemporal nerve emerges through a foramen located on the anterior wall of the temporal fossa. This foramen is actually behind the lateral orbital rim posterior to the zygoma at the approximate level of the lateral canthus (Fig. 9.16).

The injection technique involves sliding a $1\frac{1}{2}$ inch 27 gauge needle behind the concave portion of the lateral orbital rim. It is suggested that this area should be closely examined on a model skull prior to attempting this injection as it will facilitate understanding of the anatomy and make the technique simpler. To orient for this injection it is necessary to palpate the lateral orbital rim at the level of the frontozygomatic suture (which is frequently palpable). With the index finger in the depression of the posterior lateral aspect of the lateral orbital rim (inferior and posterior to the frontozygomatic suture), the operator places the needle just behind the palpating finger (which is about 1 cm posterior to the frontozygomatic suture (Fig. 9.16). The needle is then 'walked' down the concave posterior wall of the lateral orbital rim to the approximate level of the lateral canthus. After aspirating, 1–2 mL of 2% lidocaine (lignocaine) is injected in this area with a slight pumping action to ensure deposition of the local anesthetic solution at or about the foramen. Again, it is important to hug the back concave wall of the lateral orbital rim with the needle when injecting.

Blocking the zygomaticotemporal nerve causes anesthesia in the area superior to the nerve, including the lateral orbital rim and the skin of the temple from above the zygomatic arch to the temporal fusion line (see ZT on Fig. 9.17).

Zygomaticofacial nerve

The zygomaticofacial nerve exits through a foramen (or foramina in some patients) in the inferior lateral portion of the orbital rim at the zygoma. If the surgeon palpates the junction of the inferior lateral portion of the lateral orbital rim, the nerve emerges several millimeters lateral to this point. By palpating this area and injecting just lateral to the finger, this nerve is successfully blocked with 1–2 mL of local anesthetic (Fig. 9.18). Blocking this nerve

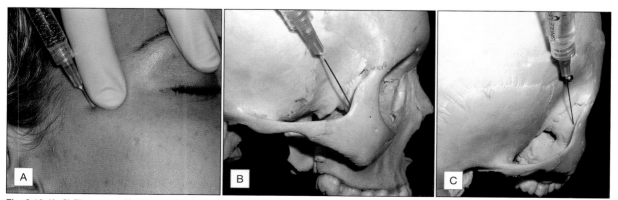

Fig. 9.16 (A–C) The zygomaticotemporal nerve is blocked by placing the needles on the concave surface of the posterior lateral orbital rim

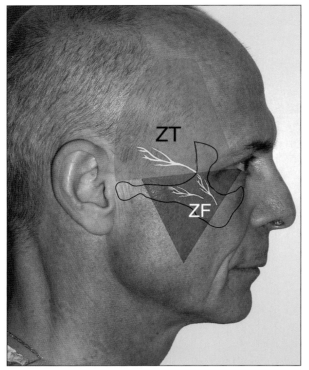

Fig. 9.17 The anesthetized areas form the zygomaticotemporal (ZT) and the zygomaticofacial (ZF) nerves

will result in anesthesia of a triangular area from the lateral canthus and the malar region along the zygomatic arch and some skin inferior to this area (see ZF on Fig. 9.17).

MENTAL NERVE BLOCK

The mental nerve exits the mental foramen on the hemi-mandible at the base of the root of the second premolar (many patients may be missing a premolar due to orthodontic extractions). The mental foramen is on average 11 mm inferior to the gum line (Fig. 9.19). There is variability with this foramen (like all foramina), but by injecting 2–4 mL of local anesthetic solution about 10 mm inferior to the gum line or 15 mm inferior to the top of the crown of the second premolar tooth the block is usually successful. In a patient without teeth, the foramen is often times located much higher on the jaw and can sometimes be palpated. This block is performed more superiorly in the denture patient. As stated earlier, the foramen does not need to be entered as a sufficient volume of local anesthetic solution in the general area will be effective. By placing traction on the lip and pulling it away from the jaw, the labial branches of the mental nerve can sometimes be seen traversing through the thin mucosa. The mental nerve gives off labial branches to the lip and chin (Fig. 9.20).

Alternatively, the mental nerve may be blocked through the skin of the cheek with a facial approach, aiming for the same target.

When anesthetized the distribution of numbness will be the unilateral lower lip to the midline and laterally to the mentolabial fold, and in some patients the anterior chin and cheek depending on the individual furcating anatomy of that patient's nerve (Fig. 9.21).

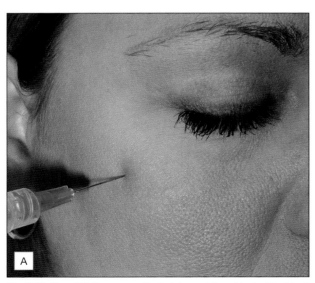

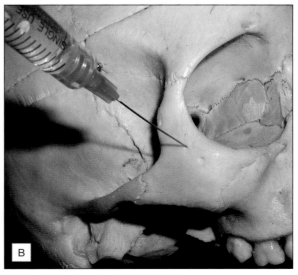

Fig. 9.18 (**A** and **B**) The zygomaticofacial nerve(s) are blocked by injecting the inferior lateral portion of the orbital rim

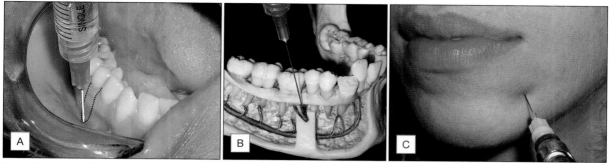

Fig. 9.19 The mental foramen is approached intraorally below the root tip of the lower second premolar (**A** and **B**) or from a facial approach (**C**)

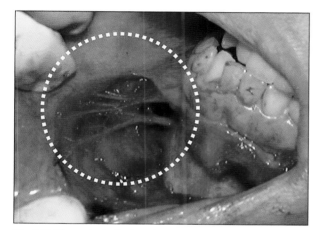

Fig. 9.20 The vast arborization of the distal branches of the mental nerve (in circle) are visualized intraoperatively in a genioplasty incision

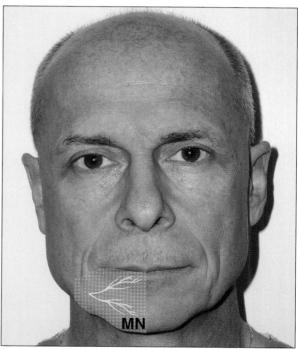

Fig. 9.21 The anesthetized areas from a unilateral mental nerve block. Owing to various anatomic factors, the area below the mentolabial fold or at the midline may share other innervation

The author after performing hundreds of facial blocks for filler injection now uses a simple infiltration technique. Instead of blocking the infraorbital and mental nerves, the author first places topical anesthetic on the maxillary and mandibular vestibule from the canine tooth on one side to the canine tooth on the other side. After several minutes, a 32 gauge needle is used to inject 1/4 cc of local anesthetic solution at the depth of the maxillary and/or mandibular vestibule. The vestibule is defined as the junction of the attached gingiva (gum) and the lip mucosa. These injections are made just above the periosteum in 4 or 5 spots between the upper or lower canine teeth. This technique provides remarkable anesthesia suitable for filler injection and is often easier for the doctor and patient than nerve blocks. This technique is shown in Figure 9.22. Figure 9.23 shows the approximate area of anesthetized tissue with this infiltration. Profound numbness (10/10 is seen in the central portion of the lips and the degree of anesthesia tapers off toward the oral commisures 7/10.

To increase the depth of anesthesia at the lateral lip, the injections need to be carried to the premolar area.

An additional block of the anterior maxilla is one that is convenient for removing telangectasias or other lesions from the perinasal area nostrils. This is a common area for ectatic vessels and is very sensitive without anesthesia. Using a 32 gauge, $^1/_2$ in needle, 0.25 cc of local anesthesia is injected into the junction of the columella and upper lip. The injection pain is mitigated by pinching the upper lip and columella with the noninjecting hand while injecting. Figure 9.24 shows this technique. This local anesthetic

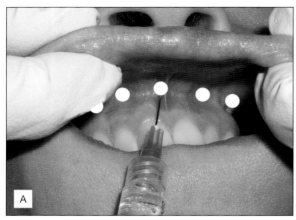
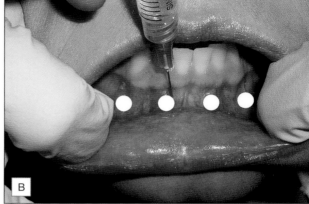

Fig. 9.22 (**A** and **B**) Submucosal lip infiltration can be used to augment or in place of bilateral mental nerve block to treat the lower lip. Very small volumes will create adequate anesthesia. The solution is injected across the entire lip. The same technique can be used on the upper lip as well

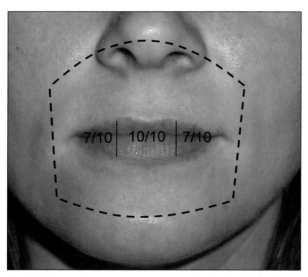

Fig. 9.23 Shows the approximate area anesthetized by this method. Numbness is profound in the midportion of the lip and tapers off laterally

infiltration will anesthetize the central portion of the upper lip, columella, nasal sill and the lower portion of the nostrils.

CONCLUSION

As advances are made in the science of facial fillers more products and indications will become available for these minimally invasive, highly effective esthetic procedures. This chapter outlines some of the more basic anatomy and techniques for anesthetizing the common areas of the face amenable to injectible fillers.

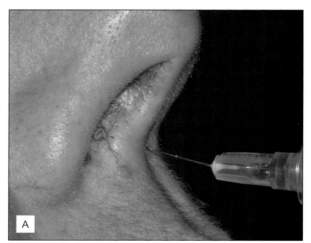
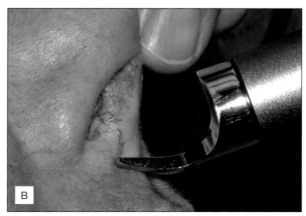

Fig. 9.24 (**A** and **B**) A simple local anesthetic injection with a 32 gauge needle at the base of the columella will provide adequate anesthesia for such procedures as lesion removal, ablation of telangectasias or fillers of this area

FURTHER READING

Aceves J, Machne X 1963 The action of calcium and of local anesthetics on nerve cells and their interaction during excitation. Journal of Pharmacology and Experimental Therapeutics 140:138–148

Alster TS, Lupton JR 2002 Evaluation of a novel topical anesthetic agent for cutaneous laser resurfacing: a randomized comparison study. Dermatologic Surgery 28:1004–1006

Bucalo BD, Mirikitani EJ, Moy RL 1998 Comparison of skin anesthetic effect of liposomal lidocaine, nonliposomal lidocaine, and EMLA using 30-minute application time. Dermatologic Surgery 24:537–541

Covino BG, Vassalo HG 1976 Chemical aspects of local anesthetic agents. In: Kitz RJ, Laver MB (eds) Local anesthetics: mechanism of action and clinical use. Grune & Stratton, New York, pp 1–11

Fink BR 1988 History of neural blockade. In: Cousins MJ, Bridenbaugh PO (eds) Neural Blockade in Clinical Anesthesia and Management of Pain, ed 2. JB Lippincott, Philadelphia, pp 3–21

Friedman PM, Fogelman JP, Nouri K, Levine VJ, Ashinoff R 1999 Comparative study of the efficacy of four topical anesthetics. Dermatologic Surgery 25:950–954

Gray H 1918 Anatomy of the human body, 13th edn. Lea & Febiger, Philadelphia, 1158–1169

Hadda SE 1962 Procaine: Alfred Einhorn's ideal substitute for cocaine. Journal of the American Dental Association 64:841–845

Hersh EV 2000 Local anesthetics. In: Fonseca RJ (ed.) Oral and Maxillofacial Surgery. WB Saunders, Philadelphia, pp 58–78

Hersh EV, Condouis GA 1987 Local anesthetics: a review of their pharmacology and clinical use. Compendium of Continuing Education in Dentistry 8:374–382

Hollins M, Roy EA, Crane SA 2003 Vibratory antinociception: effects of vibration amplitude and frequency. Journal of Pain 4:381–391

Jastak JT, Yagiela JA, Donaldson D 1995 Local anesthesia of the oral cavity. WB Saunders, Philadelphia

Kakigi R, Shibasaki H 1992 Mechanisms of pain relief by vibration and movement. Journal of Neurology, Neurosurgery and Psychiatry 55:282–286

Kosten TR, Hollister LE 1998 Drugs of abuse. In: Katzung BG (ed.) Basic and clinical pharmacology, 7th edn. Appleton & Lange, Norwalk, CT, pp 516–531

Lathers CM, Tyau LSY, Spino MM, Agarwal I 1988 Cocaine-induced seizures, arrhythmias, and sudden death. Journal of Clinical Pharmacology 28:584–593

Lener EV, Bucalo BD, Kist DA, Moy RL 1997 Topical anesthetic agents in dermatologic surgery. A review. Dermatologic Surgery 23:673–668

Malamed SF 1997 Handbook of local anesthesia, 4th edn. Mosby, St Louis, MO

Mendel N, Puterbaugh PG 1938 Conduction, infiltration and general anesthesia in dentistry, 4th edn. Dental Items of Interest Publishing Company, p. 140

Niamtu J 2005 Simple technique for lip and nasolabial fold anesthesia for injectable fillers. Dermatologic Surgery 31:1330–1332

Niamtu J 2005 Local anesthetic blocks of the head and neck for cosmetic facial surgery. Part V: Techniques for the head and neck. Cosmetic Dermatology 18:65–68

Niamtu J 2004 Local anesthetic blocks of the head and neck for cosmetic facial surgery. Part IV. Techniques for the lower face. Cosmetic Dermatology 17:714–720

Niamtu J 2004 Local anesthetic blocks of the head and neck for cosmetic facial surgery. Part III. Techniques for the maxillary nerve. Cosmetic Dermatology 17:645–647

Niamtu J 2004 Local anesthetic blocks of the head and neck for cosmetic facial surgery. Part II. Techniques for the upper and midface. Cosmetic Dermatology 17:583–587

Niamtu J 2004 Local anesthetic blocks of the head and neck for cosmetic facial surgery. Part I. A review of basic sensory neuroanatomy. Cosmetic Dermatology 17:515–522

Smith KC, Comite SL, Balasubramanian S, et al 2006 Vibration anesthesia: A noninvasive method of reducing discomfort prior to dermatologic procedures. Dermatology Online Journal 10:1 (accessed 15 July 2006) http://dermatology.cdlib.org/102/therapy/anesthesia/comite.html

Stricharatz D 1976 Molecular mechanisms of nerve block by local anesthetics. Anesthesiology 45:421–441

Yagiela JA 1991 Local anesthetics. In: Dionne RA, Phero JC (eds) Management of Pain and Anxiety in Dental Practice. Elsevier, New York, pp 109–134

Zide BM, Swift R 1998 How to block and tackle the face. Plastic and Reconstructive Surgery 101:840–851

10 Injectable Fillers in Skin of Color

Pearl E. Grimes, Julius W. Few

INTRODUCTION

Skin color and its characteristic physical defining traits are important factors in cosmetic surgery. Phrases commonly used to describe darker racial/ethnic groups include ethnic, dark, black, brown and/or skin of color. People of color constitute the majority of the global population. They include Hispanics, Latinos, Africans, African-Americans, Caribbeans, Native Americans, Pacific Islanders, East Indians, Pakistanis, Eskimos, Koreans, Chinese, Vietnamese, Filipinos, Japanese, Thais, Cambodians, Malaysians and Indonesians. Such individuals are often classified as having Fitzpatrick skin types IV–VI.

The United States Census Bureau data from 2000 estimated that the total resident population included 33 million Hispanic Americans (12%), 34 million African-Americans (13%), 11 million Asians and Pacific Islanders (4%), and 2 million Native Americans, Eskimos and Aleuts (1%). Statistical projections suggest continued substantial growth of the nonwhite United States population, with Hispanics having the most significant growth rate. By the year 2050, at least 50% of Americans will represent people of color.

According to statistical data from the American Society for Aesthetic and Plastic Surgery for 2005, the overall number of cosmetic surgical procedures in the United States increased 544% since 1997. There was a 764% increase in nonsurgical procedures during the same period. People of color accounted for 20% of all cosmetic procedures. Of this group, 9% were Hispanic, 6% African-American, 4% Asian and 1% represented other groups.

Hyaluronic acid fillers were the third most commonly performed nonsurgical procedure following botulinum toxin (Botox) injections and laser hair removal. There was a 35% growth in such agents in 2005 compared to data from 2004.

The popularity of injectable fillers in people of color is increasing substantially in cosmetic practices in the United States and globally. The most frequently used products include bovine and human collagen, hyaluronic acid products (HA) polylactic acid, calcium hydroxylapetite and autologous fat. Despite the increasing popularity of injectable fillers, there is a dearth of published data in skin types IV through VI. This chapter will review skin structure and aging in skin of color, clinical efficacy and safety, anesthesia, injection techniques and complications of fillers in people of color.

THE AGING FACE OF THOSE WITH DARKER SKIN TYPES

Deeply pigmented skin is characterized by an increased content of epidermal melanin and large, singly dispersed melanosomes within melanocytes. Melanosomes are distributed throughout the epidermis in black skin, whereas in white skin, they are limited to the basal and lower malphigian layer of the epidermis. Melanin serves as a significant filter to block the deleterious effects of ultraviolet light hence the incidence of skin cancers and photodamage is less in those with darker skin types. However, melanocytes in dark skin show labile responses to cutaneous injury. As reported in Fitzpatrick et al, Rhine & Campbell, Phillips & Smuts, Halder & Nootheti and Matory, conditions such as post-inflammatory hyperpigmentation and melasma are common.

Black skin has a thicker and more compact dermis compared to Caucasian skin. Fibroblasts are large and numerous, suggesting active biosynthesis and turnover of collagen. Comparison of soft tissue measurements in American blacks, whites, Japanese and a mixed South African population show that facial soft tissue measurements are thicker in blacks in the upper and lower face. The dermal and soft tissue characteristics of dark skin may indeed slow the aging process. However, heightened activity of fibroblasts predispose the skin to hypertrophic scars and keloids. In general, the aging face is an amalgam of photodamage and intrinsic aging changes. In Caucasians, photodamage encompasses a significant component of the aging process. It is characterized by wrinkles, laxity, dyschromia and textural alterations. In contrast according to Matory, in darker skin types, the aging process is predominantly characterized by soft tissue and gravitational changes of intrinsic aging (Fig. 10.1).

Soft Tissue Augmentation

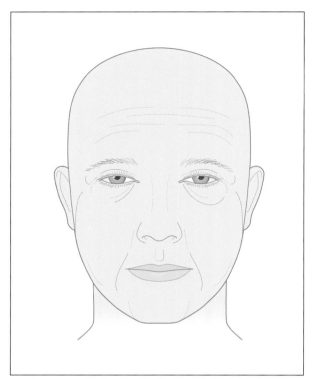

Fig. 10.1 Diagram demonstrating intrinsic aging of the upper, mid, and lower face including brow furrows, eyelid ptosis and laxity, tear trough deformity, nasolabial lines and jowl formation in an African-American

Table 10.1 Key indicators for use of injectible fillers in skin of color
Glabeller lines
Nasolabial lines
Jowls/sagging cheeks
Tear trough deformities
Lip augmentation*
Marionette lines
Perioral rhytides
*Minimal interest among African-Americans

augmentation. Many of the aforementioned signs of aging are indeed amenable to correction and/or augmentation by injection of temporary or permanent fillers. An understanding of the features and patterns of facial aging are essential in achieving desired esthetic outcomes with injectable fillers.

PATIENT SELECTION AND EVALUATION

Key indicators for use of injectable fillers in skin of color are listed in Table 10.1. Often the cultural esthetic ideal dictates protocols and procedures used for restoration of facial volume and symmetry in darker racial ethnic groups. Detailed consultations are important for the patient interested in injectable fillers. Following assessment, the treating physician or health care provider should have a detailed discussion with the patient regarding selection of the appropriate filler, i.e. temporary versus a longer lasting product. Temporary fillers should be considered in patients who have never undergone tissue augmentation. The amount of filler necessary for optimal correction should also be discussed with the patient. In addition, patients should be advised that optimal correction is predicated on the volume or quantity of filler injected. For example, in patients with severe nasolabial lines, one syringe of an HA filler will not provide optimal correction.

ANESTHESIA

As in Caucasians, similar methods of anesthesia are used for injection of filling substances. These include topical anesthesia with agents such as lidocaine 2.5% and prilocaine 2.5% (EMLA), cryoanesthesia with ice, infiltrative anesthesia and nerve blocks. To avoid patient discomfort, one of the authors (PEG) prefers to inject each NLF with 0.3–0.4 cc of xylocaine 1% immediately prior to injection of the filling substance. Nerve blocks are indeed beneficial when injecting the lips. However, experience and physician preference also dictate the choice of topical anesthesia.

Facial aging occurs due to loss of hard and soft tissues, including bone remodeling, fat atrophy and the gravitational redistribution of the skin and subcutaneous tissue. Matory and Harris report that dark-skinned individuals have a tendency to age prematurely in some areas and late in others because of adipose tissue atrophy, bone remodeling and gravitational redistribution of soft tissue. Patients with darker skin, particularly African-Americans, tend to manifest signs of aging in the deeper muscular layers of the face, with sagging of the malar fat pads toward the nasolabial folds (NLFs). NLFs become prominent and there is also sagging of the cheeks. In the middle and lower face the classic signs of aging include tear trough deformity, infraorbital hollowing, and ptosis of the subcutaneous adipose tissue in the malar region. Given the thicker dermis and subcutaneous tissue of some darker racial ethnic groups combined with infraorbital hypoplasia, midface aging can occur at an earlier age. In some instances it is pronounced.

In the lower face, darker racial ethnic groups may experience jowl formation and pronounced marionette lines. Lower face alterations also occur later in dark-skinned patients and are less pronounced than in the white races. According to Grimes (2005), the voluminous lips of blacks show minor aging changes, hence few show interest in lip

INJECTION TECHNIQUES

It is important to have well documented digital photography available prior to injection. Close-up, frontal and fronta–lateral views should be taken. The treating injector needs to make note of pigment irregularities prior to treatment, as filling of a depression may increase visibility of a pigment irregularity which was hidden by a recess and shadow. There are many safe and effective ways to inject fillers in individuals with skin of color (Fig. 10.2). An effort should be made to use the least number of epidermal injections to achieve appropriate outcomes. Deep-dermal injection depth has been shown to be beneficial in skin of color. Linear threading uses the full length of the needle inserted into the center of the wrinkle. Antegrade and/or retrograde techniques are appropriate. The technique can be used along areas such as the NLF. Fanning and/or crosshatching can also be used to maximize results while minimizing epidermal trauma. For optimal correction, fanning and crosshatching are important techniques for patients with moderate to severe and extreme NLFs (Fig. 10.3A and B). The fanning injection technique can be used to maximize injection without withdrawing the tip of the needle from the skin. Fanning shows maximal efficacy in the nasal triangle. Crosshatching involves placement of a series of linear threads into the dermis 5–10 mm from each other and a new series of threads are then injected at right angles, at a slightly different skin depth. HA fillers should be injected slowly to avoid overcorrection. Serial puncture has been reserved for deep-set commissures and/or isolated depressions such as a scar, understanding the potential trade-off of increased epidermal injury.

EFFICACY AND SAFETY STUDIES

From a historical perspective, darker skin types have been substantially underrepresented in clinical trials assessing the efficacy and safety of filling substances for soft tissue augmentation. Recent clinical trials have included skin types IV through VI. Given the unique structural and aging differences in people of color, clinical trials have attempted to address myriad issues regarding the use of fillers in this group. Are injectable fillers safe and efficacious? Are there differences in longevity of filling substances? Are conditions such as postinjection hyperpigmentation, keloids and hypertrophic scars major complications?

Grimes et al assessed the efficacy and safety of a variety of filling substances for correction of NLFs and marionette lines in 66 African-Americans. Their mean age was 52 years; 61 were female and five were male. Injected fillers included bovine collagen (25) Restylane (20), human collagen (15) and avian hyaluronic acid (5). Of the subjects, 60% achieved excellent correction while 40% had moderate correction (Figs 10.4–10.6). Four patients experienced post-inflammatory hyperpigmentation at the

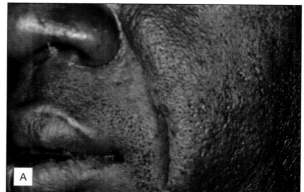

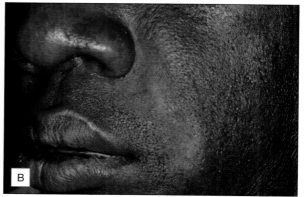

Fig. 10.3 (A) Baseline, severe NLFs in an African-American male. **(B)** Immediately after three syringes of avian hyaluronic acid injections. (Courtesy of Dr PE Grimes)

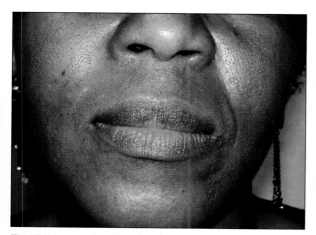

Fig. 10.2 45-year-old African-American woman presenting for correction of NLFs. The right NLF has been treated to demonstrate the immediate effect. Note that 0.6 cc Restylane was injected into the right side, using serial threading placed in deep dermis. (Courtesy of Dr Julius Few)

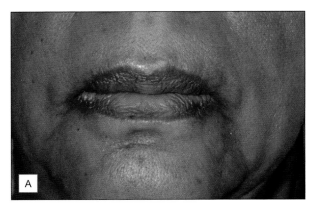

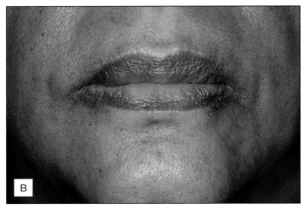

Fig. 10.4 (A) Baseline, frontal view of marionette lines in an African-American patient. **(B)** Melomental correction with Restylane (one syringe). (Courtesy of Dr PE Grimes)

injection site, which resolved with topical steroids and hydroquinone 4%. None experienced hypertrophic scars or keloids at the injection site. Preliminary data from the Vitiligo & Pigmentation Institute in African-Americans show persistence of HA fillers beyond 1 year in many patients.

A new family of hyaluronic acid-based fillers (Juvéderm family) was recently approved by the FDA for use in the United States. One unique attribute of this new family of HA fillers is the patented Hylacross technology, which allows the filler to be formulated with a higher concentration of HA and a higher amount of crosslinked HA compared to other HA products available in the United States. The Juvéderm family of fillers include Juvéderm (J)30, J24HV and J30HV. Juvéderm 30 is a highly crosslinked formulation for subtle correction of facial wrinkles and folds. Juvéderm 24 HV is a highly crosslinked formulation for even more versatility in contouring and volumizing of facial wrinkles and folds. Juvéderm 30 HV is the most highly cross-linked and robust of the Juvéderm family. It is used for deeper folds and wrinkles. A multi-center, double-blind randomized trial evaluated the efficacy and safety of the Juvéderm-based family

of products compared with bovine collagen in Caucasians and nonCaucasian subjects. A total of 420 patients completed the 24-week split face study.[12] Of that group, 26% were nonCaucasian including 11% African-American; 12% Hispanic; 2% Asian and 1% other. One of 3 Juvéderm fillers was injected in one fold and bovine collagen (Zyplast) in the opposite fold. Compared with bovine collagen, the Juvéderm products resulted in significantly longer-lasting results compared to bovine collagen. At 24 weeks, all of the Juvéderm family of fillers (J30, J24HV and J30HV) had nasolabial scores of mild, significantly less than bovine collagen. Efficacy was similar in Caucasians and nonCaucasians (Fig. 10.7). Safety and tolerability was assessed in detail for both groups. No patients experienced hypertrophic scars or keloids. In addition the nonCaucasian subjects did not show a higher incidence of post-inflammatory hyperpigmentation.

A 12-week double-blind, randomized study of 439 people compared the efficacy and safety of avian hyaluronic acid (hylaform) to bovine collagen in both Caucasians and nonCaucasians. Of the 423 subjects who completed this study, the median age was 47 for Caucasians and 49 for nonCaucasians. In this study the avian-based HA was found to be superior to bovine collagen for correction of nasolabial lines. There were no significant differences in efficacy scores in Caucasians and nonCaucasians. In addition there were no statistically significant differences in adverse events including hyperpigmentation. None of the subjects developed hypertrophic scars or keloids.

Odunze et al assessed the efficacy of an HA (Restylane) in skin types I, II, and III and compared them to skin types IV, V and VI. The average age for all patients was 56 years with greater than 90% of the patients being female. All patients received herpes simplex virus prophylaxis when indicated. Anesthesia included topical agents and/or intra-oral regional block. Serial threading techniques were used whenever possible. The injected material was placed deep within the dermis in skin of color because the Northwestern University group felt that a deeper level of injection would minimize potential disruption of the dermis-epidermis junction, which minimizes the risk of hyperpigmentation. A total of 60 patients, 40 in group I and 20 in group II were followed for a mean of 331 days. During treatment, emphasis was placed on minimizing the number of skin injections/perforations with the needle. The NLFs, forehead rhytides, marionette lines, tear trough, perioral rhytides, and/or contour/scar defects were treated in both groups. Patients were re-evaluated within 6 weeks of the treatment. The authors reported substantial efficacy in individuals with skin types IV through VI (Fig. 10.8). There were no reported short- or long-term cases of post inflammatory hyperpigmentation or related adverse events. Overall satisfaction between the groups was equal at greater than 90%. Of the test subjects, 83% had only one injection during the study period with persons of color reporting a longer longevity that was not statistically significant compared to those with lighter skin types.

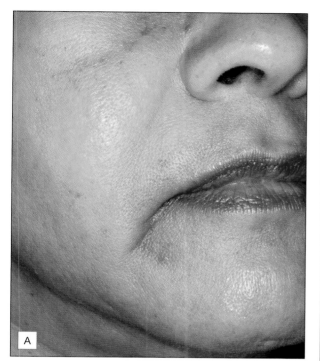

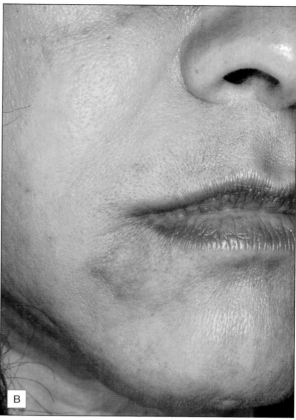

Fig. 10.5 (A) Baseline, side view of marionette line in an African-American patient. **(B)** Melomental correction with human collagen Cosmoplast. (Courtesy of Dr PE Grimes)

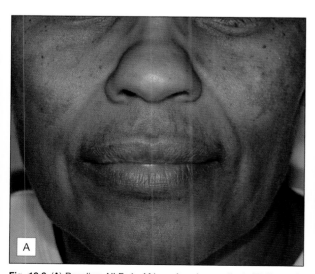

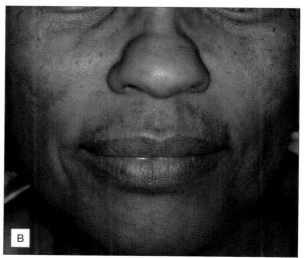

Fig. 10.6 (A) Baseline, NLFs in African-American patient. **(B)** Correction with hyaluronic acid injection (Juvéderm 30 HV) to NLFs, 6 months post treatment. (Courtesy of Dr PE Grimes)

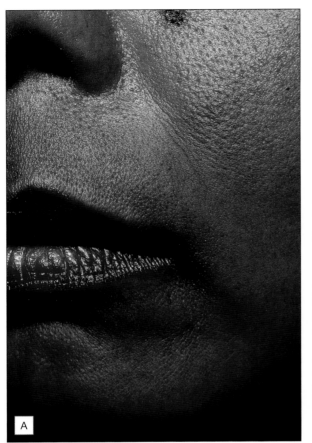
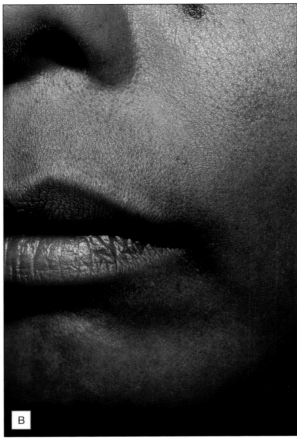

Fig. 10.7 (**A**) Baseline, nasolabial folds of an African-American patient. (**B**) Nasolabial correction and cheek augmentation with Restylane (three syringes). (Courtesy of Dr PE Grimes)

AUTOLOGOUS FAT INJECTIONS

The concept of injecting fat has been in existence since 1922. Visibility of fat in dermal applications can be highly variable and repeat treatments are often necessary. The primary advantage is abundant available tissue, with complete compatibility and great potential for dynamic change. The disadvantages include donor site needs, extended recovery, overcorrection and reabsorption. Fat injections can be performed under local anesthesia (Fig. 10.9). The lower abdomen and flank/hip regions are the typical donor sites. The technique for harvesting fat includes injecting into the donor site Tumescent local, 60 cc 1% lidocaine with epinephrine 1 : 100,000 diluted into 250 cc of normal saline plus 10% bicarb. Accordingly, the recipient site is anesthetized with 1% lidocaine with epinephrine 1 : 100,000 concentrated to the area of the fold or depression. Fat is aspirated utilizing the Byron aspiration system (Byron Medical in Tucson, Arizona), which offers graded cannulae. The harvested fat is then concentrated and purified by centrifuge or on a Telfa pad prior to injection. A 30–40% overcorrection is made in anticipation of absorp-

tion. For the lower facial area, typical injection volumes range from 5–10 cc, however this can be greater depending on the needs of the patient. Care is taken to avoid bolus injections as this may lead to increased risk of fat necrosis. An effort is made to place the fat in microdroplet form with frequent passes to minimize soft tissue trauma and bolus injection. In skin of color, the fat is typically placed in the deep subcutaneous areas. If fine lines exist a combination treatment can be utilized with additional fillers such as hyaluronic acid.

COMPLICATIONS

There is a paucity of literature looking at filler complications in skin of color. Post-inflammatory hyperpigmentation is common in darker skin types following even minor trauma. Hyperpigmentation can last months to years. Areas of pre-existing hyperpigmentation appear to be at a greater risk for further darkening with repeat trauma and unprotected sun exposure. A unique propensity for scar formation makes injectable fillers an appealing alternative

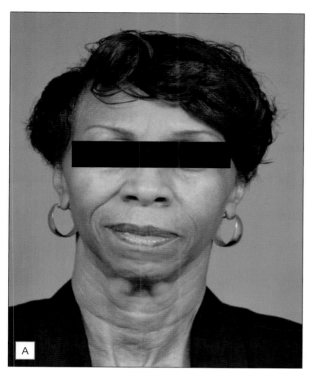

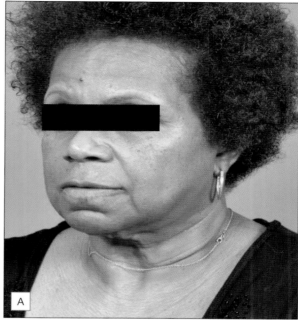

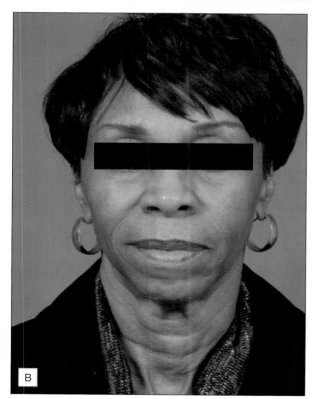

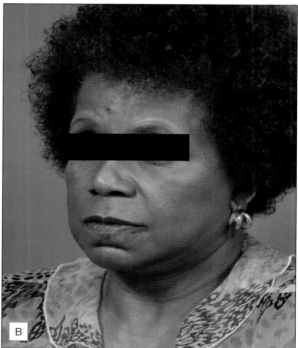

Fig. 10.9 60-year-old woman before (**A**) and after (**B**) short scar face lift with smasectomy and fat injection to the NLF and oral region. (Courtesy of Dr Julius Few)

Fig. 10.8 65-year-old African-American woman with aging facial changes who refuses facial rejuvenation surgery. The patient was treated with Restylane to glabella, NLF, commissure, marionette, 2 syringes and Botox to glabella (25 u). (Courtesy of Dr Julius Few)

to more invasive surgical techniques. To the authors' knowledge, there have been no reported cases of keloid scar formation post filler injection using a small caliber (less than 18 gauge needle) injection. There is a greater potential for scarring with fat injection using larger, 14 gauge or greater, needles. The authors have avoided suture use in these cases and favored Steri-Strips for their closure. Hypersensitivity complications have been reported at an incidence of less than 1% in larger European studies. The studies of skin of color suggest an equal or better safety profile. Fat injection in skin of color also has risks of fat necrosis, reabsorption, infection, irregularity, and donor complications. In the authors' experience, this risk is less than 2%. Meticulous technique and an attempt to minimize blood accumulation are vital components for minimizing complications. Fortunately, most of the fillers discussed are very user friendly and very forgiving. The most frequent side effects of collagen and hyaluronic acid fillers include temporary erythema and edema at the injection site, which resolves in several days in most patients. In rare cases of severe reaction, a short course of oral antibiotics and medium to high potency topical steroids are most efficacious. If HA injections are placed too superficial in the dermis, a Tyndall effect can occur. One of the authors (PEG) has had success in treating this complication by puncturing the skin with a 20 gauge needle and expressing the filler with a comedone extractor. Excellent results have been achieved.

Fillers are not a replacement for surgery but can be a powerful adjunct. In addition, patients of color unwilling to consider surgery due to risks described earlier have a viable alternative to surgery.

SUMMARY

In summary, injectable fillers are indeed increasing in popularity in skin of color. The authors' current database suggests that agents such as collagen and hyaluronic acid products offer substantial efficacy with minimal complications. Patient satisfaction is substantial. This database does not show a higher incidence of post inflammatory hyperpigmentation, keloids, or hypertrophic scars following filler injections. However, it is essential that the authors expand the published database regarding use of injectable fillers in people of color.

FURTHER READING

Andre P 2004 Evaluation of the safety of a non-animal stabilized hyaluronic acid (NASHA – Q-Medical, Sweden) in European countries: a retrospective study from 1997 to 2001. Journal of the European Academy of Dermatological Venereology 18:422–425

Bruning P 1914 Contributions a l'etude des greffes adipeuses. Bulletin of the Academy of Royal Medicine Belgigue 28:440

Broder KW, Cohen SR 2006 An overview of permanent and semipermanent fillers. Plastic and Reconstructive Surgery 118:7s–14s

2004 Cosmetic Surgery National Data Bank statistics. (The American Society for Aesthetic Plastic Surgery) at *http://www.surgery.org/download/2004-stats.pdf*

Fitzpatrick TB, Szabo G, Wick MM Biochemistry and physiology of melanin pigment.

Gendler E, Manheit G, Bauman L, Grimes PE 2006 The Efficacy and Safety of Hylaform in Caucasians and non Caucasian. Presented Poster Exhibit American Academy of Dermatology. San Francisco

Grimes PE 2005 Fillers in Darker Racial Ethnic Groups presented American Academy of Dermatology meeting New Orleans, LA

Grimes PE, Thomas JA, Murphy DK, Walker PS 2006 Efficacy and Safety of Novel Hyaluronic Acid-Based Fillers and Crosslinked Bovine Collagen in Caucasians and Persons of Color. Presented Poster Exhibit American Academy of Dermatology San Diego, CA

Grimes PE 2007 Structural and physiologic differences in the skin of darker racial ethnic groups. In: Grimes PE (ed.) Cosmetic Surgery in Darker Racial Ethnic Groups. Lippincott, (in press)

Halder RM, Nootheti PK 2003 Ethnic skin disorders overview. Journal of the American Academy of Dermatology 48(6 Suppl): S143–S148

Harris MO 2004 The aging face in patients of color: minimally invasive surgical facial rejuvenation – a targeted approach. Dermatologic Therapy 17:206–211

Lowe NJ, Maxwell CA, Lowe P, Duick MG, Shah K 2001 Hyaluronic acid skin fillers: adverse reactions and skin testing. Journal of the American Academy of Dermatology 45:930–933

Matory WE 1998 Aging in people of color. In: Matory WE (ed.) Ethnic considerations in facial aesthetic surgery. Lippincottt-Raven, Philadelphia, PA, pp 151–170

Nordlund JJ, Abdel-Malek ZA 1988 Mechanisms for post-inflammatory hyperpigmentation and hypopigmentation. Advances in Pigment Cell Research 219–236

Odunze M, Cohen A, Few JW Restylane and skin of color. Plastic and Reconstructive Surgery (in press)

Phillips VM, Smuts NA 1996 Facial reconstruction: utilization of computerized tomography to measure facial tissue thickness in a mixed racial population. Forensic Science International 83:51–59

Rhine JS, Campbell HR 1980 Thickness of facial tissues in American blacks. Journal of Forensic Science 25:847–858

US Census Bureau, Population Division, April 12, 2000

11 Complications of Soft Tissue Augmentation

Sue Ellen Cox, Naomi Lawrence

FILLER COMPLICATIONS

All fillers are associated with the risk of both early and delayed complications. Early side effects that can be expected include swelling, bruising and erythema at the injection site.

Prior to treatment the patient is educated and accepts these risks. Technique-associated risks are generally apparent after a couple of weeks and relate to placement of the filler. These include too superficial injections contributing to the appearance of the implant under the skin, palpability of the implant and asymmetric placement of the filler. Necrosis, intravascular injections and infection can be partially but not entirely technique dependent. Late adverse events include immunologic phenomena such as delayed type hypersensitivity reactions and foreign body granulomatous reactions. Unrealistic expectations and undertreatment due to not using enough product can also create an unhappy patient.

• General principles

Currently, implantation of dermal fillers is a minimally traumatic event. The gauge of the needle required to implant the product contributes to the extent of the trauma. A more viscous product or one with a large particle size necessitates a lower gauge, larger diameter needle. In this scenario there is a larger epithelial tear or puncture, greater disruption of dermal structures such as capillaries, resulting in more significant edema and stimulation of inflammatory cascades. A multiple puncture, rapid injection technique is also more traumatic than a limited puncture, slow injection technique. Another purely technical source of expected adverse events is the location of product implantation. Implantation immediately above or beneath a muscle such as in the lip or tear drop sulcus area can result in higher intensity and propensity (for) swelling and bruising due to the vascular nature of the muscle.

Patients respond to trauma within a range of bruising and swelling inherent to their natural tendencies. Oral anticoagulants in medicines, nutritional supplements, and food can exacerbate the normal response to trauma.

• Bruising and swelling

Immediately after injection of a dermal filler all patients experience the normal expected adverse events: needle marks, swelling, and bruising. The extent of these adverse reactions fall along a bell curve in a range of magnitude and duration expected for that particular filler. In addition there are technical variables and patient variables that can augment or detract from these adverse events.

SWELLING

Study of the inflammatory and edematous response in traumatic, irritant, and burn wounds reported by Bonelli et al, Rikimaru et al and Boykin et al has shown that release of both histamine and prostaglandin E_2 play a critical role in the early mediation of the inflammatory response. In forensic science the prevalence of mast cells can help distinguish between vital, antemortem and postmortem wounds. In burn wounds the application of cold water may significantly reduce histamine release therefore reducing generation of remote edema formation. According to Boykin et al, in animal models, pretreatment with a H2 histamine receptor antagonist such as cimetidine can mimic the cold water effect. Similarly, pretreatment and post-treatment with ice can decrease the swelling and bruising response associated with cosmetic filler injection.

BRUISING

The intensity and extent of bruising secondary to trauma can vary from patient to patient. It is well known that a number of orally injested medications and nutritional supplements prolong bleeding time and increase bruising post surgical trauma (Table 11.1). The most common mechanism is inhibition of platelet aggregation. Any inherent abnormality in coagulation such as coagulation factor

Table 11.1 Anticoagulants

Anticoagulant medicinal herbs/supplements			
Multi-vitamins	Arthra G	Feverfew	Oxyprozin
Bilberry	Artropan	Fiorinal	Pamprin
Chamomile	A.S.A.	Flurbiprofen	Pepto-Bismol
Chondroitin	Ascodeen	Froben	Percodan
Clove	Ascriptin	4-way cold tabs	Persantine
Echinacea	Aspergum	Gelpirin	Phenaphen
Ephedra	Aspirin	Genpril	Phenylbutazone
Vitamin E	BC Powder	Genprin	Piroxicam
Valerian	Baby Aspirin	Goody's Body Pain	Ponstel
Fish oil	Bayer	Haltrin	Prednisone
Garlic	Brufen	Halfprin	Quagesic
Garlic capsules	Bufferin	Ibuprin	Relafen
Ginger	Burazolidin	Ibuprofen	Rexolate
Ginko Biloba	Cephalgesic	Ibuprohm	Robasissal
Ginseng	Cheracol Caps	Indameth	Roxiprin
Glucosamine	Children's Aspirin	Indocin	Rufin
Grape seed	Choline salicylate	Indomethacin	Saleto
Herbal teas	Clinoril	Ketoprofen	Salflex
Horseradish	Congesprin	Ketorolac	Salaslate
Kava	Cope	Lortab ASA	Salsitab
Licorice	Coricidin	Magan	Sine-off
Willow bark	Corticosteriods	Magnesium salicylate	Sine-Aid
St. John's Wort	Coumadin	Meclofenamate	Sodium thiosalicylate
Goldenseal	Darvon ASA	Meclofen	Soma Compound
Milk Thistle	Darvon Compound	Medipren	Sulindac
Saw Palmetto	Daypro	Mefenamic acid	Synalgos DC
	Depakote	Menadob	Tanacetum
Anticoagulant medicinal herbs/supplements	Dexamethasone	Midol	Tolecrin
Advil	Diclofenac	Mobidin	Tolmetrin
Aleve	Dipyridamole	Monogesic	Toradol
Alcohol	Disalcid	Motrin	Trandate
Alka-Seltzer	Divalproex	Nabumetone	Trendan
Amigesic	Doan's pills	Nalfon	Trental
Anacin	Dolobid	Naprosyn	Trigesic
Anaprox	Dristan	Naproxen	Trilisate
Anaproxin	Easprin	Norgesic	Tusal
Ansaid	Ecotrin	Norwich	Vanquish
APC	Empirin	Nuprin	Voltaren
Argesic	Emprazil	Ocufen	Warfarin
	Endodan	Orudis	Zactrin
	Excedrin	Oruvail	Zorprin
	Feldene	Oxyphenburazone	
	Fenoprofen	Oxyburazone	

deficiency or platelet abnormalities increase post-surgical bruising and often are diagnosed for the first time postoperatively. According to Talwar et al, as the skin ages the dermis atrophies and provides less support for the constituent blood vessels. This leads to easy bruising post minor trauma (Fig. 11.1).

Use of home remedies to accelerate and improve healing are extremely common. These can be difficult to evaluate for efficacy since the body naturally resorbes bruising and swelling progressively in the early postoperative period. Seely et al recently published an elegant study on the effect of homeopathic Arnica Montana on bruising in face lifts. Arnica is probably the most common agent used by clinicians to lessen bruising in the postoperative period. It is an herbaceous perennial of the family asteraceace. Sinecca (Alpine Pharmaceuticals, San Rafael,

CA) is the retail formulation. The concept of homeopathic treatment is controversial and based on the teaching of Hippocrates in the 'law of similiars'. In homeopathy the basic tenant is 'like is cured by like'. That is, any substance that can create symptoms in a higher dose can also cure those symptoms in an unhealthy person in a repeated smaller dose. In the study by Seely, 29 white female, nonsmoking patients had elective rhytidectomy. The patients were given 12 doses of Arnica beginning with the first on the morning of surgery and continuing every 8 hours for a total of 4 days. The investigators developed a novel evaluation tool using 35 mm slides converted to digital images, Adobe Photoshop software, and the concepts of reflectance photometry. They were able to precisely measure both the degree of color change from bruising and the amount of surface area affected. They

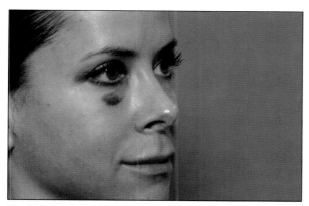

Fig. 11.1 Bruising 5 days after hyaluronic acid injection for tear trough deformity

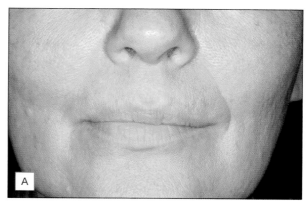

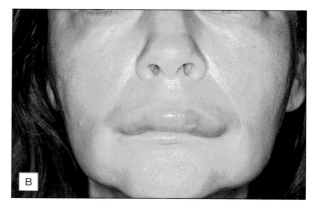

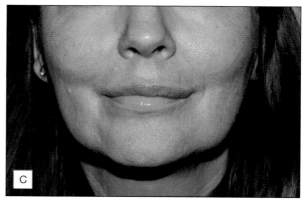

found no objective difference in degree of color change. Patients on Arnica Montana had a smaller area of ecchymosis on postoperative days 1, 5, 7 and 10. This difference was only statistically significant on postoperative day 1 (PL 0.005) and day 7 (PL 0.001). There was also a trend towards less edema. Interestingly, both the patients and physician staff noted no subjective difference, which may indicate that the improvement although statistically significant may not be enough in magnitude to be clinically relevant.

• Immediate and delayed hypersensitivity reactions

The terminology and classification of hypersensitivity reactions to injectable fillers is confusing. This is most likely because hypersensitivity reactions are rare for most fillers (0–5%) and therefore most of our information comes from sporadic case reports. The impediment to determining the best potential classification is that hypersensitivity reactions don't have a unique morphology. The difference between a hypersensitive, allergic, or abnormal response is often one of magnitude rather than morphology. Swelling and induration are normal after filler injections. The physician considers a swelling response abnormal if it is more exaggerated and longer in duration than typical adverse injection site events. This is not a difficult diagnosis in a case such as the author (NL) and colleagues reported in which the patient had an immediate, massive angioedematous reaction to hyaluronic acid (Fig. 11.2A–C). However, the author has seen two lesser cases that were not reportable but may similarly have been a lesser manifestation of the same reaction.

Classification by etiology is equally elusive as it is difficult to assess the etiology of hypersensitivity reactions from the literature. Are they pure allergic reactions? Mechanical or direct stimulation of mast cell degranulation? Idiosyncratic reactions? Lack of uniform morphology, low case numbers, difference in temporal onset, and deficiency of confirmatory scientific evidence such as skin

Fig. 11.2 (**A**) Before lip augmentation. (**B**) Immediately after hyaluronic acid lip injection. (**C**) 12 days after hyaluronic acid lip augmentation

tests, biopsies or circulating antibodies makes it difficult to clearly identify etiology.

• Hyaluronic acid fillers

Lupton and Alster reported the first case of a patient developing acute hypersensitivity to hyaluronic acid gel. It occurred after the third treatment. They felt the hypersensitivity reaction was most likely due to an impurity in bacterial fermentation. The clinical manifestation was multiple tender red nodules. The nodules were polymorphous and contained some yellow stringy material and others were indurated and fibrotic. No pathogenic bacteria were cultured from these nodules. Micheels reported eight adverse reactions derived to hyaluronic acid fillers from 1995–2001. He described the patients' clinical picture as redness, pruritis, and painful swelling of the treated areas manifesting after one or more treatments. The onset in his case series ranged from 2 days to 11 months after implantation. Two patients had what was referred to as a 'nettle type' skin eruption. He used antibody titers, lymphocyte transformation on tests, intradermal challenges, and biopsies to confirm hypersensitivity in these patients. Furthermore, since this case series, the manufacturing of nonanimal stabilized hyaluronic acid (NASHA) gel has changed (mid 1999) to lower trace protein 6-fold and greatly decrease adverse reactions.

In 2002 Friedman et al reviewed the worldwide adverse event data for NASHA. The data was obtained from a retrospective review of manufacturers' data for 1999 and 2000. As of 1999 there was an estimated 144,000 patients treated. There were 104 cases of hypersensitivity (incidence 0.07%), which was defined as swelling, erythema, and tenderness shortly after injection. In the 2000 data there were 52 cases of hypersensitivity of 262,000 patients treated (incidence 0.02%). The decline in hypersensitivity was attributed to changes in the processing of NASHA to decrease trace protein. These authors relate that in several of the hypersensitivity cases IgE and IgG antibodies and were measured and found to be normal.

In conclusion, hypersensitivity to both NASHA and animal-derived hyaluronic acid is rare and often self-resolving. The most clearly identifiable morphology is immediate swelling and erythema at the implantation site. Although one case series in Lupton and Alster reviewed found evidence of immunologic mediation of this reaction, this had not been clearly elucidated. Another reasonable explanation given in Leonhardt et al is stimulation of direct mast cell degranulation.

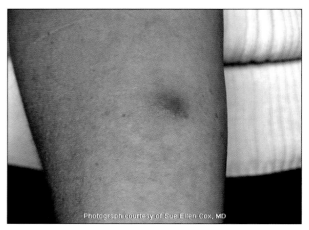

Fig. 11.3 Positive collagen skin test; hypersensitivity reaction

steroid treatment. They reported successful treatment of one patient with short course cyclosporine (5 mg 11 cc/day for 18 days) Moody and Sengelmann described the use of 0.1% topical tacrolimus after a short course of oral corticosteroids with near resolution within 14 days.

• Human collagen

In 2003, the human collagen implants, CosmoDerm and CosmoPlast (Inamed Corp Toronto, Ont/Allergan Corp.) were FDA approved. Baumann and Halem showed no allergic reactions in a trial of 400 patients. Since the introduction there has been one case report of two hypersensitivity reactions to CosmoDerm (Inamed Aesthetics, Santa Barbara, CA, USA). Both patients had been previously exposed to bovine collagen. One had simply had a single skin test (without adverse reaction) and the other an allergic response to Zyplast. As reported by Stolman, both responded to topical treatment with Protopic ointment (TM Fujisawa Healthcare, Inc. Deerfield, IL, USA).

• Bovine collagen

As reported in Naoum and Dasiou-Plakida, and Chen et al, bovine collagen was approved by the FDA for use in the US in the early 1980s. Allergy to bovine collagen has an incidence of 3% in the population (Fig. 11.3). Two skin tests are recommended prior to treatment as Watson et al confirm that 1.2% of people will develop hypersensitivity after their first exposure. Hypersensitivity reactions are most commonly pain, redness and swelling at injection sites. Occasionally systemic symptoms and sterile abscesses can develop. Paradoxically, the allergic reaction has been reported by Zyderm/Zyplast literature and Tolleth to last up to 2 years, long after the normal host would have any clinical evidence of product. Treatment of these reactions can prove challenging according to Baumann and Kerdel as patients tend to rebound with symptoms after cortico-

• Poly-L-lactic acid

Injectable poly-L-lactic acid (Sculptra, Dermik Laboratories, Bridgewater, NJ) available in Europe as New-fill since 1999 and in the US market since August 2004 has a significant history of complications. The early usage of Sculptra was practiced with low volume (2 cc) reconstitution and higher volume of total product injected. This coupled with closely spaced treatment sessions led to frequent nodule formations. According to Vleggaar, many European injectors rejected this product as high risk for complications. The product is composed of particulate matter – microbeads of PLA and mannitol – which is prone to clump, extrude, and form small nodules even without an adverse host immune response. Lam et al recently published new guidelines for PLA injection: 8–12 cc dilutant (i.e. 5–10 cc sterile water and 2 cc 1% lidocaine with epinephrine) and a minimum of 12 hours for reconstitution. In addition they recommended no more than 2 vials for injection into the subcutaneous fat, and spacing sessions at least 6 weeks apart. These authors in Salyan report granulomatous nodules in 0.2–12% incidence, which occurs as a delayed hypersensitivity phenomenon.

Poly-L-lactic acid differs from the other fillers in that it is dependent on the host immune/reparative response to accomplish filling. Other similar products include silicone and polymethyl-metracrylate (neither is currently FDA approved for soft tissue augmentation). Unfortunately this mechanism of action for augmentation has two potentially negative effects inherent to the nature of the response: (1) the host immune system can respond less than optimally causing less augmentation then desired; or (2) the host immune system can respond overexuberantly creating granulomas. In the mouse model histologic evaluations at 1 month has shown: (1) polylactide surrounded by 100 μm thick capsule; (2) mononuclear cells, macrophages, fibroblasts with increased collagen; and (3) mature vascularized fibrous capsule. As reported by Gogoleski et al, at 3 months there are: (1) Decreased cell numbers and increased collagen fibers with a capsule thickness of 80 μm. At 6 months the cell numbers decreased and the capsule thickness is only 60 μm. Lemperle studied the histologic reaction in his own forearm to poly-L-lactic acid. At 1 month there was fine capsule around implant. At 3 months the PLLA microspheres were intact, and surrounded by macrophages and lymphocytes. At 6 months the PLLA microspheres were degraded and deformed, and surrounded by macrophages and giant cells. At 9 months the PLLA microparticles completely degraded and there was no detectable scar tissue. Poly-L-lactic acid is a filler in which mechanism of augmentation has been proposed but not proven. Beljaards et al report the histology from complications has shown fibroblast giant cell granulomas but no new collagen. The immune system has an intergral role in fibroblast behavior so the response to this product in the immune-competent population might be quite different to that of the immunocompromised (HIV) population. The mechanism of augmentation for this product, particularly the short- and long-term tissue effects in immunocompetent patients, needs to be better characterized by further study.

• Necrosis

Injection site necrosis is extremely rare. Nairns et al show extrapolation of the incidence based on estimated usage is less than 0.001% worldwide. Necrosis has been reported for every type of filler. Locations at risk for necrosis include the glabella, cheeks (with injections into acne scars) and lips.

Necrosis develops due to pressure occlusion of the cutaneous vessels or cannulation and direct injection into vessels producing occlusion and ischemia (Fig. 11.4). Pressure due to an emerging hematoma will not produce arterial occlusion but can still result in necrosis of the

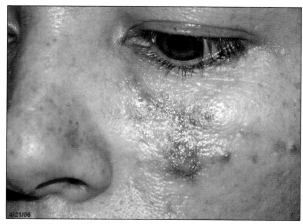

Fig. 11.4 Erosion following intravascular injection of hyaluronic acid filler to acne scars

overlying dermis. The process is slower and does not produce either the immediate pain or blanching that characterizes an intra-arterial injection. Intradermal bleeding will produce a gradual area of darkening. Immediate pressure should be applied until the bleeding stops. Ice can also be applied to help with vasoconstriction and reduce the risk of necrosis.

Arterial occlusion is characterized by immediate pain and blanching. Any filler injected into a vessel can produce occlusion. The risk of intravascular injection is partially but not entirely technique dependent. The following algorithm for management of arterial occlusion has been outlined by Narins et al. First stop the injection. Blanching may resolve immediately or last for several hours prior to the development of a dusky appearance to the skin. Massage the area to help dissipate the product. Post massage erythema may develop and indicate resolution of the occlusion. Finally if the blanching or dusky appearance continues 2% nitroglycerine paste should be applied to the overlying skin. Priority is to re-establish circulation to the ischemic tissue. Warm compresses may also be used to produce local vasodilatation. If sloughing of skin occurs it is generally within a couple days to a week. This should be treated with gentle wound care including antibiotic ointment or Vaseline and daily acetic acid soaks to prevent crusting. Typically these wounds heal without scarring. Primary surgical repair is always a last resort that will result in a scar.

Collagen products have a procoagulant effect that can result in propagation of occlusion. Most of the cases of necrosis seen are in the midline area and have been due to Zyplast injections (Fig. 11.5). Speculation regarding why this is a high risk location include: vascular compression or poor collateral circulation of the supra trochlear vein. Zyderm I, Cosmoderm I, or hyaluronic acids are the preferred products in this area. Superficial injection technique and small quantities of material lessen the risk of

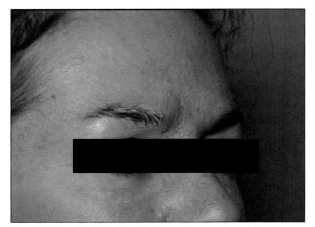

Fig. 11.5 Re-epithelialization with impending scar formulation 2 months after Zyplast injection into glabellar crease

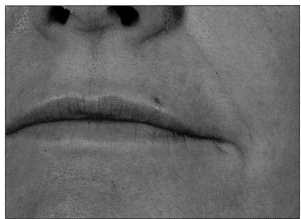

Fig. 11.6 Active infection at the skin site of filler placement is a contraindication. Patient with herpes simplex virus of the upper lip. (Courtesy of Dr Joel Cohen)

necrosis. Hyaluronic acids are more viscous and pliable, allowing for dispersion with massage. The most dreaded filler complication is blindness. This is due to retinal artery embolization and has been reported with a variety of fillers. Fat, bovine collagen, cadaveric dermis and hyaluronic acid fillers have all been reported to cause either temporary or permanent loss of vision.

• Infection

Infection at the site of soft tissue filler is rare. It can be avoided, although not completely by properly cleaning the skin prior to placing the filler. To help prevent inoculation of bacteria into the skin with injectable fillers, all make-up should be removed and the skin cleansed with alcohol. Injectable fillers have a lower risk of infection than solid implantable fillers such as expanded polytetrafluoroethylene (ePTFE). The infection rate for ePTFE in one study reported in Wall et al was 4%. When placing a solid implant sterile technique is mandatory. Prophylactic antibiotics should be started 2 days prior to the procedure and continued 3 days postoperatively. If infection is suspected the implant should be immediately removed. If a patient has a history of oral herpes simplex virus prophylactic antiviral medication should be started prior to solid or injectable fillers to prevent reactivation. The prophylactic dose of valaciclovir commonly used is 500 mg bid. Active infection at the site of desired filler placement is a contraindication. If a herpes or bacterial infection is present at the site the patient should be treated with the appropriate therapy and treatment rescheduled for when there is no active infection (Fig. 11.6).

Early infections can be indistinguishable from a normal inflammatory response. Bacterial microorganisms associated with the skin include *Streptococcus* and *Staphylococcus aureus*. Patients presenting with single or multiple erythematous and/or fluctuant nodules, should be treated

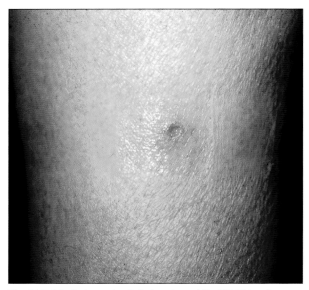

Fig. 11.7 A typical mycobacteria (courtesy of Dr. Phil Eichorn)

with a short course of antibiotics. Prior to starting antibiotics if the nodules are fluctuant it is prudent to do a bacterial culture to help guide the antibiotic choice. While awaiting culture results broad-spectrum antibiotic therapy should be initiated. Antibiotics of choice include Keflex, amoxicillin, Levaqin, minocycline and Biaxin.

If the lesions do not respond or continue to develop 2 weeks after systemic antibiotics, atypical mycobacterium should be suspected. Patients will present with a firm, mildly tender erythematous papule or nodule (Fig. 11.7). Systemic reactions have also been reported by Lowe et al. The atypical mycobacterium may be due to contamination from tap water or exist on the facial skin. Possible culprits include *Mycobacterium* sp. such as *chelonae, fortuitum,* or *abscessus.* It is prudent at this point to obtain a 2 mm punch biopsy to be sent for atypical mycobacterium culture and if possible one for routine bacteria and fungal tissue culture. Successful tissue identification requires a highly specialized laboratory and the authors have found success when specimens are sent to The University of Texas Health Center Pathology Microbiology AFB Lab in Tyler Texas. The specimen should be labeled with the patient's name and a completed Pathology AFB referral requisition to accompany the specimen. The specimen needs to be placed in a sterile leak-proof container with a small amount of sterile saline. The specimen container should then be placed in an additional container to help prevent any leakage or loss of contents. Do not add fixative. Special stains are performed with a high level of success by this laboratory. Without proper identification the physician cannot be certain of an effective antibiotic regimen. These patients often require an antibiotic course of 6 months or longer and the patient may lose faith in the physician if there is uncertainty in the effectiveness of the treatment. The regimen may include up to four different antimicrobial agents depending on the culture result and the severity of the infection. Biaxin 500 mg bid for several weeks has activity against some atypical mycobacterial infections. This is a good choice to empirically use while awaiting the culture results, which may take several weeks. Optimal treatment of rapidly growing mycobacterial infections remains poorly established. A recent study reported by Uslan et al compared clinical features and susceptibility patterns and treatments for skin infections due to *Mycobacteria fortuitum, M. chelonae,* and *M. abcessus.* In this study of 63 patients 100% of their isolates for *M. fortuitum* were susceptible to amikacin. Clarithromycin appears to be reliably active against *M. chelonae* and *M. abcessus,* although its activity against *M. fortuitum* is less predictable. Combination therapy seems prudent because of concerns about acquired resistance. Physicians should have a high index of suspicion if a patient has prolonged erythematous papules or fluctant nodules at the site of soft tissue augmentation. Although atypical mycobacterial infection is uncommon it has occurred with a variety of fillers including fat, hyaluronic acid, and silicone injections according to Butterwick, Uslan et al and Fox et al, respectively.

• Implant palpability and visibility

Malposition of both injectible and solid implants is the underlying cause for visible and/or palpable implants. The appearance of the implant papule will depend on which filler has been chosen. The nodules should be noninflammatory, therefore lower suspicion for infection.

Collagen, both human and bovine, is white in color; if collagen is placed too superficially the skin will appear to have a whitish, papular appearance. This is most common with the thin skin of the lower eyelids. Beading or clumping can also occur due to overcorrection. A 10–20% over-

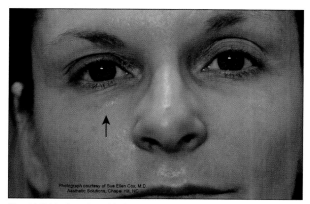

Fig. 11.8 Hyaluronic acid placement too superficial producing the 'Tyndall effect'

correction with bovine collagen (Zyderm I and Zyderm II) is sought due to the physiochemical properties of these products. Overcorrection can lead to lumping; massaging the area allows for dispersion of the product. If this is not successful the bumpy appearance does resolve as the collagen degrades over a 4–6-month period.

Hyaluronic acid products are clear, colorless viscous gels. When these products are placed too superficially they will produce a Tyndall effect. The Tyndall effect gives a light blue glass-like appearance to the skin that can be distressing to the patient (Fig. 11.8).

This effect can occur in any location, however the thin skin of the lower eyelids is most common. Physician's hesitancy to place the implant layered on the periosteum results in a higher risk for visible papules. The bluish bumps are extremely resistant to the normal process of isovolumetric degradation that occurs with these hydrogels. A patient in the authors' practice experienced persistence of the papules for more than 18 months. The most successful treatment for reabsorption of the bumps is the use of hyaluronidase (Fig. 11.9 A and B). Hyaluronidase is a soluble protein enzyme that acts at the site of local injection to break down and hydrolyze hyaluronic acid. It splits the glucosaminidic bond of glucuronic acid. According to Brody this temporarily decreases the viscosity of the intercellular cement, promoting diffusion and absorption. The author has had successful resolution of nodules with an injection of hyaluronidase 15 u to the area of excess. Resolution is reported within 2 days of the injection. Other treatment options include nicking the papule and gently squeezing the redundant product out.

Patients with very thin skin also can be difficult to correct as the implant is more likely to be visible or create an undesired palpable linear elevation even with correct dermal placement.

Microlipoinjections can also be associated with contour irregularities. Uncorrectable irregularities are uncommon with judicious placement in experienced hands. Firm,

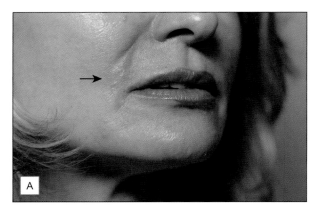

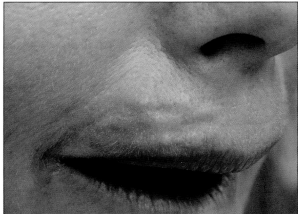

Fig. 11.10 Perioral nodules from Sculptra injections

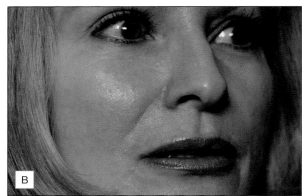

Fig. 11.9 (A) 'Tyndall effect;' hyaluronic acid placement too superficial. **(B)** Dissolution of the 'Tyndall effect' after placement of hyaluronic acid

hard nodules represent sterile fat cysts or calcified fat that may respond to dilute intralesional triamcinalone injections or rarely incisional removal.

Poly-L-lactic acid (Sculptra) is an injectable bioabsorbable material that is purported to be immunologically inert. US Food and Drug Administration (FDA) approval came in 2004 and is specifically indicated for treatment of HIV lipoatrophy. Duration of correction is not completely known but is thought to be over 2–3 years as reported by Moyle et al. In one of the largest studies to date the European VEGA study reported by Valantin et al evaluated 50 patients with severe lipoatrophy over 96 weeks. Of the patients included, 44% had palpable but not visible subcutaneous nodules, with a reported spontaneous resolution in only six patients at 96 weeks. In the author's (SEC) experience nodularity is more common if the material is placed too superficially or in the periocular or perioral locations (Fig. 11.10). Placement should be deep to the subcutaneous plane. With 6–8 cc of sterile water and 2 cc of plain lidocaine also helps decrease the risk of papule formation. Mixing the product at least 24 hours in advance and placing it in a warm bath just before using helps prevent clumping of the particles. Discarding pre-

cipitate at the bottom of the syringe is recommended, due to the higher concentration of particles that could induce granuloma formation. Not injecting the final content of the syringe also prevents inadvertent placement of product in the dermis on withdrawal. This author (SEC) has experienced persistence of the papules more often in the nonHIV population. This could be due to the normal immunologic response that is more likely to trigger an inflammatory response and foreign body granulomas. Because of this it is important to educate patients regarding this side effect. These papules may or may not be visible, and are small and extremely firm. In one patient without HIV, papules persisted over 18 months and were distressing. Removal was unsuccessful with both dilute steroid injections and Nokor needle subcission. Surgical excision of each papule was necessary. The specimen was sent for histopathology and revealed foreign body granuloma formation. Therefore, injectable poly-lactic acid cannot be considered to be completely biologically inert (Figs 11.11 and 11.12). Cosmetic patients without HIV who do not have severe lipoatrophy may not tolerate the side effects of palpable papules. Thorough informed consent regarding this risk is crucial.

Solid implants can also result in visual papule formation. The correct placement of solid implants such as expanded polytetrafluoroethylene is of utmost importance. Revision rates for this material have been noted by Cox to be as high as 100% in the lips (Fig. 11.13). Most physicians have significantly decreased their use of this product. A newer product – Advanta – was reported by Hanke to provide better esthetic results for those patients desiring a permanent option.

Migration can also cause a visible or palpable nondesired effect. This is more common in areas of excessive movement due to muscular activity. If the implant is pushed by muscular activity superiorly above the nasolabial fold this can accentuate the convex portion or the mound worsening the appearance of the fold. This occurs

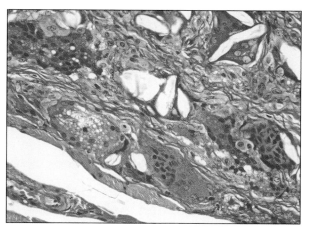

Fig. 11.11 In the dermis, there is foreign material with birefringent properties. This is surrounded by an inflammatory reaction including histiocytes

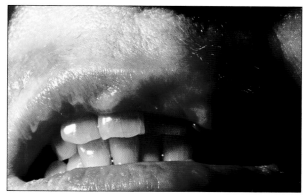

Fig. 11.13 Nodularity in the lip due to Gortex

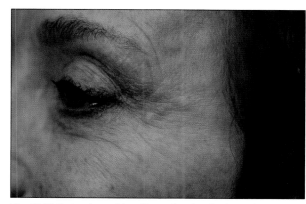

Fig. 11.12 Periocular nodules 18 months after Sculptra injections

with injectable and solid fillers. It is best with injectable fillers to place the product inferior to the mound and in a criss-cross fashion to facilitate blending between the cosmetic units.

UNREALISTIC EXPECTATIONS

The most common reason for an unhappy patient who has had fillers is due to undertreatment. It is important for the physician to educate the patient regarding the volume necessary to get good or complete correction. In some cases the number of syringes may be cost prohibitive. Patients that have very deep nasolabial folds or who have strong muscular-dermal attachments are difficult to treat. For patients who have these dermal attachments consider either nasolabial fold subcision or injection of 1–2 u of

botulinum toxin into the levator labii superiorus alequa nasi muscle just lateral to the pyraform aperature. These patients need to be chosen carefully as this can lengthen the upper lip.

FURTHER READING

American Academy of Dermatology 1996 Guidelines of care for soft tissue augmentation: collagen implants. Journal of the American Academy of Dermatology 34:698–702

Baumann LS, Kerdel F 1999 The treatment of bovine collagen allergy with cyclosporine. Dermatologic Surgery 25:247–249

Bonelli A, Bacci S, Vannelli B, Norelli A 2003 Immunohistochemical localization of mast cells as a tool for the discrimination of vital and postmortem lesions. International Journal of Legal Medicine 117:14–18

Boykin JV Jr, Erriksson E, Sholley MM, Pittman RN 1980 Histamine-mediated delayed permeability response after scald burn inhibited by cimetidine or cold-water treatment. Science 209:815–817

Brody H 2005 Use of hyaluronidase in the treatment of granulomatous hyaluronic acid reactions or unwanted hyaluronic acid misplacement. Dermatologic Surgery 31:893–897

Baumann LS, Halem ML 2003 Soft tissue augmentation with human bioengineered collagen. Cosmetic Dermatology 16:39–42

Beljaards RC, DeRoos KP, Bruins FG 2005 NewFill for skin augmentation: A new filler or failure? Dermatologic Surgery 31:772–776

Butterwick K 2005 Fat autograft muscle injection (FAMI): New technique for facial volume restoration. Dermatologic Surgery 31:1488–1495

Chen JT, Perkins SW, Hamilton MM 2002 Office based procedures in facial plastic surgery. Otolaryngology Clinics of North America 35

Cox SE 2005 Who is still using expanded polytetrafluoroethylene? Dermatologic Surgery 31:1613–1615

Dinehart SM, Henry L 2005 Dietary supplements: altered coagulation and effects on bruising. Dermatologic Surgery 31:819–826

Donofrio L 2005 Panfacial volume restoration with fat. Dermatologic Surgery 31:1496–1505

Fox LP, Geyer AS, Hussain S, et al 2004 *Mycobacterium abcessus* cellulites and multifocal abcesses of the breast in a transsexual from illicit intramammary injections of silicone. Journal of the American Academy of Dermatology 50:450–454

Friedman PM, Mafong EA, Kauvar ANB, Geronemus RG 2002 Safety data of injectable nonanimal stabilized hyaluronic acid gel or soft tissue augmentation. Dermatologic Surgery 28:491–494

Gogoleski S, Jovanovic M, Perren SM, et al 1993 Tissue response and in vivo degradation of selected polyhydroxyacids: poly-lactides (PLA), poly(3-hydroxybutyrate) (PHB), and poly (3-hydroxybutyrate-co-3-hydroxyvalerate) (PHB/VA). Journal of Biomedical Materials Research 27:1135–1148

Hanke CW, Hingley HR, Jolivette DM, Swanson NA, Stegman SJ 1991 Abscess formation and local necrosis after treatment with Zyderm or Zyplast collagen implant. Journal of the American Academy of Dermtology 25:319–326

Hanke W 2005 Commentary. Dermatologic Surgery 31:1615

Klein AW 2001 Skin filling. Collagen and other injectables of the skin. Dermatology Clinics 19:491–508, ix

Lam SM, Azizzadeh B, Graivier M 2006 Injectable poly-L-lactic acid (Sculptra): technical considerations in soft-tissue contouring. Plastic and Reconstructive Surgery 118:55s–63s

Lemperle G, Morhenn V, Charrier U 2004 Human histology and persistence of various injectable filler substances for soft tissue augmentation. Aesthetic Plastic Surgery Epub 2004 Jan 14

Leonhardt JM, Lawrence N, Narins RS 2005 Angioedema acute hypersensitivity reaction to injectable hyaluronic acid. Dermatologic Surgery 31:577–579

Lowe N, Maxwell A, Patnaik R 2005 Adverse reactions to dermal fillers. [Review] Dermatology Surgery 31:1616–1625

Lupton JR, Alster TS 2000 Cutaneous hypersensitivity reaction to injectable hyaluronic acid gel. Dermatology Surgery 26:135–137

Meyers H, Brown-Elliott BA, Moore D et al 2002 Clinical Infectious Disease 34:1500–1507

Micheels P 2001 Human anti-hyaluronic acid antibodies: is it possible? Dermatologic Surgery 27:185–191

Moody BR, Sengelmann RD 2001 Topical tacrolimus in the treatment of bovine collagen hypersensitivity. Dermatologic Surgery 27:789–791

Moon SY, Chang GY 2004 A complication of Cosmetic Surgery. New England Journal of Medicine 350:1549

Moyle GJ, Lysakova L, Brown S, et al 2004 A randomized open label study of immediate vs. delayed polylactic acid injections for the cosmetic management of facial lipoatrophy in persons with HIV infection. HIV Medicine 5:82–97

Narins R, Jewell M, Rubin M, Cohen J, Strobos J 2006 Clinical Conference: Management of Rare Events Following Dermal Fillers-Focal Necrosis and Angry Red Bumps. Dermatologic Surgery 32:426–434

Naoum C, Dasiou-Plakida D 2001 Dermal filler materials and botulinum toxin. International Journal of Dermatology 40:609–621

Rikimaru T, Nakamura M, Takafumi Y, et al 1991 Mediators, initiating the inflammatory response, released in organ culture by full-thickness human skin explants exposed to the irritant, sulfur mustard. Journal of Investigative Dermatology 96:888–897

Salyan Z 2003 Facial fillers and their complications. Aesthetic Surgery Journal 23:221

Seely BM, Denton AB, Ahn MS, Maas CS 2006 Effect of homeopathic Arnica Montana on bruising in face-lifts. Archives of Facial Plastic Surgery 8:54–59

Siegle RJ, McCoy JP, Schade W, Swanson NA 1984 Intradermal implantation of bovine collagen: humoral responses associated with clinical reaction. Archives in Dermatology 120:183

Stegman SJ, Chu S, Armstrong RC 1988 Adverse reactions to bovine collagen implant: clinical and histologic features. Journal of Dermatologic Surgery and Oncology 14:39–48

Stolman LP 2005 To the Editor: Human collagen reactions. Dermtologic Surgery 31:1634

Talwar HS, Griffiths CEM, Fisher GJ, Hamilton TA, Voorhees JJ 1995 Reduced type-I and Type-III procollagens in photodamaged adult human skin. Journal of Investigative Dermatology 105:285–290

Temourian B 1988 Blindness following fat injections. Plastic and Reconstructive Surgery 80:361

Tolleth H 1985 Long-term efficacy of collagen. Aesthetic Plastic Surgery 9:155–158

Toy BR, Frank PJ 2003 Outbreak of Mycobacterium abcessus infection after soft tissue augmentation. Dermatologic Surgery 29:971–973

Uslan D, Kowalski T, Wengenack N, et al 2006 Skin and soft tissue infections due to rapidly growing mycobacteria. Archives of Dermatology 142:1287–1292

Valantin MA, Aubron-Olivier C, Ghosh J, et al 2003 Polylactic acid implants (Newfill) to correct lipoatrophy in HIV-infected patients: results of the open-label study VEGA. AIDS 17:2471–2474

Vleggaar D 2005 Facial volumetric correction with injectable poly-L-lactic acid. Dermatologic Surgery 2005;31:1511–1518 and Saylan Z [Counterpoint to above article] Dermatologic Surgery 2005;31:1517–1518

Wall S, Adamson P, Baily D, Van Norstrand P 2003 Patient satisfaction with expanded polytetrafluoroethylene implants to the perioral region. Archives of Facial Plastic Surgery 5:320–324

Watson W, Kay RL, Klein A, Stegman S 1983 Injectable collagen: A clinical overview. Cutis 31:543–546

Zyderm/Zyplast package insert

Synthetic Fillers: Carboxymethyl Cellulose, Polyethylene Oxide Dermal Filler

Philippa Lowe, Samuel Falcone, Richard Berg, Nicholas J. Lowe

BACKGROUND

In this chapter a novel dermal filler (DF) composed of carboxymethyl cellulose (CMC), and polyethylene oxide (PEO) and its use, is described for soft tissue augmentation. The DF was designed using measurements of the viscoelastic and physical properties of marketed DFs composed of cross-linked hyaluronic acid (HA). A total of 12 patients with moderate or severe nasolabial folds (NLFs) were randomized to contralateral treatments of similar volumes of DF or Restylane. Both DF and Restylane were effective in providing clinical correction for up to 6 months. Related adverse events were similar for both products and typical of DF products. The results from this study indicate that a DF composed of a solution of CMC, and PEO was similar to Restylane in safety and effectiveness, providing NLF correction for up to 6 months. Subsequently 15 additional patients were treated with NLF injection and/or lip augmentation with DF without complication other than transient expected mild edema of 1–2 days' duration.

INTRODUCTION

HA is a naturally occurring polysaccharide, consisting of linear chains of alternating D-glucuronic acid and N-acetyl-D-glucosamine residues, which is present in the skin and connective tissues. HA has an identical sequence of disaccharide subunits across species and tissues and, if cross-linked for stabilization, makes a suitable candidate for a biocompatible polymer from which to manufacture medical devices such as DFs.

Other polycarboxylic acids can be formulated to have rheological properties similar to cross-linked HAs. In particular, CMC in solution, without cross-linking, behaves as a viscoelastic gel with dynamic and rotational properties that are similar to cross-linked HAs according to Falcone and Berg. The CMC- and PEO-based DF described here has a CE mark and this study is a post-market study of this DF. This chapter describes the results of the post

market study and additional experiences with patient treatment.

NOVEL CMC DERMAL FILLER CHARACTERISTICS

The DF is composed of CMC and PEO at a concentration of 35 mg/mL in physiological saline containing calcium chloride. The filler has the appearance of a clear viscoelastic gel and is packaged sterile in 3 mL polypropylene syringes. The gel can easily be injected through a 30 gauge needle. A comparison of the rheological properties of DF and Restylane are given in Table 12A.1. Restylane is composed of cross-linked particles of HA. DF is a solution of two pharmaceutical grade polymers that are not cross-linked. Restylane has a higher complex viscosity than DF and is much less compliant. The two gels are similar in terms of the percent elasticity indicating that they have similar apparent stiffness.

CLINICAL STUDY

A 6-month study was performed in the UK with recruited subjects seeking soft tissue augmentation for correction of bilateral NLFs. The study design was a single treatment session with bilateral, randomized, treatment of NLFs with DF on one side and Restylane on the contralateral side, followed by an evaluator-blind 6-month follow up.

Following initial screening, including a forearm skin test with DF, each patient received DF or Restylane on contralateral sides of the face after peroral anesthetic nerve injection with Xylocaine 1% allowing intra-patient comparison of treatment outcomes. Treatment allocation could not be concealed from the treating investigator. Both the patient and the evaluating investigator were unaware of treatment allocation, thus ensuring that a blinded study design was maintained.

Injection technique of both fillers was similar, i.e. tunneling with a 30 gauge needle followed by filler injection on retraction of needle.

Table 12A.1 Rheological properties, at 0.0628 (rad/s) of hyaluronic acid-based dermal fillers

Product	η* (Pas)	G* (Pa)	J*(1/Pa)	tan(δ)	% Elasticity
Restylane	4264	267.9	0.0037	0.395	71.7
DF	369	23.5	0.0432	0.459	68.5

The two dermal fillers were analyzed using a Thermo Haake RS300 Rheometer, fitted in the cone and plate geometry. All measurements were performed with a 35 mm/1° titanium cone sensor at 25°C. Oscillation measurements were acquired over a frequency range of 0.01–100 Hz (0.62–628.3 rad/s^{-1}).
Presented in the table are the complex viscosity, the complex modulus, the compliance, the tan(δ), and the percent elasticity at low frequency, 0.0628 rad/s. The percent elasticity is calculated as 100*G'/(G' + G''). Although Restylane has a higher complex viscosity and lower compliance than DF, the percent elasticity of these two materials are very similar. The percent elasticity is an important property that is often related to the persistence of a dermal filler (Falcone et al, 2006)

The response to the initial injection of DF or Restylane was evaluated after 2 weeks for adverse events. Patients were evaluated at 1 month, 3 months, and 6 months post treatment. Because DF had limited clinical exposure prior to this study, subjects participating in the study were required to have a skin test 28 days prior to treatment that was negative prior to treatment in all patients. This is not our practice in nonstudy patients.

Photographs for baseline Wrinkle Severity Rating Scale (WSRS) scoring were taken of each patient using Canfield clinical photography. Each side of the patient's face was randomized with respect to treatment procedure. Follow-up visits were at 1 month, 3 months, and 6 months post-treatment.

A masked, trained evaluator determined Wrinkle Severity Rating Scale (WSRS) scoring using a 5-point scale. In addition to the masked, trained evaluator, the patient and the treating investigator determined scores using the Global Aesthetic Improvement Scale (GAIS).

• Exclusionary medications

❖ Prescription facial wrinkle therapies (e.g. Renova etc.) or topical steroids applied in the treatment area within 4 weeks before treatment and for 6 months after treatment

❖ Immunosuppressive medications or systemic steroids (i.e. oral prednisone) within 6 months before treatment or 6 months after treatment

❖ Drugs or therapies which may affect thrombin or platelet formation within 72 hours prior to study treatment (e.g. aspirin, aspirin-containing products, nonsteroidal anti-inflammatory drugs, vitamin E, estrogen preparations and herbal supplements known to affect coagulation)

❖ Anticoagulant therapy, including coumadin, 2 weeks prior to or during the treatment phase.

• Exclusionary procedures/treatments

❖ Facial injections of botulinum toxin products (e.g. Botox injections, etc.) in the facial treatment areas within 6 months before treatment and for 6 months after treatment

❖ Nonpermanent cosmetic filler-type products (e.g. Zyplast, Zyderm, Hylaform, Cosmoplast, etc.) in the facial area within 12 months before treatment and for 6 months after treatment.

❖ Permanent or long-lasting cosmetic filler-type products in the facial area at any time prior to or during the study

❖ Superficial dermal resurfacing procedures in the facial area including chemical peel, dermabrasion, or microderm treatments within 6 weeks before treatment and for 6 months after treatment.

Clinical efficacy assessments were conducted independently by the trained, masked evaluator at 1, 3 and 6 months after the treatment session. Efficacy comparisons between study treatments were made on the mean change from baseline in the WSRS (reported by Day et al) of the NLFs as determined by the masked evaluator at all follow-up time points. The WSRS has demonstrated its robustness in previous clinical trials reported by Narins et al and Lindqvist et al of intradermal fillers. Scoring of wrinkle severity is based on visual comparison of the length and apparent depth of the NLF against an agreed set of reference photographs of NLFs. The WSRS is an absolute 5-point scale with scale values of 1 (absent), 2 (mild), 3 (moderate), 4 (severe) or 5 (extreme). The range of scores (1–5) covered by this scale represents visibly distinct and hence clinically significant gradations in fold severity.

In addition, the overall change in appearance of the NLF from its pretreatment condition was determined at each follow-up visit during the double-blind phase using the GAIS reported by Narins et al. The GAIS is a relative 5-point scale with scale values of 1 (worse), 2 (no change), 3 (improved), 4 (much improved) or 5 (very much improved) from pretreatment. Both the patient and the treating investigator scored the patient using the GAIS. An archival (pretreatment) photograph was kept for each patient and this was used as the reference image at each follow-up visit.

Safety assessments were based on observed and spontaneously reported adverse events occurring throughout the study.

The primary efficacy analysis was based on the patient response rate defined as the proportion of patients showing a [3]1-grade improvement in evaluator-assessed WSRS score from pre-treatment value at 1, 3 and 6 months post treatment.

Secondary efficacy analyses were based on the investigator- and patient-assessed GAIS rating at 1, 3 and 6 months post treatment.

For each of these scales, a masked evaluator assessed each side. For the WSRS, the score of the DF and Restylane sides were subtracted from the baseline score. For the GAIS, the score of the DF and Restylane side are presented.

CLINICAL RESULTS

A total of 12 patients were recruited for the study. All 12 patients completed 6 months' follow up. The average volume of gel implanted in either NLF was 1.81 mL DF and 1.75 mL Restylane. The results from this study indicated that DF was effective in providing a clinical correction for up to 6 months. The WSRS scores for all 12 patients are plotted in Figure 12A.2. The data demonstrate that both products were effective for up to 6 months. The number of patients was too small to determine the level of statistical significance for a comparison of the two products. The Global Assessment Scores were also determined from the responses of both the patient and the treating physician and the results are plotted in Figure 12A.3. These results from the patients and the treating investigator indicate that the correction is noticeable by the patient and the investigator at 3 and 6 months for both treatments. The mean baseline score for both groups was 3.4 and both fillers demonstrated measurable clinical correction at 6 months.

All safety analyses were performed on all 12 subjects who received a treatment. The safety profile of both products was similar. The adverse events were similar and consisted of swelling and firmness at the injection site. One patient experienced a localized reaction of redness and itching within 2 minutes on the side treated with DF. This type of reaction has been observed in the past with Restylane as reported by Klien and Elson, and Andre et al. The localized redness was treated with ice and topical hydrocortisone and improved within 2 hours. It completely resolved within 24–48 hours, the patient completing the study and maintaining clinical correction for 6 months. Localized redness, swelling, bruising, and induration are common adverse events for DFs as reported by Andre et al. Based on similarity to other cross-linked HA

DFs, DF is considered to be safe. Induration involving the injection site affected most of the patients for both groups and generally resolved within 1 week. Importantly there were no delayed-onset local reactions during the study.

Since the study was concluded a total of 15 additional patients have been treated with DF. In the 15 patients (9 nasolabial only/6 nasolabial and lips) now treated outside the study the authors have observed no side effects except for transient (1–2 days) post injection swelling in most patients, similar to that experienced with HA fillers.

To date of writing (October 2006) over 1500 patient treatments have been conducted in Europe without any significant adverse events (data on file, Fziomed).

See Figure 12A.1A, B, C, D.

DF DISCUSSION

Numerous substances have been tested over the years for augmenting soft tissue of the face to improve cosmesis. DFs may have various tissue responses in the dermis from phagocytosis to foreign body reactions, and even granulomas, depending on the material. The ideal DF temporarily augments the dermis to correct the surface contour of the skin without producing an unacceptable inflammatory reaction, hypersensitive reactions or foreign body reaction. One of the first materials to be used for dermal augmentation was Zyplast, derived from bovine collagen. However, bovine collagen was found to be associated with delayed hypersensitivity in a small percentage of patients as reported by Charriere et al. Another material used for this application is cross-linked HA, which was considered to be an improvement on biocompatibility over bovine collagen. One such product is Restylane, which is composed of cross-linked HA derived from bacteria-produced HA. Restylane has been compared with Zyplast in human clinical studies reported by Narins et al and Restylane was found to provide longer-lasting cosmetic improvement than the cross-linked bovine collagen Zyplast.

Both CMC and HA are high molecular weight polysaccharides. Since CMC and cross-linked HA have similar viscoelastic properties, an evaluation of DF for the correction of facial wrinkles was merited. Restylane is considerably more viscous than DF. However, its stiffness as determined by percent elasticity, is similar to DF. Since its effectiveness is similar to DF, viscosity itself is not clearly associated with increased clinical persistence.

CMC and PEO are biocompatible polymers that have been extensively used as surgical implants in both animal studies and clinical experience reported by Kim et al and Lundorf et al. The unique properties of the combination of these polymers make DF a novel DF. DF is synthetic, not derived from animal or bacterial sources, and is noninflammatory. Clinical safety for the use of DF in the treatment of NLF wrinkles in humans is supported by this study.

Cross-linked HA displays longer tissue retention than natural HA and is less immunogenic than bovine collagen according to Larsen et al, Friedman et al and FDA P20023.

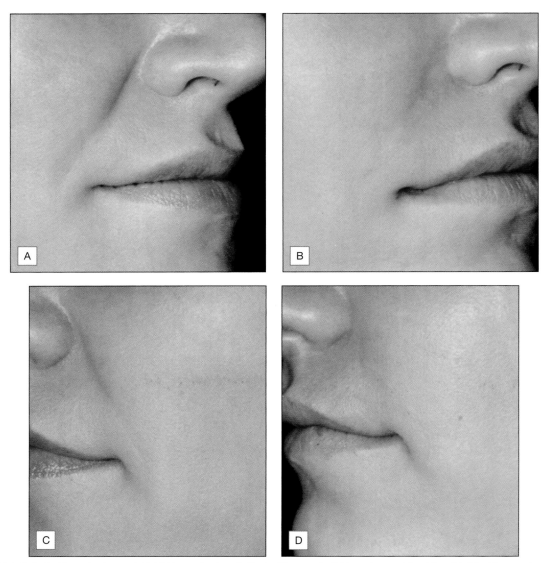

Fig. 12A.1 Patient with moderate nasolabial folds pre-treatment. She had Laresse to NLFs and upper lateral lips. A total of 1 cc each side was injected.1% Xylocaine nerve block was administered prior to treatment

As reported by Duranti et al and FDA PO30032, HAs are all produced from animal or bacterial systems providing the possibility of contamination with antigens from the source. Clinical experience in Piacquadio et al and Duranti et al indicates that cross-linked HA provides good initial efficacy in correcting facial wrinkles and folds. Cross-linked HA products including Restylane have acceptable biocompatibilities in most cases detailed in Lowe, Maxwell and Lowe; Andre et al; and Lowe et al). Reports such as in Micheels have questioned the safety of cross-linked HA fillers.

Chemical cross-linking of HA results in the formation of a water-insoluble polymer that has higher elasticity than un-cross-linked HA and improved resistance to enzymatic degradation. Because of the requirement to crosslink HA, HA DFs are all particulate with various sizes of gel particles. In some cases the particles are large enough to appear lumpy to the touch after implantation. CMC, a polysaccharide similar to HA, is not subject to enzymatic degradation and does not require cross-linking to have dynamic physical properties similar to cross-linked HA. CMC is a true polymeric solution and therefore if it is as persistent as cross-linked HA, it could have advantages over cross-linked DFs. One advantage is the absence of gel particles, which makes it smoother to the touch and easier to inject, and a second advantage is a lack of poten-

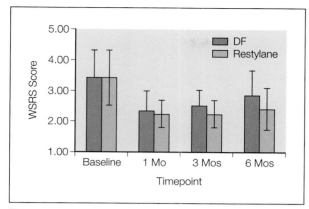

Fig. 12A.2 The WSRS results of a feasibility study of 12 patients treated with DF and Restylane in a blinded bilateral comparison study. The values are the average and the bars are the standard deviation

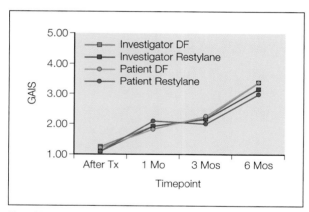

Fig. 12A.3 Average Global Assessment scores

tial irritancy from unreacted cross-linkers remaining in the cross-linked HA DF or released as the filler is degraded.

The absence of cross-linkers and the similarity in safety and effectiveness to HA fillers, suggests that DF is a promising, novel, DF. Currently an improved version of DF is available in the European Community under the trade name Laresse. See Figures 12A.1A, B, C, D.

FURTHER READING

Andre P, Lowe NJ, et al 2005 Adverse reactions to dermal fillers: a review of European experiences. Journal of Cosmetic Laser Therapy 7:171–176

Charriere G, Bejot M, et al 1989 Reactions to a bovine collagen implant. Clinical and immunologic study in 705 patients. Journal of the American Academy of Dermatology 21:1203–1208

Day DJ, Littler CM, et al 2004 The wrinkle severity rating scale: a validation study. American Journal of Clinical Dermatology 5:49–52

Duranti F, Salti G, et al 1998 Injectable hyaluronic acid gel for soft tissue augmentation. A clinical and histological study. Dermatologic Surgery 24:1317–1325

Falcone SJ, Berg RA (in preparation) Crosslinked hyaluronic acid dermal fillers: A comparison of rheological properties

Falcone SJ, Berg RA (in preparation) Novel dermal fillers based on sodium carboxycellulose (CMC)

Falcone SJ, Palmeri DM, et al 2006 Biomedical applications of hyaluronic acid. American Chemical Society Symposium Series, Washington DC

FDA 2003 Summary of Safety and Effectiveness Data; Restylene Injectable Gel (P20023).

FDA 2004 Clinical Review P030032 Hylaform Viscoelastic gel

Friedman PM, Mafong EA, et al 2002 Safety data of injectable non-animal stabilized hyaluronic acid gel for soft tissue augmentation. Dermatologic Surgery 28:491–494

Kim KD, Wang JC, et al 2003 Reduction of radiculopathy and pain with Oxiplex/SP gel after laminectomy, laminotomy, and discectomy: a pilot clinical study. Spine 28:1080–1087, discussion 1087–1088

Klein AW, Elson ML 2000 The history of substances for soft tissue augmentation. Dermatologic Surgery 26:1096–1105

Larsen NE, Pollak CT, et al 1993 Hylan gel biomaterial: dermal and immunologic compatibility. Journal of Biomedical Materials Research 27:1129–1134

Lindqvist C, Tveten S, et al 2005 A randomized, evaluator-blind, multicenter comparison of the efficacy and tolerability of Perlane versus Zyplast in the correction of nasolabial folds. Plastic and Reconstructive Surgery 115:282–289

Lowe NJ, Maxwell CA, Lowe PL, et al 2001 Hyaluronic acid skin fillers: adverse reactions and skin testing. Journal of the American Academy of Dermatology 45:930–933

Lowe NJ, Maxwell CA, Patnick R 2005 Adverse reactions to dermal fillers: review. Dermatologic Surgery 31:1616–1625

Lundorff P, Donnez J, et al 2005 Clinical evaluation of a viscoelastic gel for reduction of adhesions following gynaecological surgery by laparoscopy in Europe. Human Reproduction 20:514–520

Micheels P 2001 Human anti-hyaluronic acid antibodies: is it possible? Dermatologic Surgery 29:185–191

Narins RS, Brandt F, et al 2003 A randomized, double-blind, multicenter comparison of the efficacy and tolerability of Restylane versus Zyplast for the correction of nasolabial folds. Dermatologic Surgery 29:588–595

Olenius M 1998 The first clinical study using a new biodegradable implant for the treatment of lips, wrinkles, and folds. Aesthetic in Plastic Surgery 22:97–101

Piacquadio D, Jarcho M, et al 1997 Evaluation of hylan b gel as a soft-tissue augmentation implant material. Journal of the American Academy of Dermatology 36:544–549

Schwartz HE, Blackmore JM, et al 2005 Compositions of polyacids and polyethers and methods for their use in reducing adhesions. FzioMed, Inc.

12 B
Synthetic Fillers: BioAlcamid

David J. Goldberg

INTRODUCTION

In the early 1990s, after a long period of using bovine collagen, hyaluronic acids (HA) started to be the most commonly used biodegradable filler used in both dermatology and plastic surgery. Currently HA are very popular for both soft tissue augmentation and facial volume restoration.

Dermal filler HA have a high water retention capacity and are both effective tissue volume correctors and well tolerated. In addition to the highly popular HA, other European fillers, some not available in the United States, are either nondegradable or slowly degradable. They have now been used for 30 years for the correction of facial volume wasting.

An ideal biomaterial must be nonallergic, inert, sterile nonpyogenc, noncancer producing, stable, incapable of migrating, and most importantly biologically compatible with the host tissue. The latter factor is required because it impacts on the ability of the filler to coexist with surrounding tissues without either stimulating the immune system or causing persistent inflammatory reactions.

Current dermal fillers can be divided into those that are short acting, intermediate in duration and permanent (Table 12B.1). BioAlcamid is a permanent filler.

BIOALCAMID

BioAlcamid, a synthetic polyalkylamide manufactured by Polymekon in Italy, is a permanent implant that fulfills some, but certainly not all, of the aforementioned requirements.

• Clinical studies

In a clinical study performed by Protopapa et al, 80 BioAlcamid implants were injected into 73 subjects between the ages of 16 and 48 years (40 females and 33 males) (Table 12B.2). All patients were HIV-positive and suffered from lipodystrophy syndrome to varying degrees. Individuals with uncompromised diabetes mellitus, psychiatric disorders and pregnant women were excluded from the study. No prior skin tests were given. Initial implants were placed in the face. Ultimately three patients requested further corrections to the buttocks; four patients requested corrections to their limbs. The BioAlcamid was injected into the subcutaneous layer.

Facial deformities received up to 35 mL of the product; correction of buttock deficits required up to 1600 mL of the biopolymer. In over 90% of cases, a second injection of BioAlcamid was carried out 4 weeks after the first injection to optimize implant appearance. Injection of material into the face was carried out with 19 gauge needles; 16 gauge needles were used in the buttocks and legs. No more than 15 mL was injected at any site. Multiple injections were undertaken until total correction of the deficit was obtained. All patients were given antibiotics after injection of the prosthesis.

All patients were evaluated at 4 weeks, 2 months and 1 year following implantation. Three patients were followed for 3 years. Immediately after injection, the material appeared soft. Post-injection edema disappeared in 3–4 days after treatment.

In assessing clinical results, the investigators considered the degree of patient satisfaction (modest, fair, average, good or excellent), the degree of observed clinical improvement, short- or long-term complications, and the possible need for implant removal. Improvement was deemed to be excellent by both physician and patient. No implant dislocation, implant migration, or other adverse reactions were noted.

In order to assess the biocompatabilty of BioAlcamid, skin biopsy specimens were taken from human volunteers subjected to BioAlcamid implants. Seven healthy male and female volunteers between the ages of 19 and 37 years were evaluated. Each subject was injected with 0.5–1.0 cc of BioAlcamid in the subcutaneous layer of the abdominal wall. Skin biopsy specimens were obtained 3 months after implantation. Light microscopic analysis of the skin specimens revealed fibroblasts located in the subcutaneous

Table 12B.1 Fillers		
Short lasting	**Longer lasting**	**Permanent**
Hyaluronic acid	Calcium hydroxyapatite	Beaded hyaluronic acid
Collagen	Poly-L-lactic acid	Beaded collagen
		Silicone
		Acrylic gel
		Alkylamide gel

Table 12B.2 BioAlcamid reported injection sites	
Location	**Authors**
Face, legs, buttocks	Protopapa, C
Face	Treacy

layer. These fibroblasts were arranged around a central amorphous core, representing the injected biomaterial, and were surrounded by a normal intercellular matrix showing no signs of inflammation. In the treated skin, the epidermis, dermis and subcutaneous tissue adjacent to the filler were normal and identical to that of controls. Of great interest to the investigators were the observed connective fibrils that appeared to anchor the biomaterial to the deeper fibroblastic layer of the capsule that had formed at the capsule–implant interface. There were virtually no signs of neutrophil or monocyte tissue infiltration around the implant. The authors felt this confirmed that BioAlcamid was a material highly compatible with human skin.

The authors further noted that BioAlcamid was a permanent substance, without toxicity, was insoluble in tissue fluids, radiotransparent, and because of its high water content did not alter tissue consistency. Though permanent in nature, they suggested the implant could be removed from human skin months to years after implantation.

In another study, 11 subjects with severe facial lipodystrophy secondary to HIV-infection were evaluated. All but one were male, the mean age was 48 (±7) years, and the mean HIV duration was 17 (±11) years. The subjects were randomly selected from patients seeking treatment for HIV Associated Lipoatrophy (HLS). They came from differing countries, including the United States, United Kingdom, Ireland, and Spain. All of the subjects had a full hematologic evaluation including full blood count, biochemistry, liver function, lipids, glucose, lactate, viral load and CD4 cell count. All subjects had not received prior treatment for their HLS. Patients who were receiving anticoagulant therapy, steroids, or diclofenac were not excluded from the study. Each of the subjects was injected bilaterally with 15–30 cc of BioAlcamid into the subcutaneous regions of their buccal, malar, and temporal areas of the face. During the procedure, care was taken to inject the polymer superficially to the superficial musculoaponeurotic system (SMAS). Regional injected anesthesia was used in conjunction with topical anesthesia in all treated subjects. The treated area was sculptured to obtain the best esthetic appearance. At the end of the treatment, each patient received amoxicillin and clavulanate potassium (GlaxoSmithKline, Dublin, Ireland) or clarithromycin (Abbott Laboratories, Dublin, Ireland) for 3 days to prevent infection. All of the subjects were first esthetically assessed and then digitally photographed prior to injection after written informed consent had been obtained. The endpoint of treatment was achieved whenever the physician, nursing staff and the subject all noted, and agreed, that the changes in facial contour had reached an optimal esthetic outcome by visual observation. In addition to photographic documentation, all treated subjects had evaluation of their quality of life and psychological consequences of lipodystrophy investigated before and after treatment with a specifically designed social interaction questionnaire using a modified Beck Depression Scale. Clinical improvement was evaluated 3 and 18 months after treatment.

The subjects had a mean CD4 = 632/μl (±247), with a viral load below limit of detection in 73% of the cases. Every treated subject noted that their quality of life improved dramatically 3 months after treatment. Four of the subjects felt that they had been able to obtain different employment as a direct result of the procedure. None of the subjects expressed regret at having had the procedure. All of the subjects showed a significant positive improvement in their social functioning ($P = 0.03$), and the modified Beck Depression Scale showed a mean overall score decrease from 14.57 to 10.21 after the procedure ($P = 0.1$). Almost all of the subjects reported that the results of the permanent filler became more natural in the weeks following the procedure. No treated subject reported any evidence of migration or nodules 3 months

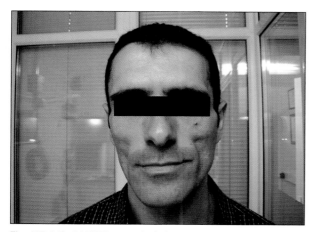

Fig. 12B.1 Facial HIV lipoatrophy before treatment with BioAlcamid

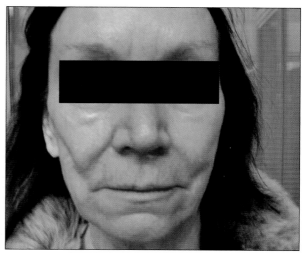

Fig. 12B.3 Facial HIV lipoatrophy before treatment with BioAlcamid

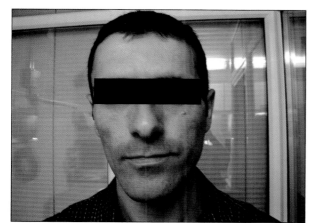

Fig. 12B.2 Facial HIV lipoatrophy after treatment with BioAlcamid

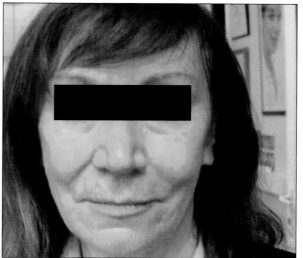

Fig. 12B.4 Facial HIV lipoatrophy after treatment with BioAlcamid

after treatment. The benefits of the biopolymer persisted at the 18-month evaluation (Figs 12B.1–4).

• Treatment technique

The ideal patient for BioAlcamid treatment is a patient with significant facial lipoatrophy who seeks a permanent injectable treatment modality (Fig. 12B.5). BioAlcamid is marketed as a frozen 4% acrylic alkylamide gel dissolved in 96% sterile water. It currently has CE clearance in Europe, and although approved in Canada, has yet to receive FDA clearance in the United States.

Anesthesia is usually provided through localized nerve blocks (Fig. 12B.6). Currently used BioAlcamid polyalkyl-imide gel, although injected into deep dermal and subcutaneous tissue, appears to be different from other dermal fillers in that once implanted it becomes covered by a very thin collagen capsule (0.02 mm), This completely surrounds the gel, isolating it from the host tissues and making it a type of endogenous prosthesis. According to Polymekon, the Italian manufacturer, the encapsulated prosthesis has the potential for later extraction from surrounding tissue. To date, reactions to polyacrylamide gels appear to be rare and have not been reported in HLS-treated patients. The compound has been used since 2000 in over 20 countries and does not require any sensitization test as no allergic reaction has been reported. Although the gel has been extensively evaluated in a 2000 patient study that demonstrated its safety, efficacy and biocompatibility, there have been reports of occasional poorly

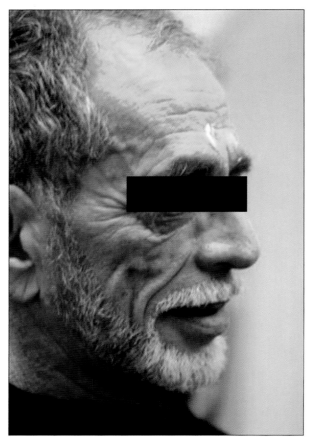

Fig. 12B.5 Ideal BioAlcamid patient with significant lipoatrophy

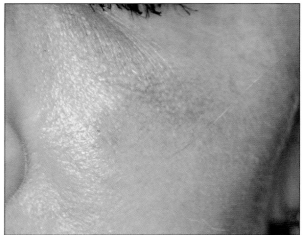

Fig. 12B.7 Permanent nodules after BioAlcamid injection

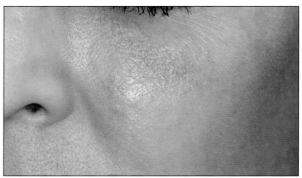

Fig. 12B.8 Permanent nodules after BioAlcamid injection

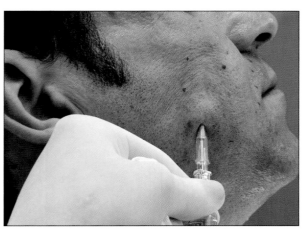

Fig. 12B.6 BioAlcamid injection into the mid malar region
(Photograph courtesy of Dr Jean Carruthers)

defined adverse reactions (Figs 12B.7–8). These reactions present as delayed hard nodular lesions that can only be removed with surgery.

• Advanced topic

Once implanted BioAlcamid forms a true permanent endoprosthesis, encompassed in a thin (0.02 mm), yet continuous fibrous capsule separating it from the host tissue. Although some have suggested that the prosthesis is easily removed, one must assume that with encapsulation prosthesis removal may become increasingly more difficult.

What also has yet to be determined is whether this prosthesis is totally nonbiodegradable. Nonspecific free radical processes are always functioning in the skin. Further safety studies will be required to determine if there is specific enzymatic degradation of the prosthesis.

FURTHER READING

Ascher B, Bui P, Halabi A 2006 Fillers in Europe. In: Goldberg DJ (ed.) Dermal Fillers. Taylor & Francis, London

Formigli L, Zecchi S, Protopapa C, et al 2004 BioAlcamid: An electron microscopic study after skin implantation. Plastic and Reconstructive Surgery 113:1104–1106

Guaraldi G, Orlando G, De Fazio D 2004 Prospective, partially randomized, 24-week study to compare the efficacy and durability of different surgical techniques and interventions for the treatment of HIV-related facial lipoatrophy. 6th Lipodystrophy Workshop (6th IWADRLH), Washington. Abstract 12. Antiviral Therapy 9:L9

Pacini A, Ruggiero S, Morucci B, Cammarota SS, Protopapa B, Gulisano M 2002 BioAlcamid: A novelty for reconstructive and cosmetic surgery. Italian Journal of Anatomy and Embryology 107:209–214

Pacini S, Ruggiero M, Cammarota N, et al 2004 BioAlcamid, a novel prosthetic polymer, does not interfere with morphological and functional characteristics of human skin fibroblasts. Plastic and Reconstructive Surgery 113:1104–1106

Protopapa B, Sito G, Caporale G, and Cammarota N 2003 BioAlcamid in drug-induced lipodystrophy. Journal of Cosmetic Laser Therapy 5:226–230

12 C Synthetic Fillers: Bioinblue

Jean Carruthers, Alistair Carruthers

INTRODUCTION

Bioinblue (Polymekon Research, Brindisi, Italy) is a bio-degradable synthetic hydrogel filler consisting of highly purified polyvinyl alcohol (PVA; 8%) and nonpyrogenic water (92%). Commercially available in Europe since 2002, PVA hydrogel is available in two forms: Bioinblue Lips (for lips and other fine rhytides), and Bioinblue DeepBlue (for deeper wrinkles, folds and grooves, as well as tissue augmentation) and is becoming well accepted as an effective and long-lasting dermal filler for correction of facial deficits. In the United States, PVA is approved for biomedical but not cosmetic uses.

CLINICAL EFFICACY

Although only recently used for facial augmentation, PVA has been widely used in medicine for a number of applications. Among others, PVA has been proposed as a base for blood plasma substitute agents and is used as a carrier of therapeutic substances and as an immobilization matrix. PVA membranes have been developed as artificial pancreas and for use in hemodialysis as reported in Young et al and Paul and Sharma, respectively.

Cross-linked by freeze-thawing cycles, PVA hydrogel is a strong, elastic, and resistant gel with a three-dimensional structure and similar to soft tissue in high water content (92%), mechanical properties, softness, oxygen permeability, and high biocompatibility. PVA hydrogels have been proposed as promising biomaterials to substitute damaged articular cartilage and have been used in tendon injury repair, and as controlled drug delivery systems according to Stammen et al, Kobayashi et al and Li et al, respectively. Recent research involves the use of PVA hydrogel for ophthalmologic and cardiovascular applications as reported in Maruoki et al and Uchino et al, and Millon et al, respectively.

Clinical data for the use of PVA hydrogel in cosmetic applications are scarce. Unlike other three-dimensional gels, PVA hydrogel is biodegradable and reversible and is indicated for injection into the mid-to deep dermis and/or subcutaneous layer of the face for the correction of moderate to severe wrinkles or folds (deficits of the cheeks, chin, sunken and post-acne scars, nasolabial folds, lip volume deficit, and correction of labial profile and harelip). Immediate effects last for at least 7 months and up to 18 months before undergoing degradation and clearance. Treatment tightens and smoothes the skin, restoring a sense of youth and lending a natural appearance.

SIDE EFFECTS OR COMPLICATIONS

Since PVA hydrogel is composed entirely of synthetic material and contains no animal protein, allergy tests are not required prior to injection. To date, there has been no indication of allergic reaction or serious complications, but side effects associated with any tissue augmentation can occur. Side effects may include persistent erythema, tissue damage from injection (subcutaneous bleeding, infection, abscesses, nerve damage, necrosis, and broken veins), pain and/or discoloration at the injection site. Temporary swelling or flushing may occur for 12–24 hours after treatment. Swelling rarely lasts for more than a few days but has been reported for up to 1 month, sometimes accompanied by itching. Swelling, hardening, sclerosis, contusions, and discoloration at the injection site have persisted for several months in rare cases.

FURTHER READING

Kobayashi M, Toguchida J, Oka M 2001 Development of polyvinyl alcohol-hydrogel (PVA-H) shields with a high water content for tendon injury repair. Journal of Hand Surgery 26:436–440

Koo KM, Ting YP 2001 Polyvinyl alcohol as an immobilization matric – a case of gold biosorption. Water Science and Technology 43:17–23

Li JK, Wang N, Wu XS 1988 Poly(vivyl alcohol) nanoparticles prepared by freezing-thawing process for protein/peptide drug delivery. Journal of Control Release 56:117–126

Maruoka S, Matsuura T, Kawasaki K, et al 2006 Biocompatibility of polyvinylalcohol gel as a vitreous substitute. Current Eye Research 31:599–606

Millon LE, Mohammadi H, Wan WK 2006 Anisotropic polyvinyl alcohol hydrogel for cardiovascular applications. Journal of Biomedical Materials Research B Applied Biomater 79:305–311

Paul W, Sharma CP 1997 Acetylsalicylic acid loaded poly(vinyl alcohol) hemodialysis membranes: Effect of drug release on blood compatibility and permeability. Journal of Biomedical Science Polymer Ed 8:755–764

Rybacki E, Stozek T 1980 Substancje pomocnicze w tecnologii postaci leku. PZWL 50–51

Stammen JA, Williams S, Ku DN, Guldberg RE 2001 Mechanical properties of a novel PVA hydrogel in shear and unconfined compression. Biomaterials 22:799–806

Uchino Y, Shimmura S, Miyashita H, et al 2006 Amniotic membrane immobilized poly(vinyl alcohol) hybrid polymer as an artificial cornea scaffold that supports a stratified and differentiated corneal epithelium. Journal of Biomedicine Materials Research B Applied Biomater. [Epub ahead of print]

Young TH, Chuang WY, Yao NK, Chen LW 1998 Evaluation of asymmetric poly(vinyl alcohol) membranes for use in artificial islets. Biomaterials 40:385–397

Index

As the subject of this book is soft tissue augmentation, all index entries refer to this unless otherwise stated.

Page numbers in **bold** refer to information in tables or boxes: those in *italics* refer to figures.

vs. indicates a comparison.

A

ablative laser resurfacing
  nasolabial folds 109
  perioral rejuvenation 51–52, 60, *60*
abscesses, collagen injections 29
Achyal 49
acne scarring, liquid injectable silicone 92, *93*
AdatoSil 5000 19, 94, 121
Advanta 158
aging face *see* facial aging
Alloderm 21
amethocaine 129
anesthesia *see* pain control/anesthesia
anterior superior alveolar nerve 133
antibiotics 157
  prophylactic 156
anticoagulants **152**
'apple dumpling' effect 51
Aptos Threads 109, *111, 112*
Arnica Montana 4, 54, 152–153
Artecoll *see* ArteFill
ArteFill 22, 84–86
  allergic reactions 123
  blanching effect 123
  collagens *vs.* 84
  complications 84–86, 123
  duration of action 84
  history 84
  indications 84
  injection depth 7
  lip enhancement 85
  lip lumpiness *85*
  mechanism of action 84
  nasolabial folds 84, 85, 121–123, *122*
    injection technique 123
  patient selection 85
  perioral rejuvenation 51
  side effects 123
Arteplast 83, 84
arterial occlusion 155
Atelocollagen 21
atypical mycobacteria *156,* 156–157
auriculotemporal nerve 129

B

beading, liquid injectable silicone 96, 97, **98,** 111
Beletero 49
betacaine 129
biaxin 157
blepharoplasty correction, fat augmentation 74
botulinum toxin (Botox)
  with collagen injections 26–27
  crow's feet 28
  fat augmentation 69
  with Restylane 8
botulinum toxin A (BTX-A)
  nasolabial fold management 108, *110*
  perioral rejuvenation
    benefits 52
    Glogau photoaging type 3 58
    Glogau photoaging type 4 60, *60*
    patient selection 51
bovine collagen 4, 22–23
  adverse reactions 154
  disadvantages 4
  glabellar complex 28
  history 19–20
  hypersensitivity 23, 29, 154, *154*
  malpositioning 157
  nasolabial folds 114–116
  overcorrection 157
  Restylane *vs.* 35, *36*
  skin of color 146
  skin testing 23, 154
brow, fat augmentation 73–74, *74*
bruising 151–153, *153*
  coagulation abnormalities 151–152
  home remedies 152–153
  hylan injections 46
buccal fat pad
  aging 14–15
  augmentation 75, *75*
buccal nerve 129

C

calcium hydroxylapatite (CaHA) 6, *6,* 87
  injection depth 7
  nasolabial fold 118–119
  post-procedure management 8
  see also Radiesse
Captique 34, **35**
  lips 42
  Marionette lines 45
  nasolabial fold 45

Carruthers' Facial Lipoatrophy Severity Scale *95*
centistoke (cs) 90
centrifuge, fat augmentation 70
cephelexin 71
cheek(s)
    aging 14–15, *15*
    fat augmentation 74–75, *75,* 79
    hylan injection contouring 48–49
chemical peels, perioral rejuvenation 60
chin
    contouring, hylan injections 48–49
    drooping 56–57, *57*
    fat augmentation 76, *77*
cimetidine 151
ciprofloxacin 71
clarithromycin 157
coagulation abnormalities 151–152
cold compresses 8
    hylan injection 42
collagens, injectable 19–30
    anesthesia 24–25
    bovine *see* bovine collagen
    complications 25, *25,* 28–29, **29,** 150, 154
    FDA-approved 22–24, **23**
    human *see* human collagen
    hylans *vs.* **32**
    hypersensitive reactions 29
    indications 25
    lip augmentation *see* lips
    malpositioning 157
    nasolabial fold *see* nasolabial fold (NLF)
    patient education 24
    patient selection 24
    porcine 21, 116
    preinjection considerations 24, **24**
    pretreatment preparations 24–25
    products 21–22, **23**
    scars 25
    storage 22
    treatment guidelines 24–29
    see also individual preparations
combination therapy 8–9
complications 151–160
corticosteroids 85, 154
CosmoDerm **23,** 24
    glabellar complex treatment 28
    hypersensitivity 154
    injection depth 7
    lip augmentation 54–55
    nasolabial folds 116, *117*
CosmoPlast **23,** 24
    hypersensitivity 154
    nasolabial folds 27, 116, *117*
Coumadin 3–4
cross-hatching injection technique
    facial contouring 48
    hylans 41, *43*
    skin of color 145, *145*
crow's feet, collagen injections 28
    with Botox 28

cryoanesthesia 130–131
    benefits 131
    lips 131
    mechanism of action 130
    technique 130, *130*
Cupid's bow
    age-related changes 17, *17*
    collagen injections 26
cyclosporine 29, 154
Cymetra 21

D

dermabrasion, perioral rejuvenation 60
Dermadeep 49
Dermalive 49
Dermalogen 21
dermatomes, head and neck 128, *128*
diazepam 71
dimpling 8
drool area, collagen injections 26
drool lines *see* Marionette lines
dyschromia, liquid injectable silicone **98**

E

ecchymosis
    fat transplantation 68
    liquid injectable silicone 97, **98**
ectropion 14
edema
    fat augmentation 68, 77–79
    lip augmentation 55
    liquid injectable silicone 97, **98**
ELA-Max 129
Endoplast-50 22
entropion 14
erythema, liquid injectable silicone 97
erythromycin 71
ethylmethacrylate (EMA) 49
Eutectic Mixture of Local Anesthetics (EMLA)
    129
Evolence 8, 21, *22*
    nasolabial folds 116, *117*
expanded polytetrafluoroethylene (ePTFE) 156
expectations, unrealistic 159

F

facial aging 63–66, *65*
    anatomical approach 13–17, *14*
        lower third 15–17
        middle third 14–15
        upper third 13–14
    animation 63, 66, *66*
    etiology 11–12
    'hills and valleys' 63
    lean face 63, *65*
    skin of color 143–144, *144*
    suborbital area 63
facial appearance, esthetic 11
facial contouring, chin/cheeks 48–49
facial expression lines 1

facial foramina 132, *133*
facial markings
  fat augmentation 70–71, *71*
  liquid injectable silicone 95, *96*
  upper eyelid filling 71
fanning injection technique
  facial contouring 48
  hylans 41, *43*
  Marionette lines 45–46
  mouth corners 57, *57*
  nasolabial fold 45–46, 115, *115*
  skin of color 145, *145*
fat augmentation 4–5, *5,* 63–82
  alternative approaches 77–79
  anesthesia 72–73, 148
  with Botox 69
  combination therapy 8–9
  complications 77–79, 150
  contraindications 66
  entry sites *73*
  equipment 70, 73, *73*
  expected benefits 66–68, *68*
  extraction *see* fat extraction
  facial markings 70–71, *71*
  follow up 79–81
  forehead 73, *74*
  frozen fat use 81, *81*
  injection depth 7
  lateral facial 75
  malpositioning 157–158
  patient interviews 69–70, **70**
  patient preparation 71
  patient selection 66, *67*
  photographs, preoperative 69, *70*
  postoperative course 79–81
  reasons for 69
  rebalancing 66, 77
  retention rates 68, *78,* 79, *79, 80*
  side effects 77–79
  skin of color 148, *149*
  suborbital *see* suborbital fat augmentation
  surgical errors/pitfalls 77, **77**
  techniques 70–81, *73*
  touch up procedures 79–81
  treatment approach 68–69
  volumes used 77
fat autograft muscle injection (FAMI) 124, *124*
fat cysts, sterile 79
fat extraction 71–72, *72,* 148
  anesthesia 68
  equipment 72, *72*
  microliposuction 76–77
  tumescent fluid 72, **72**
fibroblasts, autologous 21
fillers
  biodegradable **4,** 4–5
  blepharoplasty substitute 2
  characteristics **20**
  choice of **4,** 4–6
  combination therapy 8–9

complications 8, 151–159
contraindications 4
esthetics 11–18
  approaches to 17–18
fibroplast-inducing 83–104
history 1, 19–20, **20**
indications 1–3
injection depth 7, *8*
limitations 8
materials 20–23
needle length comparison 131, *131*
needle size 151
new developments 8
nonbiodegradable **4,** 6
patient esthetic evaluation 1
photographs, preoperative 4
post-procedure management 8
pre-procedure planning 3–4
skin of color *see* skin of color
technique 6–8
  see also individual preparations
forehead
  fat augmentation 73, *74*
  nerve blocks 132–133
frontal nerve 129
frontal nerve blocks 133
frown lines *see* glabellar lines/rhytids

G

gasserian ganglion 128
'gate theory of pain control' 130, 132
gender differences, facial esthetics 11
Genzyme 6-point scale 105, *107*
Gingko Biloba 4
glabellar lines/rhytids
  collagen injections 28
  hylans 44–48, *48*
Glogau-Klein point 55
Glogau photoaging classification **12,** 12–13
  lips *see* lips
  perioral rejuvenation *see* perioral rejuvenation
  type I 12, *12*
  type II 12, *13*
  type III 12–13, *13*
  type IV 13, *14*
granuloma formation 8
  ArteFill 84–85, *85,* 123, *123*
  biodegradable fillers 4
  collagen injections 29
  hylans 118
  liquid injectable silicone 97
  nonbiodegradable fillers 5
  Poly-L-lactic acid 155

H

hematomas 38, 155
hemosiderin pigmentation 79
herpes labialis 51
herpes simplex infection 44, 156, *156*

HIV-associated lipoatrophy
    liquid injectable silicone 92–94, *94, 95*
    Radiesse 87–89, *88*
HIV-associated lipodystrophy, facial contouring 48–49
homeopathy 152
human collagen 4
    cadaveric 21
    complications 154
    malpositioning 157
    synthetic 24
    see also individual preparations
Hyacell 49
hyaluronan *see* hyaluronic acid (HA)
hyaluronic acid (HA) 5, *5,* 31–33
    gels *see* hylans
    half-life 31
    malpositioning 157
    skin of color 146, *147, 148*
    structure 31, *33*
hyaluronidase 157, *158*
hydroxyethylmethacrylate (HEMA) 49
Hylaform 33–34
    clinical trials 34
    lips 42
    nasolabial folds 117–118
    other hylans *vs.* **35**
    side effects 34, **37**
    skin of color 146
hylan B gel *see* Hylaform
Hylan Rofilan Gel 49
hylans 31–50
    anesthesia 41
    chin contouring 48–49
    collagen *vs.* **32**
    complications 150, 153–154
    contraindications **33**
    dermal depths 39–40, *40*
    dynamic viscosity 32, *33*
    other fillers containing HA 49
    implant agent choice 39–40
    implantation techniques 40–42
        injection pressure 41
        needle placement depth 41–42
        post injection 42
        resistance 42
        selected anatomical areas 42–49
    isovolemic degradation 32–33, *34*
    lips *see* lips
    Marionette lines *see* Marionette lines
    nasolabial fold *see* nasolabial fold (NLF)
    nerve blocks 41, 43
    overcorrection 42
    patient interview 38–39, **39**
    patient selection 42, 45, 46, 48
    preparations **32**
    side effects **37, 38**
    skin testing 49
    treatable conditions 31, **32**
    treatment strategy 38–40
hyperdynamic wrinkles 12
hypersensitivity 153
    bovine collagen 23, 154, *154*

collagens, injectable 29
    delayed reactions 153
    human collagen 154
    hylans *153,* 153–154
    immediate reactions 153, *153*
    lip augmentation 56
    Restylane 36–37, **37**
    skin of color 150

I
ice, cryoanesthesia 130
ice packs 8
    fat augmentation 79
    hylan injections 42
    lips augmentation 44, 45
implant migration 158–159
    liquid injectable silicone 90, 98
implant palpability 157–159
implant visibility 157–159
incisive nerve 129
infection 156–157
    liquid injectable silicone 98
    prevention 156
inferior alveolar nerve 129
infiltrative local anesthesia 132
infraorbital foramen 129, 133, *133*
infraorbital nerve 129, 133
infraorbital nerve block 133–138
    areas anesthetized 133–134, *137*
    intraoral approach 134, *135*
    lip augmentation *42,* 43, 54, 134–137
    needle insertion angle 134, *135*
    transcutaneous facial approach 134, *136*
infratrochlear nerve 133, *133*
    blocking 133, *134*
injection site inflammation, Restylane 37
injection site necrosis *155,* 155–156
Isolagen 21

J
jawline
    age-related changes 3
    fat augmentation 76, *77*
jowls 15, *16*
    infants 63, *64*
    microliposuction 77, *77*
Juvéderm **35,** 38
    facial (re)contouring 48
    glabellar lines 46–47
    lip augmentation 42, *44,* 45
    Marionette lines 45
    nasolabial fold 45, 117–118, *119*
    skin of color 146, *148*

K
'kiss the ice,' hylans 44, 45

L
labiomental crease, fat augmentation 76, *76*
lacrimal nerve 128

lateral facial fat augmentation 75
levator labii superioris 105
lidocaine 129
lid show 69, *70*
lignocaine 129
linear threading injection technique
    facial contouring 48
    glabellar lines 47
    hylans 41, *43*
    lips 43, 45
    Marionette lines 48
    nasolabial fold 45
    skin of color 145
lips
    age-related changes 16–17, *17*
        skin of color 144
    anesthesia 26, *42,* 43, 134–137, *137*
        infiltration 139, *140*
    ArteFill 85, *85*
    collagen injections 25–27, *27*
        anesthesia 26
        with Botox 26–27
        contraindications 26
        patient selection 26
        pretreatment preparation 25–26
        ptosis correction 26
        threading injections 26
    cryoanesthesia 131
    ectropion 17
    fat augmentation 75, *76*
    Glogau photoaging type 1 54–56, *56*
        complications 55–56
        layering technique 55, *56*
        serial puncture technique 54
    Glogau photoaging type 2 56–58
    hylan injection 42–44
        alternative approaches 44
        complications 44
        definition improvement 43, *43*
        equipment 42
        indications 42
        linear threading injections 43–44
        necrosis 44
        pain/blanching 44
        patient selection 42
        side effects 44, 45
        troubleshooting 44
        upper rhytids 45, *45*
        volume augmentation 44, *44*
    injection technique 7–8, *8*
    pseudoaugmentation 27, *28*
    Radiesse 87, 89
    vertical rhytides 56, *57*
lipstick lines 25, 51
liquid injectable silicone (LIS) 90–100
    adverse reactions 91, 97–98
    anesthesia 95
    anticoagulant avoidance 97
    beading 96, 97, **98**
    complications 97–98
    contraindications 90, 92
    controversies 91–92

expected benefits 92–94
    acne scarring 92, *93*
    correction/improvement 92, *92*
    rhytids 92, *92*
facial marking 95, *96*
granulomatous inflammatory reactions 97
history 90–91
HIV lipoatrophy 92–94, *93, 94*
idiosyncratic reactions 98
implant migration 90, 98
impurities 91
injection method 95–97, **97**
    pressure application 96
    treatment intervals 97
    treatment protocol 97
    volume injected 96, **96**
instrumentation 94
mechanism of action 90, *91*
microdroplet technique 91
off-label use 90–91
Orentreich microdroplet serial puncture technique
    95–97
overcorrection 97
patient preparation 95
patient selection 90, 92
side effects 97–98
storage 94
structure 90, *91*
troubleshooting **98**
usage guidelines 91
LMX-5 129
lower face, aging 3, 15–17
    skin of color 144
lumpiness 8
    ArteFill 85

M

malar eminences 15, *15*
    fat augmentation 75, *75*
mandibular fat augmentation 76, *77*
mandibular foramen 129
mandibular nerve *128,* 129
Marionette lines 3, 16, *17*
    hylan injection 45–46
        alternative approaches 46
        complications 46
        indications 45
    Radiesse 87
    skin of color 145, *146, 147*
maxillary labial frenum anesthesia 134, *137*
maxillary nerve (V2) *128,* 129
melanin 143
melanosomes 143
melolabial folds 15–16, *16*
    Glogau photoaging type 2 57, *57*
mental foramen 129, 138, *139*
mental nerve 129
mental nerve block 138–140
    areas anesthetized 138, *139*
    labial branches 138, *139*
    lip anesthetic *42,* 43, 54, 139, *140*
    supplemental infiltration *140*

microliposuction 76–77, *77*
midface
 aging 2, 14–15
  skin of color 144
 filler indications 2
morphea 1, *2*
mouth corners 51–61
 injection technique *57*
 injection techniques 57
mouth frown 51
multiple puncture technique 7
mycobacteria, atypical *156,* 156–157
Mycobacterium 157
Mycobacterium spp. 49

N
nasociliary nerve 129
nasolabial fold (NLF) 2–4, *3,* 105–126
 aging 105, *106*
 alternative procedures 106–109, *110*
 anatomy 105, *106*
 anesthesia 111–113, **113,** *113,* 118
 beading 111
 botulinum toxin A 108, *110*
 collagen injections 27–28, 114–116
  session intervals 115
  technique 115, *115*
 dynamic phase 105, *108*
 fat augmentation 76, *76,* 123–124, *124*
 filler benefits 109, **110**
 fillers used **113**
 Genzyme 6-point scale 105, *107*
 hylan injections 45–46, *47,* 117–118, *118, 119*
  alternative approaches 46
  equipment 45
  indications 45
  side effects 46, 118, *119*
  technique 45, 118
  troubleshooting 46
 lasers 109
 medial cheek ptosis 109, *111*
 moderate 105, *108*
 nonbiodegradable fillers 121, **121**
 patient interview 113–114
 patient selection 45, 105–113
 Radiance 118–119, *120*
 Restylane 35, *36*
 severe 105, *108*
 skin of color 144, 145, *145*
 treatment techniques 114–124
  consent 114
  photographs 114
  see also specific techniques
 volume depletion correction 108–109
necrosis 155–156
nerve blocks 6, 132–140
 advantages 132
 anatomic variation 132
 disadvantages 132
 fat augmentation 68
 forehead augmentation 132–133

hylans 41, 43
 preinjection aspiration 132
 skin of color 144
 see also individual types
'nettle type' skin eruption 154
New-Fill *see* Poly-L-lactic acid (PLLA)
nitroglycerin paste 47
nodule formation
 ArteFill 85
 fat augmentation 79
 hylans 154
 Poly-L-lactic acid 102, 154
 Radiesse 87, 89
 silicone 121, *122*
nonablative laser resurfacing
 nasolabial folds 109
 perioral rejuvenation 52, 59, *59*
nonanimal stabilized hyaluronic acid (NASHA) 34, 154
nose, aging 15, *15*

O
ophthalmic nerve (V1) *128,* 129
oral commissure lines *see* Marionette lines

P
pain control/anesthesia 6–7, 127–141
 collagens, injectable 24–25
 expected benefits 127–129
 fat augmentation 72–73, 148
 fat extraction 68
 lip augmentation *see* lips
 liquid injectable silicone 95
 nasolabial fold 111–113, **113,** *113,* 118
 nerve blocks *see* nerve blocks
 patient selection 127
 perioral rejuvenation 53, 58
 sensory dermatomes 128, *128*
 skin of color 144
 topical anesthesia 129
 vibratory anesthesia 132
Paris Lip 42
perioral region
 aging 51, *52*
 fat augmentation 75
perioral rejuvenation 51–61
 anesthesia 53, 58
 approach **53**
 Botox *see* botulinum toxin A (BTX-A)
 complications 59
 expected benefits **52,** 52–53
 Glogau photoaging classification **53, 55**
  type 1 54–56
  type 2 56–58
  type 3 *58,* 58–59, *59*
  type 4 59–60
 laser resurfacing 51–52, 53, 59, *59,* 60, *60*
 patient interview 53–54, **54**
 patient selection 51–52
 problems treated 51
 skin testing 51
 techniques **54,** 54–60

treatment strategy 53–54
undercorrection 59
periorbital region
aging 14, *14*
collagen injections 28
fat augmentation retention 79
Perlane **39**
facial contouring 48
injection depth 39, *40*
lips 42
Marionette lines 45
nasolabial folds 45
uses *40*
Permacol 21
philtrum
age-related changes 16–17
hylan injection 43–44
photoaging 11, 12–13
classification **12,** 12–13
lips *see* lips
photodamage 143
photorejuvenation 58
polyacrylamide hydrogel 8
polydimethylsiloxane *see* liquid injectable silicone
Poly-L-lactic acid (PLLA) 101–104
combination treatments 102, *103–104*
complications 102, 154–155
dilution technique 101, 154–155
duration of effect 101
facial lines/hollows 101
FDA approval 83, 101
history 101
HIV patients 155
immune response 155
indications 101
injection techniques 101–103, *102,* 120
malpositioning 158, *158, 159*
massage, post-treatment 102
mechanism of action 101, *102,* 155
nasolabial fold 120
side effects 120
volume filling 120, *121*
results 102
polymethylmethacrylate (PMMA) 5–6, 83
ArteFill 84, 121–123
polytetrafluoroethylene 159
porcine collagen 21, 116
post-inflammatory hyperpigmentation 145–146, 148
fat augmentation 79
prednisone 55, 71
pressure application, post-treatment 131, *132*

R

Radiance *see* Radiesse
Radiesse 83, 87–89
clinical efficacy 87–89, *88*
complications 87, 89
correction duration 89
history 87
HIV-associated lipoatrophy 87–89, *88*
indications 87, *88*

lips 87, 89
mechanism of action 87
Resoplast 22
Restylane 34–38
bovine collagen *vs. 36*
clinical trials 35, *35*
correction persistence 35, *36*
facial contouring 48
glabellar lines 46–47
hypersensitivity 36–37
injection depth 39–40, *40*
lip augmentation 42, 45, 54
Marionette lines 45
nasolabial folds 45, 117–118
other hylans *vs.* **35**
perioral rejuvenation 58
preparation comparison **39**
side effects 35–37, **37**
skin of color 146, *149*
uses *40*
Zyplast *vs.* 35, *36*
Restylane Fine Lines **39**
glabellar lines 46–47
injection depth 39, *40*
lip augmentation 54
upper lip rhytids 45
uses *40*

S

S-Caine peel 129
scalp nerve blocks 132–133
scars/scarring
acne 92, *93*
collagen injections 25
skin of color 148–150
Sculptra *see* Poly-L-lactic acid (PLLA)
semilunar ganglion 128
serial puncture injection technique
glabellar lines 47
hylans 41, *43*
lip augmentation 43–44, 54–55
Marionette lines 45–46
nasolabial fold 115, *115*
biodegradable collagens 115, *115*
hylans 45–46
Orentreich microdroplet technique 95–97
upper lip rhytids 45, *45*
silicone 6, 90
adverse reactions 6
history 19, **20**
injection techniques 83
nasolabial folds 121
see also liquid injectable silicone (LIS)
siliconomas 97
Silikon-1000 19, 94
history 90–91
nasolabial folds 121
skin of color 143–150
anesthesia 144
complications 148–150
efficacy studies 145–146

facial aging 143–144, *144*
filler popularity 143
hypersensitivity 150
indications **144**
injection techniques 145, *145*
patient evaluation 144
patient selection 144
pigment irregularities 145
pretreatment photos 145
safety studies 145–146
temporary fillers 144
skin slough
arterial occlusion 25
collagen injection side effect 25, *25*
skin testing
bovine collagen 23, 154
hylans 49
nasolabial fold management 113
perioral rejuvenation 51
smile lines *see* nasolabial fold (NLF)
smokers lines 25, 51
sodium hyaluronate *see* hyaluronic acid (HA)
solid implants, malpositioning 158, *159*
steroids, fat augmentation 79
Streptococcus equi 34
suborbital fat augmentation 74, *74, 75*
incisions 74
textural irregularities 74
supraorbital nerve 129, 133, *133*
blocking 133, *134*
supratrochlear nerve 129, 133, *133*
swelling 151
Restylane 36–37

T

tacrolimus, collagen injections 29, 154
tetracaine gel 129
threading injection technique 7
biodegradable collagens 115, *115*
mouth corners 57, *57*
nasolabial fold 115, *115*
topical anesthesia 6, 129
trigeminal nerve *128,* 128–129
Tyndall effect 45, 157, *157, 158*

U

ultraviolet light damage 11
The University of Texas Health Center Pathology
Microbiology AFB Lab 157
upper eyelid filling, facial markings 71

V

valaciclovir 54, 156
vascular necrosis, hylan injections 48, 156
vascular occlusion
collagen injections 29, 155–156, *156*
hylan injections 44, 48, 156
vermilion lip, aging 3
vibratory anesthesia 132
vibratory massager 132
Viscontour 49

W

wattles 15, *16*
wrinkles, hyperdynamic 12

X

xenografts 19

Y

young face 63, *64*
animation 63, *65*

Z

Zyderm I 19, 22–23, **23**
glabellar complex treatment 28
nasolabial fold 114–116
Zyderm II 19, 22–23, **23**
nasolabial fold 114–116
zygomaticofacial nerve 129, 137
zygomaticofacial nerve block 137–138, *138*
areas anesthetized 138, *138*
zygomaticotemporal nerve 129, 137
zygomaticotemporal nerve block 137, *137*
zygomaticus major 105
Zyplast 19, 22–23, **23**
nasolabial fold 27, 114–116
Restylane *vs.* 35, *36*